Implementing High-Quality Primary Care

Rebuilding the Foundation of Health Care

Linda McCauley, Robert L. Phillips, Jr., Marc Meisnere,
and Sarah K. Robinson, *Editors*

Committee on Implementing High-Quality Primary Care

Board on Health Care Services

Health and Medicine Division

A Consensus Study Report of

The National Academies of
SCIENCES · ENGINEERING · MEDICINE

THE NATIONAL ACADEMIES PRESS
Washington, DC
www.nap.edu

THE NATIONAL ACADEMIES PRESS   500 Fifth Street, NW   Washington, DC 20001

This activity was supported by contracts between the National Academy of Sciences and the Academic Pediatric Association, Agency for Healthcare Research and Quality, Alliance for Academic Internal Medicine, American Academy of Family Physicians, American Academy of Pediatrics, American Board of Pediatrics, American College of Physicians, American Geriatrics Society, Blue Shield of California, The Commonwealth Fund, Family Medicine for America's Health, Health Resources and Services Administration, New York State Health Foundation, Patient-Centered Outcomes Research Institute, Samueli Foundation, Society of General Internal Medicine, and U.S. Department of Veterans Affairs. Any opinions, findings, conclusions, or recommendations expressed in this publication do not necessarily reflect the views of any organization or agency that provided support for the project.

International Standard Book Number-13: 978-0-309-68510-8
International Standard Book Number-10: 0-309-68510-9
Digital Object Identifier: https://doi.org/10.17226/25983
Library of Congress Control Number: 2021937669

Additional copies of this publication are available from the National Academies Press, 500 Fifth Street, NW, Keck 360, Washington, DC 20001; (800) 624-6242 or (202) 334-3313; http://www.nap.edu.

Printed in the United States of America

Suggested citation: National Academies of Sciences, Engineering, and Medicine. 2021. *Implementing high-quality primary care: Rebuilding the foundation of health care.* Washington, DC: The National Academies Press. https://doi.org/10.17226/25983.

The National Academies of
SCIENCES · ENGINEERING · MEDICINE

The **National Academy of Sciences** was established in 1863 by an Act of Congress, signed by President Lincoln, as a private, nongovernmental institution to advise the nation on issues related to science and technology. Members are elected by their peers for outstanding contributions to research. Dr. Marcia McNutt is president.

The **National Academy of Engineering** was established in 1964 under the charter of the National Academy of Sciences to bring the practices of engineering to advising the nation. Members are elected by their peers for extraordinary contributions to engineering. Dr. John L. Anderson is president.

The **National Academy of Medicine** (formerly the Institute of Medicine) was established in 1970 under the charter of the National Academy of Sciences to advise the nation on medical and health issues. Members are elected by their peers for distinguished contributions to medicine and health. Dr. Victor J. Dzau is president.

The three Academies work together as the **National Academies of Sciences, Engineering, and Medicine** to provide independent, objective analysis and advice to the nation and conduct other activities to solve complex problems and inform public policy decisions. The National Academies also encourage education and research, recognize outstanding contributions to knowledge, and increase public understanding in matters of science, engineering, and medicine.

Learn more about the National Academies of Sciences, Engineering, and Medicine at **www.nationalacademies.org**.

The National Academies of
SCIENCES · ENGINEERING · MEDICINE

Consensus Study Reports published by the National Academies of Sciences, Engineering, and Medicine document the evidence-based consensus on the study's statement of task by an authoring committee of experts. Reports typically include findings, conclusions, and recommendations based on information gathered by the committee and the committee's deliberations. Each report has been subjected to a rigorous and independent peer-review process and it represents the position of the National Academies on the statement of task.

Proceedings published by the National Academies of Sciences, Engineering, and Medicine chronicle the presentations and discussions at a workshop, symposium, or other event convened by the National Academies. The statements and opinions contained in proceedings are those of the participants and are not endorsed by other participants, the planning committee, or the National Academies.

For information about other products and activities of the National Academies, please visit www.nationalacademies.org/about/whatwedo.

COMMITTEE ON IMPLEMENTING
HIGH-QUALITY PRIMARY CARE

HECTOR P. RODRIGUEZ, Henry J. Kaiser Endowed Chair, Professor of Health Policy and Management, University of California, Berkeley

MARY ROTH McCLURG, Executive Vice Dean, Chief Academic Officer, Eshelman School of Pharmacy, University of North Carolina at Chapel Hill

ROBERT J. WEYANT, Associate Dean for Dental Public Health and Community Outreach, School of Dental Medicine, University of Pittsburgh

Study Staff

MARC MEISNERE, Program Officer, Study Director

TRACY A. LUSTIG, Senior Program Officer

SARAH K. ROBINSON, Research Associate

SAMIRA ABBAS, Senior Program Assistant

MICAH WINOGRAD, Senior Finance Business Partner

SHARYL NASS, Senior Director, Board on Health Care Services

JENNIFER PUTHOTA, Christine Mirzayan Science & Technology Policy Graduate Fellow (*until April 2020*)

National Academy of Medicine Fellows

KAMERON MATTHEWS, U.S. Department of Veterans Affairs

LARS PETERSON, American Board of Family Medicine

DIMA M. QATO, University of Southern California School of Pharmacy

Consultants

JOE ALPER, Science Writer

ROBERT BERENSON, Institute Fellow, Urban Institute

RICHARD G. FRANK, Margaret T. Morris Professor of Health Economics, Department of Health Care Policy, Harvard Medical School

WILLIAM MILLER, Chair Emeritus, Department of Family Medicine, Lehigh Valley Health Network Professor of Family Medicine, Morsani College of Medicine, University of South Florida

KURT STANGE, Director, Center for Community Health Integration, School of Medicine, Case Western Reserve University

Reviewers

This Consensus Study Report was reviewed in draft form by individuals chosen for their diverse perspectives and technical expertise. The purpose of this independent review is to provide candid and critical comments that will assist the National Academies of Sciences, Engineering, and Medicine in making each published report as sound as possible and to ensure that it meets the institutional standards for quality, objectivity, evidence, and responsiveness to the study charge. The review comments and draft manuscript remain confidential to protect the integrity of the deliberative process.

We thank the following individuals for their review of this report:

RUTH BALLWEG, University of Washington
L. EBONY BOULWARE, Duke University School of Medicine
GWEN DARIEN, National Patient Advocate Foundation
KAREN DESALVO, Google Health, Google LLC
ARVIN GARG, University of Massachusetts Medical School
LAURIE G. JACOBS, Hackensack Meridian School of Medicine
CARLOS ROBERTO JAÉN, UT Health San Antonio
M. A. J. LEX MACNEIL, Midwestern University (retired)
KEDAR S. MATE, Institute for Healthcare Improvement
GLORIA J. McNEAL, National University
EUGENE RICH, Mathematica
MARTIN ROLAND, University of Cambridge
SARA ROSENBAUM, The George Washington University
PENELOPE ANN SHAW, University of Massachusetts

JEANNETTE E. SOUTH-PAUL, J. South-Paul Academic
  Consultants, LLC
SUSAN E. STONE, Frontier Nursing University

Although the reviewers listed above provided many constructive comments and suggestions, they were not asked to endorse the conclusions or recommendations of this report nor did they see the final draft before its release. The review of this report was overseen by **MARSHALL H. CHIN,** The University of Chicago, and **ANTONIA M. VILLARRUEL,** University of Pennsylvania. They were responsible for making certain that an independent examination of this report was carried out in accordance with the standards of the National Academies and that all review comments were carefully considered. Responsibility for the final content rests entirely with the authoring committee and the National Academies.

Contents

Preface

The National Academies of Sciences, Engineering, and Medicine (the National Academies) has a long history of issuing independent reports that provide evidence and recommendations from national experts that address the directions the country should take to meet challenges that confront us. The Institute of Medicine (IOM) Study of the Future of Primary Care was launched in early 1994 with the intent to influence what was a maelstrom of health care reform at that time. In 1991, the Bush administration started a conversation about health reform that became a plank of Bill Clinton's presidential campaign and a main focus of the Clinton administration's political efforts. In addition to President Clinton's proposal, more than 70 proposals from both sides of the aisle and beyond were considered before health reform foundered in 1994. Beyond the political failure to achieve consensus, considerable experimentation was happening in the marketplace that emphasized primary care. The preface to the IOM's 1996 report *Primary Care: America's Health in a New Era* speaks to the optimism and opportunity that the committee operated to influence:

> *After decades of relative neglect in a health care system that placed most of its emphasis on specialization, high technology, and acute care medicine, the value of primary care is again being recognized as part of the wave of reform that is sweeping the U.S. health care industry. There are numerous indications of the increasingly important role being played by primary care.*

By the time that report was released, political paths to health reform were closed and managed care was also in trouble. What had been fallow ground for primary care was politically salted, and the report's recommendations remained largely unimplemented. It is hard to imagine how primary care, and health care generally, would be different had even some of the 1996 report's recommendations taken root. More than a decade later, the Patient Protection and Affordable Care Act in 2010 aided primary care through expansion of federally qualified health centers, Medicaid expansion, and health information technology support, but most of the 1996 report's recommendations were still not addressed. A 2012 IOM report on integrating primary care and public health also highlighted the lack of relationships between these important community-based agents of population health and opportunities to purposefully heal this schism. The recommendations of this report also went largely unheeded.

Thus, the charge to the current committee was not to relitigate the evidence underpinning these prior reports and recommendations, nor was it simply to produce new recommendations, as is common with most consensus studies of the National Academies. Instead, this consensus committee had the unusual and specific charge to develop an implementation plan for recommendations, using the 1996 report as a starting point.

This study launched in January 2020 and ran headlong into the novel coronavirus pandemic, which quickly highlighted a host of problems in primary care:

- the perils of fee-for-service funding for supporting the health care platform where most people turn for heath advice and care;
- the dangers of the long-standing schism between public health and primary care to communicating a consistent message to the public;
- the lack of inclusion of primary care in national epidemic planning;
- the lack of understanding or inclusion of primary care in congressional COVID-19 relief bills;
- the bizarreness of not supporting telehealth prior to the pandemic; and
- the profound effect that social determinants have on the probability that a person will live or die.

In addition to the lens that the coronavirus pandemic offered to the committee, it was obvious early in the deliberations that major societal factors were framing the importance of a robust system of primary care. Several themes emerged that were critically important in our discussions with clinicians, health system experts, community advocates, and patients themselves. One major difference today compared to 1996 is the emergence of health information technology. Another change is the increased recognition that health care teams, which today are more inclusive of non-clinician team members, ought not to be bounded by clinical walls but should be able to reach into and partner with communities. Similarly, issues of unequal access, health equity, and social determinants of health were commonly used to describe the current challenges and opportunities before us. These themes all informed the committee's recommendations on how we measure, value, and support primary care's capacity to respond to these changes.

As co-chairs, we are indebted to the dedication and critical thinking of the committee members who shaped this report. The volunteer committee comprised of 20 members from a diversity of backgrounds but with a shared commitment to primary care as a common good. We are also indebted to the patients and patient advocacy groups that met with us and whose suggestions and experiences helped shape this report; we hope they see their voices in these pages.

The committee wishes to acknowledge the superb support it received from the National Academies staff. Study Director Marc Meisnere, Senior Program Officer Tracy Lustig, Research Associate Sarah Robinson, Senior Program Assistant Samira Abbas, and Sharyl Nass, Senior Director of the Board on Health Care Services, were essential to the work behind meeting our unusual charge and contributing to the management and writing of the report. The committee also appreciates the considerable help of three National Academy of Medicine fellows, Drs. Kameron Matthews, Lars Peterson, and Dima Qato.

We are sensitive to the fact that 1996 report recommendations and those of subsequent IOM reports dealing with primary care remain fallow. Primary care was reinvented in the United States in the late 1960s, embraced by the world at Alma Ata in 1978, reported on by the IOM in 1978, 1983, 1996, and 2012, and emphasized by most efforts at health reform in the United States. We believe that some of the challenges we address in this report are at the root of the major differences in population health in the United States compared to our global neighbors. The evidence is there, the public values are clear, and care teams want to change the way that they function today. All that is needed is meaningful action to begin the change. We hope that this report will provide clear guidance on the actions we need to take to provide to the public what is necessary to improve lives and promote health. If there is one key message that readers should take away from this report, it is that the committee firmly believes that primary care should be a common good, available to all and sufficiently valued and resourced to repair health equity in the United States.

Linda McCauley and Robert L. Phillips, Jr., *Co-Chairs*
Committee on Implementing High-Quality Primary Care

Acknowledgments

This Consensus Study Report would not have been possible without the invaluable contributions from many experts and stakeholders dedicated to primary care. The committee would like to thank all of the speakers and participants who played a role in the public meetings conducted for this study, as well as the many others who provided valued insight and responded to rapid requests for information to accommodate our short and demanding timeline, including the individuals who shared their personal stories from the patient perspective with the committee.

Many of these contributors, with their affiliations at the time of their presentations to the committee, are listed below:

Toyin Ajayi, Chief Health Officer and Co-Founder, Cityblock Health
Christine Bechtel, Co-Founder, X4 Health
Robert Berenson, Institute Fellow, Urban Institute
Marc Boutin, Chief Executive Officer, National Health Council
Gwen Darien, Executive Vice President for Patient Advocacy and
    Engagement, National Patient Advocacy Foundation
Doug Eby, Vice President of Medical Services, Southcentral
    Foundation
Larry Green, Professor and Epperson Zorn Chair for Innovation
    in Family Medicine and Primary Care, University of Colorado
    School of Medicine
Kelly Kelleher, Chlapaty/ADP Endowed Chair for Innovation in
    Pediatric Practice, Nationwide Children's Hospital

Barbara Leach, Family Support Specialist and Special Projects Coordinator, University of North Carolina Family Support Program

Amy Liebman, Director of Environmental and Occupational Health, Migrant Clinicians Network

Thomas Mattras, Director of Primary Care Operations, U.S. Department of Veterans Affairs

Kara Odom Walker, Secretary of Health and Social Services, Delaware

Hoangmai (Mai) Pham, Vice President of Provider Alignment Solutions, Anthem Inc.

Jennifer Purdy, Executive Director for Veterans Patient Experience, U.S. Department of Veterans Affairs

Winifred Quinn, Director of Advocacy and Consumer Affairs, AARP

Allysa Ware, Project Director, Family Voices

The committee appreciates the sponsors of this study for their generous financial support: Academic Pediatric Association, Agency for Healthcare Research and Quality, Alliance for Academic Internal Medicine, American Academy of Family Physicians, American Academy of Pediatrics, American Board of Pediatrics, American College of Physicians, American Geriatrics Society, Blue Shield of California, The Commonwealth Fund, Family Medicine for America's Health, Health Resources and Services Administration, New York State Health Foundation, Patient-Centered Outcomes Research Institute, Samueli Foundation, Society of General Internal Medicine, and U.S. Department of Veterans Affairs. The committee thanks Richard Frank for his invaluable consultation and the following individuals who provided commissioned papers: Robert Berenson, Adele Shartzer, and Roslyn Murray from the Urban Institute for their paper on primary care payment models; William Miller for his account on the history of primary care; and Kurt Stange for his paper on the effects and consequences of the COVID-19 pandemic on primary care.[1] The committee gives special thanks to Joe Alper for his writing and editing contributions and Casey Weeks for his graphic design expertise.

Finally, deep appreciation goes to staff at the National Academies of Sciences, Engineering, and Medicine for their efforts and support in the report process, especially to Joe Goodman, Andrew Grafton, Megan Kearney, Sarah Kwon, Stephanie Miceli, Maryjo Oster, Devona Overton, Tina Seliber, Lauren Shern, Leslie Sim, Cyndi Trang, Dorothy Zolandz, and the staff of the National Academies Research Center, including Christopher Lao-Scott, Rebecca Morgan, Maya Thomas, and Colleen Willis.

---

[1] The commissioned papers can be found at https://www.nap.edu/catalog/25983.

Acronyms and Abbreviations

AAFP	American Academy of Family Physicians
AAMC	Association of American Medical Colleges
AAP	American Academy of Pediatrics
ACA	Patient Protection and Affordable Care Act
ACO	accountable care organization
AHRQ	Agency for Healthcare Research and Quality
AIMS	Ambulatory Integration of the Medical and Social
AMA	American Medical Association
APRN	advanced practice registered nurse
BPHC	Bureau of Primary Health Care
CDC	Centers for Disease Control and Prevention
CDPHP	Capital District Physician Health Plan
CHGME	Children's Hospitals Graduate Medical Education
CHIP	Children's Health Insurance Program
CHIPRA	Children's Health Insurance Program Reauthorization Act of 2009
CHT	community health team
CHW	community health worker
CMMI	Center for Medicare & Medicaid Innovation (CMS Innovation Center)
CMS	Centers for Medicare & Medicaid Services
CNM	certified nurse-midwife

CPC	Comprehensive Primary Care
CPC+	Comprehensive Primary Care Plus
CTSA	Clinical and Translational Science Awards
ED	emergency department
EHR	electronic health record
FFS	fee-for-service
FQHC	federally qualified health center
GAO	U.S. Government Accountability Office
GIS	geographic information system
GME	graduate medical education
GNE	graduate nurse education
GRACE	Geriatric Resources for Assessment and Care of Elders
GRECC	Geriatric Research, Education and Clinical Center
HCC	hierarchical condition category
HHS	U.S. Department of Health and Human Services
HIE	health information exchange
HIPAA	Health Insurance Portability and Accountability Act
HIT	health information technology
HITECH	Health Information Technology for Economic and Clinical Health
HPSA	Health Professional Shortage Area
HRSA	Health Resources and Services Administration
HSR	health services research
IHS	Indian Health Service
IMPaCT	Individualized Management for Patient-Centered Targets
InCK	Integrated Care for Kids
IOM	Institute of Medicine
IPEC	Inter-professional Education Collaboration
LCSW	licensed clinical social worker
LPN	licensed practical nurse
MACRA	Medicare Access and CHIP Reauthorization Act
MAPCP	Multi-Payer Advanced Primary Care Practice
MCO	managed care organization

MedPAC	Medicare Payment Advisory Commission
MLP	Medical–Legal Partnership
MU	Meaningful Use
MUA	Medically Underserved Area
NAMCS	National Ambulatory Medical Care Survey
NCEPCR	National Center for Excellence in Primary Care Research
NCQA	National Committee for Quality Assurance
NHSC	National Health Services Corps
NIH	National Institutes of Health
NMHC	nurse-managed health center
NP	nurse practitioner
NQF	National Quality Forum
OECD	Organisation for Economic Co-operation and Development
ONC	Office of the National Coordinator for Health Information Technology
PA	physician assistant
PACE	Program of All-Inclusive Care for the Elderly
PACT	Patient-Aligned Care Team
PBRN	practice-based research network
PCIP	primary care incentive payment
PCMH	patient-centered medical home
PCORI	Patient-Centered Outcomes Research Institute
PCP	primary care physician
PCPCH	patient-centered primary care home
PCR	primary care research
PFS	physical fee schedule
PPS	prospective payments system
PRO	patient-reported outcome
RHC	rural health clinic
RN	registered nurse
ROI	return on investment
RUC	Relative Value Scale Update Committee
RVU	relative value unit

SBHC	school-based health center
SCF	Southcentral Foundation
SDOH	social determinants of health
SES	socioeconomic status
SMART on FHR	Substitutable Medical Applications and Reusable Technologies on Fast Health Interoperability Resources
THCGME	Teaching Health Center Graduate Medical Education
VA	U.S. Department of Veterans Affairs
WHO	World Health Organization

Abstract

High-quality primary care is the foundation of a high-functioning health care system and is critical for achieving health care's quadruple aim (enhancing patient experience, improving population health, reducing costs, and improving the health care team experience). High-quality primary care provides comprehensive person-centered, relationship-based care that considers the needs and preferences of individuals, families, and communities. Primary care is unique in health care in that it is designed for everyone to use throughout their lives—from healthy children to older adults with multiple comorbidities and people with disabilities. People in countries and health systems with high-quality primary care enjoy better health outcomes and more health equity.

In 1996, the Institute of Medicine released *Primary Care: America's Health in a New Era*. The report made comprehensive recommendations to improve primary care, most of which were never implemented. As a result, the current Committee on Implementing High-Quality Primary Care was charged to build on the recommendations of the 1996 report and to develop an implementation plan for high-quality primary care in the United States.

The committee's implementation plan targets primary care stakeholders, balancing national needs for scalable solutions while allowing for local fit. The implementation plan includes five objectives to make high-quality primary care available for everyone in the United States.

1. **Pay for primary care teams to care for people, not doctors to deliver services.**

2. Ensure that high-quality primary care is available to every individual and family in every community.
3. Train primary care teams where people live and work.
4. Design information technology that serves the patient, family, and interprofessional care team.
5. Ensure that high-quality primary care is implemented in the United States.

The committee's implementation plan—comprising recommended actions under each implementation objective—builds on a three-element implementation strategy:

1. An implementation framework, with three levels of change that accounts for the complexity of the U.S. health care system and its public- and private-sector actors.
2. An accountability framework that establishes a structure and process for assessing the adequacy and completeness of implementation activities.
3. A public policy framework that prioritizes developing government policy to implement high-quality primary care, consistent with its status as a common good.

The committee's implementation plan calls for appropriately scaled actions by public- and private-sector actors at the macro, meso, and micro system levels and recommends accountability structures to ensure the work gets done. The value of primary care is beyond dispute, with extensive research identifying policies and practices that facilitate high-quality primary care. The actions within this plan will promote and effectively scale those policies and practices. (See the Summary or the report for a full description and discussion of each recommended action.)

The nation deserves nothing less than high-quality primary care for all, but creating such a system requires leadership, accountability, and a clear path forward to accomplish this work. The committee hopes the work captured in this report realizes this vision sooner rather than later.

Summary

High-quality primary care is the foundation of a high-functioning health care system and is critical for achieving health care's quadruple aim (enhancing patient experience, improving population health, reducing costs, and improving the health care team experience). Primary care provides comprehensive, person-centered, relationship-based care that considers the needs and preferences of individuals, families, and communities. Primary care is unique in health care in that it is designed for everyone to use throughout their lives—from healthy children to older adults with multiple comorbidities and people with disabilities. Absent access to high-quality primary care, minor health problems can spiral into chronic disease, care management becomes difficult and uncoordinated, visits to emergency departments increase, preventive care lags, and the nation's health care spending soars to unsustainable levels. People in countries and health systems with high-quality primary care enjoy better health outcomes and more health equity.

Yet, 25 years since the Institute of Medicine (IOM) report *Primary Care: America's Health in a New Era*, this foundation remains weak and under-resourced, accounting for 35 percent of health care visits while receiving only about 5 percent of health care expenditures. Moreover, the foundation is crumbling: visits to primary care clinicians are declining, and the workforce pipeline is shrinking, with clinicians opting to specialize in more lucrative health care fields.

In addition, unequal access to primary care remains a concern, and the COVID-19 pandemic amplified pervasive economic, mental health, and social health disparities that ubiquitous high-quality primary care might have reduced. The pandemic also pushed many primary care practices to the brink of insolvency, with most practices uncertain about their financial viability.

Nonetheless, primary care is the only health care component where an increased supply is associated with better population health and more equitable outcomes. For this reason, primary care is a common good, making the strength and quality of the country's primary care services a public concern.

THE STUDY CONTEXT AND CHARGE

The 1996 IOM report made comprehensive recommendations to improve primary care, although many were never implemented. As a result, in 2019, the National Academies of Sciences, Engineering, and Medicine formed the Committee on Implementing High-Quality Primary Care. Building on the recommendations of the 1996 report, the committee's task was to develop an implementation plan for high-quality primary care in the United States.[1]

WHAT IS HIGH-QUALITY PRIMARY CARE?

High-quality primary care is the provision of whole-person, integrated, accessible, and equitable health care by interprofessional teams who are accountable for addressing the majority of an individual's health and wellness needs across settings and through sustained relationships with patients, families, and communities.

The committee based this definition on the following concepts:

- integrated, whole-person health;
- interprofessional care teams;
- foundational, sustained relationships between the interprofessional care team and patients and families;
- the critical role of communities in providing primary care;
- the importance of equitable access to primary care; and
- the diversity of settings and modalities used to deliver primary care.

This definition describes what high-quality primary care *should be*, not what most people in the U.S. experience today. The committee identified seven facilitators (see Box S-1) to help realize this definition of high-quality primary care and ensure that it is accessible to all.

---

[1] The complete Statement of Task is presented in Chapter 1 of this report.

BOX S-1
Facilitators of High-Quality Primary Care

1. **Payment Models.** Payment models that support integrated, interprofessional teams working in sustained relationships with patients will ensure that high-quality primary care is possible to implement and sustain.
2. **Accountability and Improving Quality.** Effective measurement that is not onerously burdensome and holds primary care accountable will facilitate improvement over time.
3. **Digital Health Care.** An equitable use of technology can make care more accessible and make the primary care experience more efficient, higher quality, and convenient for people and the interprofessional care team.
4. **Interprofessional Care Teams.** Care provided by teams of clinicians and other professionals fit to the needs of communities, working to the top of their skills, and in coordination leads to better health.
5. **Research.** Building the empirical evidence of the epidemiology, organization, and provision of primary care will facilitate continuous improvement within the field.
6. **Leadership.** Coordination among primary care leaders will provide a unified voice on critical issues that will guide decisions of health care organizations and government while increasing accountability.
7. **Policy, Laws, and Regulations.** Federal and state policy and regulations that are compatible with locally tailored care can enable primary care stakeholders to implement needed changes.

IMPLEMENTATION PLAN

To rebuild a strong foundation for the U.S. health care system, the committee's implementation plan includes objectives and actions targeting primary care stakeholders and balancing national needs for scalable solutions while allowing for local fit.[2] The implementation plan includes five objectives to make high-quality primary care available for everyone in the United States:

1. **Pay for primary care teams to care for people, not doctors to deliver services.**
2. **Ensure that high-quality primary care is available to every individual and family in every community.**
3. **Train primary care teams where people live and work.**
4. **Design information technology that serves the patient, family, and interprofessional care team.**

---

[2] The committee's implementation plan assumes the current realities of the U.S. insurance marketplace.

5. **Ensure that high-quality primary care is implemented in the United States.**

The committee's implementation plan—comprising recommended actions under each implementation objective—builds on a three-element implementation strategy:

1. An implementation framework, with three levels of change that accounts for the complexity of the U.S. health care system and its public- and private-sector actors (see Table S-1).
2. An accountability framework that establishes a structure and process for assessing the adequacy and completeness of implementation activities.
3. A public policy framework that prioritizes developing government policy to implement high-quality primary care, consistent with its status as a common good.

TABLE S-1 The Committee's Implementation Framework

System Level	Public		Private	
	Example Actor	Example Actions	Example Actor	Example Actions
Macro	Federal/state legislative branch	Policies; laws; funding	Coalitions; associations	Policy advocacy; Public accountability; professional standards
Meso	Federal, state, local executive branch; federal payers; public delivery systems; educators	Regulations; contracting; payment; administrative practices; training	Private delivery organizations; private payers; corporations; institutions; educators	Management policies and practices; training
Micro	Individuals and interprofessional teams delivering care in public and government health systems; individuals and families seeking care	Self-education; quality assessment and improvement; behavior practice	Individuals and interprofessional teams delivering care; individuals and families seeking care	Self-education; quality assessment and improvement; behavior practice

These elements are fundamental for overcoming barriers to implementing high-quality primary care, with supportive public policy being most important. Health care is not a functioning market in the United States, and resource allocation is subject to the concentration of political and economic power.

The current environment creates the window for such policy. While most Americans are satisfied with their own health care, they remain concerned with the system's future. As the nation recovers from the COVID-19 pandemic and considers the weaknesses it revealed, the policy response should include public health investments, heath care system strengthening, pandemic preparation and resiliency, and economic recovery. Recovery and rebuilding can constitute the political imperative required to advance the committee's policy recommendations, if skillful and committed champions in positions of influence can communicate the missed potential for primary care to assist in the pandemic and capitalize on public concerns about the future sustainability of our health care system.

For policies requiring expenditures, the relatively small proportion of health care expenses spent on primary care today becomes an opportunity. A small absolute increase in primary care spending for policies this report identifies, redistributed from the large expenses across the rest of the system, can have a high proportional effect on primary care and work to stabilize the health system overall.

The committee's implementation plan calls for appropriately scaled actions by public- and private-sector actors at the macro, meso, and micro system levels[3] and creates accountability structures to ensure the work gets done. The value of primary care is beyond dispute, with extensive research identifying policies and practices that facilitate high-quality primary care. The activities within this plan will promote and effectively scale those policies and practices.

Objective One: Pay for primary care teams to care for people, not doctors to deliver services.

Action 1.1: Payers—Medicaid, Medicare, commercial insurers, and self-insured employers—should evaluate and disseminate payment models based on the ability of those models to promote the delivery of high-quality primary care, as defined by the committee, and not on their ability to achieve short-term cost savings.

---

[3] See Appendix D for a table that organizes the committee's recommended actions by system level and actor.

Action 1.2: Payers—Medicaid, Medicare, commercial insurers, and self-insured employers—using a fee-for-service (FFS) payment model for primary care should shift primary care payment toward hybrid (part FFS, part capitated) models, making them the default method for paying for primary care teams over time. For risk-bearing contracts with population-based health and cost accountabilities, such as those with accountable care organizations, payers should ensure that sufficient resources and incentives flow to primary care. Hybrid reimbursement models should:
   a.   pay prospectively for interprofessional, integrated, team-based care, including incentives for incorporating non-clinician team members and for partnerships with community-based organizations;
   b.   be risk adjusted for medical and social complexity;
   c.   allow for investment in team development, practice transformation, and the infrastructure to design, use, and maintain necessary digital health technology; and
   d.   align with incentives for measuring and improving outcomes for attributed populations.

Action 1.3: The Centers for Medicare & Medicaid Services should increase the overall portion of spending going to primary care by:
   a.   accelerating efforts to improve the accuracy of the Medicare physician fee schedule by developing better data collection and valuation tools to identify overpriced services, with the goal of increasing payment rates for primary care evaluation and management services by 50 percent and reducing other service rates to maintain budget neutrality; and
   b.   restoring the Relative Value Scale Update Committee to the advisory nature as originally intended by developing and relying on additional independent expert panels and evidence derived directly from practices.

Action 1.4: States should implement primary care payment reform by:
   a.   using their authority to facilitate multi-payer collaboration on primary care payment and fee schedules and
   b.   measuring and increasing the overall portion of health care spending in their state going to primary care.

Implementing high-quality primary care requires committing to pay primary care more and differently given its capacity to improve population health and health equity for all society, not because it generates short-term returns on investment for payers. High-quality primary care is not a commodity service whose value needs to be demonstrated in a competitive marketplace but a common good promoted by responsible public policy and supported by private-sector action. Implementation of primary care spending policies should attend to the characteristics and practice of what constitutes high-quality primary care in accordance with the committee's definition. As the nation's largest payer, Medicare offers payment policies that set the standard for other payers and merit priority. In exchange, primary care should be accountable for developing additional capacities consistent with the committee's definition.

The committee's recommended actions are not untested. Hybrid capitation and fee-for-service (FFS) arrangements, paired with practice transformation resources and aligned across payers as described in Action 1.2, build primary care capacity consistent with the committee's definition. Medicare fee schedule changes have been recommended previously and are within the purview of the U.S. Department of Health and Human Services (HHS).

Many health systems providing primary care services through employed or contracted models have accepted global capitated payments but continue to operate and compensate primary care on an FFS model, blunting the effects of models intended to strengthen primary care. Health systems in these arrangements should honor the intentions of payers and evidence of superior performance, seeing that new payment models allocate sufficient management authority and resources to the practice of primary care.

Because primary care accounts for a small proportion of health care spending, the service price reductions noted in Action 1.3 will be minimal, help equilibrate compensation between primary care and other specialties, and make primary care a more attractive choice for medical graduates. Medicare fee schedule changes are necessary because capitation, budget rates, and compensation within health care systems, as well as relative prices set by other payers, typically rely on fee schedule calculations. States and local markets that have implemented Action 1.4 have achieved reduced cost trends and improved quality. More states should follow their lead.

Self-insured employers with in-state employment bases should follow the lead of their home states and participate in these efforts. Employers with a geographically dispersed workforce should follow Medicare's lead and prioritize and pay for high-quality primary care.

The recommended actions have not been scaled and implemented widely for two reasons. First, payment reform innovations have been evaluated against short-term savings rather than the promotion of high-quality primary care. Repeated testing of new primary care payment models in search of short-term savings has left most primary care clinicians in underpaying FFS arrangements with the wrong incentives. Attention should focus on moving more clinicians to existing models rather than testing new ones.

Second, budget neutrality or premium stability requirements mean increasing the investments in primary care, redistributing funds, and prioritizing it over other health care services. This is what the committee calls for in designating primary care as a common good. This rebalancing requires leadership, particularly in the public sector. The COVID-19 pandemic's further weakening of U.S. primary care has opened a policy window and leadership opportunity for the Centers for Medicare & Medicaid Services (CMS), employers, and more state officials to act without delay.

Objective Two: Ensure that high-quality primary care is available to every individual and family in every community.

Action 2.1: To facilitate an ongoing primary care relationship, all individuals should have the opportunity to have a usual source of primary care.
  a. Payers—Medicaid, Medicare, commercial insurers, and self-insured employers—should ask all covered individuals to declare a usual source of primary care annually and should assign non-responding enrollees using established methods, track this information, and use it for payment and accountability measures.
  b. Health centers, hospitals, and primary care practices should assume and document an ongoing clinical relationship with the uninsured people they are treating.

Action 2.2: To improve access to high-quality primary care for underserved populations, and to facilitate empanelment of uninsured people, the U.S. Department of Health and Human Services, enabled by congressional appropriations, should target sustained investment in the creation of new health centers (including federally qualified health centers, look-alikes, and school-based health centers), rural health clinics, and Indian Health Service facilities in federally designated shortage areas.

Action 2.3: To improve access to high-quality primary care services for Medicaid beneficiaries, the Centers for Medicare & Medicaid Services should:
  a. Revise and enforce its fee-for-service (section 1902) and managed care (section 1937) access standards for primary care for Medicaid beneficiaries, ensuring them adequate access to primary care as defined by the committee, and
  b. Provide technical assistance resources to state Medicaid agencies for implementing and attaining these standards, and measure and publish state performance on these standards.

Action 2.4: The Centers for Medicare & Medicaid Services should permanently support the COVID-era rule revisions and Medicaid and Medicare benefits interpretations that have facilitated integrated team-based care, enabled more equitable access to telephone and virtual visits, provided equitable payment for non-in-person visits, eased documentation requirements, expanded the role of interprofessional care team members, and eliminated other barriers to high-quality primary care.

Action 2.5: Primary care practices should move toward a community-oriented model of primary care by:
  a. Including community members with lived experience in their governance, practice design, and practice delivery and
  b. Partnering with community-based organizations.

Accreditation bodies should encourage practices to be more community oriented by revising their standards to facilitate these changes.

Successfully implementing high-quality primary care means everyone should have access to the "sustained relationships" primary care offers. The committee recognizes that this access is more likely to happen when everyone has adequate health insurance with no financial barriers to primary care. Absent that, payers can improve access by encouraging, formalizing, and supporting existing relationships between enrollees and primary care teams. Aligned payer action will reinforce the value of primary care as a common good and reduce beneficiaries' misperceptions that any one payer is limiting access to specialty care. While private primary care practices are not obligated to treat the uninsured, those that do and are able should assume an ongoing clinical relationship with them.

The Health Resources and Services Administration's (HRSA's) Health Center Program serves 1 in 11 Americans and merits additional scaling, as it improves access to high-quality primary care for people without insurance or in federally designated shortage areas.

As the nation's second-largest payer, with disproportionate numbers of children and high-needs beneficiaries, Medicaid needs a primary care strategy that addresses the low rates state Medicaid agencies and their contractors pay for primary care, which limits children's access to it. CMS should lead this strategy, and its state partners should implement and enforce it. Reforming Medicaid to mirror Medicare's payment standards may be the most straightforward path to ensuring equitable access to high-quality primary care for its beneficiaries. Short of that, modifying federal access-to-care standards for state Medicaid programs can catalyze state and managed care organization payment and coverage policies to prioritize high-quality primary care. Meeting federal and accrediting bodies' access standards will require states and their contracted managed care organizations to take the necessary actions, including increasing Medicaid rates for primary care and expanding primary care provider networks as needed.

Primary care accessibility should not be limited by the walls of the practice. The COVID-19 pandemic forced Medicare and other payers to scale the ability of patients to access their primary care teams virtually by video and telephone. The benefits of telemedicine are many, and CMS should minimize the payment and regulatory barriers to their use.

Finally, much of what improves health has little to do with medical care, and efforts by primary care teams to build relationships with community organizations and public health agencies should be fostered. These efforts should place patients, their families, and community members at the center of the design and accountability efforts for successful implementation.

Objective Three: Train primary care teams where people live and work.

Action 3.1: Health care organizations and local, state, and federal government agencies should expand and diversify the primary care workforce, particularly in federally designated shortage areas, to strengthen interprofessional teams and better align the workforce with the communities they serve.

  a. Public and private health care organizations should ensure inclusion, support, and training for family caregivers, community health workers, and other informal caregivers as members of the interprofessional primary care team.
  b. The U.S. Department of Education and the U.S. Department of Health and Human Services should partner to expand educational pipeline models that would encourage and increase opportunities for students who are under-represented in health professions.
  c. The Health Resources and Services Administration, state and local government, and health care systems should redesign and implement economic incentives, including loan forgiveness and salary supplements, to ensure that interprofessional care team members, especially those who reflect the diverse needs of the local community, are encouraged to enter primary care in rural and underserved areas.
  d. Health systems and organizations should develop a data-driven approach to customizing interprofessional teams to meet the needs of the population they serve.

Action 3.2: The Centers for Medicare & Medicaid Services, the U.S. Department of Veterans Affairs, the Health Resources and Services Administration (HRSA), and states should redeploy or augment funding to support interprofessional training in community-based, primary care practice environments. The revised funding model should be sufficient in size to improve access to primary care and ensure that training programs can adequately support primary care pipeline needs of the future.

  a. HRSA funding (via Title VII and Title VIII programs) for other health professions training should be increased and prioritized for interprofessional education.

  b. The U.S. Department of Health and Human Services, enabled by Congress as needed, should redesign the graduate medical education (GME) payment to support training primary care clinicians in community settings and expand the distribution of training sites to better meet the needs of communities and populations, particularly in rural and underserved areas. Effective HRSA models (e.g., Teaching Health Centers, Rural Training Tracks) should be prioritized for existing GME funding redistribution and sustained discretionary funding.

  c. GME funding should be modified to support the training of all members of the interprofessional primary care team, including but not limited to nurse practitioners, pharmacists, physician assistants, behavioral health specialists, pediatricians, and dental professionals.

Black, Hispanic, American Indian and Alaska Native, and Native Hawaiian and other Pacific Islander people are currently under-represented in nearly every clinical health care occupation. For care teams to address race- and ethnicity-based treatment disparities, their members should reflect the lived experience of the people and families they serve. Organizations that train, hire, and finance primary care clinicians should ensure that the demographic composition of their primary care workforce reflects the communities they serve and that the care delivered is culturally appropriate.

Developing a workforce to deliver the committee's definition of primary care requires reshaping training program expectations and the clinical settings in which that training occurs. Training primary care clinicians individually in inpatient settings will not accomplish this. Examples of team-based training in community settings exist, but scaling them requires recalibrating financial incentives to support all primary care team members. Recognizing the significance of this task, the committee recommends adopting alternative financing sources for HRSA-developed, community-based primary care training.

Objective Four: Design information technology that serves
the patient, family, and interprofessional care team.

Action 4.1: The Office of the National Coordinator for Health Information Technology and the Centers for Medicare & Medicaid Services should develop the next phase of digital health, including electronic health record, certification standards to:

a. Align with the functions of primary care—supporting the relationship between clinicians, care teams and patients; providing access and continuous contact over time; collecting and understanding the patient's story; and focusing on the patient and family rather than the disease;

b. Account for the user experience of clinicians and patients (e.g., clicks and time spent using system, data transferred without manual review, and improvements in care delivery and health outcomes) to ensure that health systems are truly interoperable;

c. Ensure equitable access and use of digital health systems that support equitable care and deliver national standards, including guidelines, measures, and decision-making functions, while allowing local tailoring;

d. Include highly usable sensemaking functionality, such as automated tools that make sense of data, identify clinically important data, and inform care;

e. Ensure base products meet certification standards with minimal need for local modification to meet requirements; and

f. Hold health information technology vendors and state and national support agencies financially responsible for failing to achieve benchmarks.

Action 4.2: The Office of the National Coordinator for Health Information Technology (ONC) and the Centers for Medicare & Medicaid Services (CMS) should plan for and adopt a comprehensive aggregate patient data system to enable primary care clinicians and interprofessional teams to easily access comprehensive patient data needed to provide whole-person care.

a. This data source needs to be usable by any certified digital health tool for patients, families, clinicians, and care team members.

b. ONC and CMS could accomplish this through a centralized data warehouse, individual health data card, or distributed sources connected by a real-time, functional health information exchange. Each approach has its own challenges, and an initial effort would need to decide on the right national approach.

Digital health, and electronic health records in particular, create opportunities for improving care coordination and person-centeredness. However, digital health is a major source of professional dissatisfaction and clinician burnout. The committee supports federal standards setting but current certification requirements are a barrier to high-quality primary care. The recommended elements for new certification requirements will require additional planning before adoption along with new policies and authorizations to enforce standards. Aggregated patient data systems can benefit primary care's coordinating functions and reduce the chances of data being used for personal or organizational profit. The experience of local and regional health information exchanges can inform this effort. Creating and implementing these changes requires innovation by vendors and state and national support agencies, and accomplishing these goals will not be easy to ascertain.

Objective Five: Ensure that high-quality primary care is implemented in the United States.

Action 5.1: The U.S. Department of Health and Human Services (HHS) Secretary should establish a Secretary's Council on Primary Care to enable the vision of primary care captured in the committee's definition.
   a. Council members should include the Centers for Medicare & Medicaid Services Administrator; the Directors of the Center for Medicare & Medicaid Innovation, the Health Resources and Services Administration, and the Agency for Healthcare Research and Quality; the Assistant Secretary for Planning and Evaluation at HHS; and the National Coordinator for the Office of the National Coordinator for Health Information Technology.
   b. The council should coordinate primary care policy across HHS agencies with attention to the following responsibilities: (1) assess federal primary care payment sufficiency and policy; (2) monitor primary care workforce sufficiency including training financing, production and preparation, incentives for federally designated shortage areas, and federal clinical assets/investments (health centers, rural health clinics, the Indian Health Service, and the U.S. Department of Veterans Affairs); (3) coordinate and assess the adequacy of the federal government's research investment in primary care; (4) address primary care's technology, data, and evidence needs, including interagency collaboration in the use of multiple data sources; (5) promote alignment of public and private payer policies in support of high-quality primary care; and (6) establish meaningful metrics for assessing the quality of primary care that embrace person-centeredness and health equity goals. Additionally,

the council should coordinate implementing the committee's recommended actions that target federal agencies.

c. As part of its coordination role, the council should verify adequate budgetary resources are allotted in respective agencies for fulfilling these responsibilities.

d. The council should annually report to Congress and the public on the progress of its implementation plan and performance on each of these six responsibilities.

e. In all its work, the Secretary's Council on Primary Care should be informed through regular guidance and recommendations provided by a Primary Care Advisory Committee, created by the HHS Secretary under the Federal Advisory Committee Act, that includes members from national organizations that represent significant primary care stakeholder groups, such as patients, certifying boards, professional organizations, health care worker organizations, payers, and employers.

Action 5.2: The U.S. Department of Health and Human Services should form an Office of Primary Care Research at the National Institutes of Health and prioritize funding of primary care research at the Agency for Healthcare Research and Quality, via the National Center for Excellence in Primary Care Research.

Action 5.3: To improve accountability and increase chances of successful implementation, primary care professional societies, employers, consumer groups, and other stakeholders should assemble, and regularly compile and disseminate a "high-quality primary care implementation scorecard," based on the five key implementation objectives identified in this report. One or more philanthropies should assist in convening and facilitating the scorecard development and compilation.

Appendix E contains the committee's proposed scorecard, which aggregates a small number of already compiled state- and national-level measures for each implementation objective in this report.

Successfully implementing recommendations rests in part on clear accountability. Lack of accountability hampered efforts to implement many recommendations in the 1996 IOM report. Thus, the committee's task would be incomplete without recommending an accountability system for implementing the above actions, for which federal leadership and responsibility are essential. As the nation's two largest payers, Medicare and Medicaid shape the nation's health care delivery system. Medicare payment policy's incompatibility with high-quality primary care has weakened primary care. In addition, federal payments and policies determine priorities for health care workforce training and medical and health care services research.

A Secretary's Council on Primary Care at HHS is the appropriate entity for coordinating the federal role and agency activity called for in these actions. The council should be accountable for monitoring and aligning private-sector activities that support primary care and ensuring that federal policy supports the committee's vision. Senior Secretary–level coordination is necessary given the widespread agency-level activities affecting primary care, including HRSA's workforce training and safety net funding, CMS's payment and benefits policy, health information technology within the Office of the National Coordinator for Health Information Technology, and the Agency for Healthcare Research and Quality's (AHRQ's) health services research. No one agency can shoulder the task of coordination, which would continue to be in the public interest beyond the scope or term of a special task force, another accountability mechanism the committee considered and rejected.

The HHS Secretary should give this council authority to ensure the appropriate agencies devote adequate spending to implement the actions in this report. A key task for the Secretary's Council will be overseeing the establishment of accountability measures for providing primary care consistent with the committee's definition. These measures can change expectations for what constitutes high-quality primary care as defined by the committee, if done judiciously and with stakeholder input, and they can facilitate learning and improved population health. Public reporting will also increase accountability.

Primary care research funding has suffered relative to other health services, so the committee recommends establishing a National Institutes of Health Office of Primary Care Research, with functions similar to its Office of Emergency Care Research. This new entity, coupled with funding for AHRQ's National Center for Excellence in Primary Care Research, could foster a system of learning and improvement that would help make the committee's vision of high-quality primary care a reality for all.

To increase the chances for successful implementation, actors should be held publicly accountable for their responsibilities. Evidence abounds for what is needed to achieve high-quality primary care for all, but organized support for this work is lacking. The professional diversity of high-quality primary care teams is their clinical strength but political and economic weakness, for while other health care services have a single voice advocating for public policy change, primary care lacks a similar voice. The committee's recommended Federal Advisory Committee to the Secretary's council on primary care could serve this function. Organizing primary care clinicians, consumer groups, employers, and other stakeholders (from the variety of settings in which primary care is delivered) to assess implementation of the activities the committee recommends will hold the named actors accountable, increase the likelihood of successful implementation, and catalyze a common agenda to achieve a vital common good.

The nation deserves nothing less than high-quality primary care for all, but creating such a system requires leadership, accountability, and clear steps to accomplish this work. The committee hopes the work captured in this report realizes this vision sooner rather than later.

1

A New Vision for Primary Care

High-quality primary care is the foundation of a robust health care system, and perhaps more importantly, it is the essential element for improving the health of the U.S. population. High-quality primary care is a critical component to achieve the quadruple aim of health care—enhancing patient experience, improving population health, reducing costs, and improving the health care team experience—and it can both make health care more personal and address the inequities that currently plague the U.S. health care system (Bodenheimer and Sinsky, 2014; Christian et al., 2018; Kringos et al., 2013; Macinko et al., 2003; Park et al., 2018; Phillips and Bazemore, 2010; Starfield et al., 2005). Absent access to high-quality primary care, minor health problems can spiral into life-altering chronic disease, chronic disease management becomes difficult and uncoordinated, visits to emergency departments increase, and preventive care lags.

Yet, in large part because of chronic underinvestment, primary care in the United States is slowly dying. Indeed, U.S. investment has fallen short of that needed to make high-quality primary care accessible throughout the nation (Martin et al., 2020; Reiff et al., 2019). Today, more than 35 percent of all health care visits are to primary care physicians (Johansen et al., 2016), yet primary care receives about 5 percent of all health care spending (Martin et al., 2020) (see Figure 1-1) and less than 5 percent of Medicare spending (Reid et al., 2019). Evidence also shows that primary care's share of total health care spending has decreased in a majority of states (and overall) in recent years (Kempski and Greiner, 2020). In contrast, Organisation for Economic Co-operation and Development (OECD) countries devote an average of 7.8 percent of all health care spending to

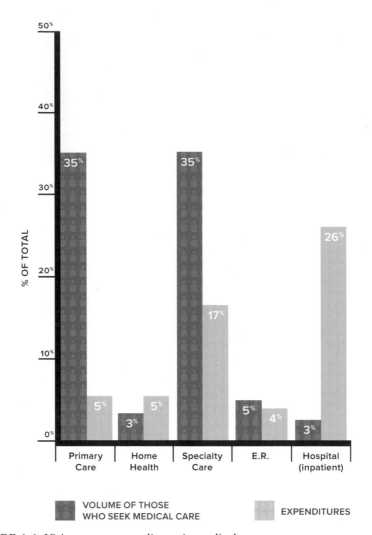

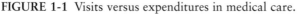

FIGURE 1-1 Visits versus expenditures in medical care.
NOTES: Visit volume data comes from the 2012 Medical Expenditure Panel Survey (MEPS), while the financing comes from 2016 MEPS data. Expenditures include direct payments for care (insurance payments or out-of-pocket payments). Primary care and specialty care include office-based and outpatient clinics. Primary care data include physicians in family medicine, general practice, geriatrics, general internal medicine, and general pediatrics only. Nurse practitioner, physician assistant, and midwife data were not broken down by setting and are not represented in this figure. Home health includes both formal (i.e., paid) and informal (i.e., unpaid) care. Informal care includes only individuals who live outside the house. All categories are not included in the figure and thus do not add up to 100 percent.
SOURCES: Johansen et al., 2016; Martin et al., 2020.

primary care (OECD, 2019). The upshot of this underinvestment in the United States is a disjointed health care enterprise that creates inequities in care, misallocates resources between primary and specialty care, burns out clinicians, generates financial pressure on primary care practices, limits the relationships that clinicians and patients can develop, produces suboptimal care for too many U.S. residents, has the United States slowly falling behind the rest of the developed world in population health outcomes, and is even beginning to lead to regression in mortality gains of the past 100 years (NRC and IOM, 2013).

On top of these well-documented negative effects of underinvestment, the COVID-19 pandemic amplified pervasive economic, mental health, and social health disparities (Dorn et al., 2020; Smith, 2020) that might have been alleviated if high-quality primary care were ubiquitous nationwide (Baillieu et al., 2019; Basu et al., 2016, 2017; Koller and Khullar, 2017; MedPAC, 2008). The pandemic has also pushed many primary care practices to the brink of insolvency. A May 2020 survey of nearly 3,000 primary care clinicians in all 50 states found that 42 percent of the respondents had laid off or furloughed staff and 51 percent were uncertain about their financial viability over the following month (The Larry A. Green Center and PCC, 2020).

Nevertheless, in the United States, primary care remains the largest platform for continuous, person-centered, relationship-based care that considers the needs and preferences of individuals, families, and communities and whose value is demonstrated with markedly stable usage patterns for more than 50 years (Green et al., 2001; Johansen et al., 2016; White et al., 1961). Regardless of a rapid growth of specialty care, a large percentage of health care visits have consistently taken place in primary care settings. Despite no universally accepted definition of which professions are considered "primary care," it is generally agreed that they include those practicing in family medicine, general internal medicine, general pediatrics, geriatrics, and other professions that fulfill general health needs. As seen in Figure 1-1, of those who seek medical care in a given month, 35 percent will visit a primary care physician but only 3 percent will be admitted to a hospital (Johansen et al., 2016). Other data sources show that of the 900 million U.S. office visits 2016, more than half were to primary care clinicians (Rui and Okeyode, 2016). In 2018, 76 percent of U.S. adults had a usual source of care; 70 percent of those found it outside of a hospital, usually in an office setting (CDC, 2019).

However, some evidence indicates that fewer people are going to a primary care office than a decade ago (see Chapter 3 for a more detailed discussion). Between 2008 and 2016, visits per person to primary care clinicians fell 6–25 percent, depending on the data source (Ganguli et al., 2019, 2020) (see Figure 1-2), with the sharpest declines in metropolitan areas and

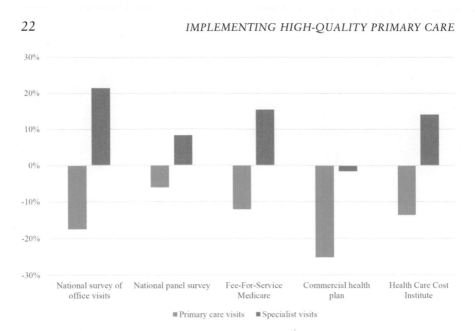

FIGURE 1-2 Change in per capita primary care and specialty visit rates between 2008 and 2016.
SOURCE: Ganguli et al., 2019.

among individuals earning 200 percent or less of the federal poverty level (Ganguli et al., 2020). Primary care visits by commercially insured children and adolescents have also fallen by approximately 13 percent over the same period, with problem-based visits dropping 24 percent and preventive care visits increasing 10 percent (Ray et al., 2020), contrasting with increases in specialty visits.

While the value of primary care has remained steady, the U.S. system is in crisis and being eroded by many forces, including inadequate investment in and chronic under-resourcing of services; incompatible payment models; diminished trainee interest; increased opportunity for subspecialty training; the challenges of rural access; the decreasing scope or comprehensiveness of primary care in many settings; and the lack of integration with health systems, community-based services, and public health (Basu et al., 2019; Casalino et al., 2014; Chen et al., 2013; Christakis et al., 2001; Coker et al., 2013; Cooley et al., 2009; Coutinho et al., 2019; IOM, 2012a; Liaw et al., 2016; Long et al., 2012; MedPAC, 2014; Mostashari, 2016; Phillips et al., 2009).

This is not to say that high-quality primary care does not exist in the United States or that it is beyond the reach of all Americans. In fact, numerous practices and health care systems deliver high-quality primary care, but these are far from the rule. Health centers,[1] for example, deliver high-quality primary care based on an integrated, interprofessional team-based model (HRSA, 2020a,b). This is by design, supported by federal policy, payment, and practice transformation support (Rittenhouse et al., 2020). Overall, however, the country can—and must—do better, for without shoring up its primary care system, the fragile foundation that primary care represents today may continue to crumble and the nation's health will suffer.

PROJECT ORIGIN AND STATEMENT OF TASK

In July 2018, the Health and Medicine Division[2] of the National Academies of Sciences, Engineering, and Medicine (the National Academies) convened a planning meeting to discuss the current and future role of primary care in the United States and how the National Academies could address some of the current challenges in the field. The Board on Health Care Services hosted the meeting, with financial support from the American Board of Family Medicine Foundation.

The planning meeting sought to answer the following questions:

- What is the current and future role of primary care in the United States?
- What can the United States learn from primary care successes and failures from around the world?
- How can the National Academies advance progress and address the challenges facing primary care in the United States and internationally, and what questions should a National Academies consensus study or workshop address?

Meeting participants included a diverse set of stakeholders and primary care experts, including representatives from government agencies, international health organizations, private foundations, academic institutions, primary care researchers, interest groups, and a member of the committee that authored *Primary Care: America's Health in a New Era* (IOM, 1996).

Participants generally agreed that primary care in the United States needed transformative action and that a National Academies consensus study would allow for a committee to carefully develop an action plan that

---

[1] Health centers, as defined by section 330 of the Public Health Service Act (42 U.S.C. § 254b), include outpatient clinics in federally designated underserved areas that qualify for specific reimbursement systems under Medicare and Medicaid.

[2] As of March 2016, the Health and Medicine Division of the National Academies of Sciences, Engineering, and Medicine continues the consensus studies and convening activities previously carried out by the Institute of Medicine (IOM). The IOM is used to refer to publications issued prior to July 2015.

could affect the future of primary care. This study was also deemed to be timely given that the World Health Organization and others were preparing to revisit the 1978 Alma-Ata Declaration[3] and a global recommitment to primary health care. The planning committee was clear that there was no need to re-litigate the evidence for the value of robust primary care, and the potential Statement of Task for a consensus study was instead focused on an action plan to strengthen primary care.

With the support of a broad coalition of sponsors (see Box 1-1), the study officially launched in October 2019. The National Academies formed the Committee on Implementing High-Quality Primary Care with the charge to revisit previous National Academies' reports on primary care, examine the current state of primary care in the United States, and develop an implementation plan to build on the recommendations of the 1996 IOM report (see Box 1-2).

BOX 1-1
Study Sponsors

- Academic Pediatric Association
- Agency for Healthcare Research and Quality
- Alliance for Academic Internal Medicine
- American Academy of Family Physicians
- American Academy of Pediatrics
- American Board of Pediatrics
- American College of Physicians
- American Geriatrics Society
- Blue Shield of California
- The Commonwealth Fund
- Family Medicine for America's Health
- Health Resources and Services Administration
- New York State Health Foundation
- Patient-Centered Outcomes Research Institute
- Samueli Foundation
- Society of General Internal Medicine
- U.S. Department of Veterans Affairs

---

[3] The Declaration of Alma-Ata was adopted at the International Conference on Primary Health Care in what was then known as Alma-Ata in the Soviet Socialist Republic (today, it is known as Almaty, Kazakhstan). The conference and declaration called for national and international action to strengthen primary health care throughout the world (International Conference on Primary Health Care, 1978). The Declaration is available at https://www.who.int/publications/almaata_declaration_en.pdf (accessed October 5, 2020).

BOX 1-2
Study Statement of Task for the Committee on
Implementing High-Quality Primary Care

An ad hoc committee, under the auspices of the National Academies of Sciences, Engineering, and Medicine, will examine the current state of primary care in the United States and develop an implementation plan to build on the recommendations from the 1996 Institute of Medicine report *Primary Care: America's Health in a New Era* to strengthen primary care services in the United States, especially for underserved populations, and to inform primary care systems around the world. The implementation plan will consider

- Barriers to and enablers of innovation and change to achieve high-quality, high-value primary care;
- The expanding scope of comprehensive primary care integration to address the needs of individuals, families, and communities;
- The role of primary care in achieving population health outcomes and health equity goals;
- The role of team-based interprofessional practice and the range of primary care providers, including those with oral health, lifestyle, and integrative medicine expertise;
- The evolving role of technological and other innovations in delivering patient-centered primary care;
- Education and training needs for the changing workforce in primary care;
- The evolution and sustainability of care delivery and payment models across different communities and care settings;
- Efficient approaches to meaningful measurement and continuous improvement of care quality;
- Changing demographics and the primary care needs and access of different patient populations, including rural and other underserved populations;
- Identifying and addressing behavioral and social determinants of health and delivering community-oriented, whole-person care; and
- The infrastructure (workforce, data, and metrics) needed to evaluate effectiveness of innovation and its impact on health outcomes and to support data-informed decision making.

To develop the implementation plan, the committee will consider successes and limitations of prior efforts to innovate in primary care, as well as the increasing demands and stresses on the primary care system, and will recommend ways to effectively scale and implement successful innovations and programs in U.S. health care settings.

STUDY APPROACH

The Committee on Implementing High-Quality Primary Care consisted of 20 members with a broad range of expertise, including clinical care, health care systems and administration, the health care workforce, health care policy, implementation science, health information technology, health care quality, health professional education, patient-centered outcomes research, community-oriented primary care, and health care payment. Appendix A presents brief biographies of the committee members, fellows, and staff.

The committee deliberated during five 2-day meetings and many conference calls between January 2020 and November 2020. At two of the meetings and one public webinar, outside speakers were invited to inform the committee's deliberations, and members of the public were given the opportunity to provide questions, comments, and suggestions. The speakers provided valuable input on a broad range of topics, including primary care payment and policy, delivery innovations, implementation, and patient experiences and perspectives. During the webinar, invited patients and representatives from patient advocacy organizations presented their thoughts and experiences on what primary care meant to them and how it could be improved. In addition, a number of experts provided written input on a range of topics, and the committee commissioned three papers on the following topics: payment models in primary care, the COVID-19 pandemic and what it has revealed about primary care, and the historical transformation of primary care since 1981. The committee also completed an extensive search of the peer-reviewed literature, ultimately considering more than 6,000 articles and targeting English-language articles published since 2010 concerning primary care delivery, innovations, and implementation. The committee also reviewed gray literature, including publications by private organizations, government, and international organizations, with a focus on implementation strategies and successes.

While this report fully embraces the unique roles of all members of the interprofessional primary care team, the majority of published literature and data regarding primary care in the United States is physician-centric and often does not consider the many professions that are part of an interprofessional primary care team. The literature included in this report reflects the state of primary care research (PCR) today. Additionally, while the following chapters discuss the roles and responsibilities of many of the professions that can be part of an interprofessional primary care team, it was beyond the scope of this report to define these roles for every profession in the context of primary care delivery. Similarly, challenges and arguments around scope of practice issues for the various professions in primary care have been the focus of other National Academies reports (IOM, 2011a,b;

NASEM, 2016) and the committee purposefully chose to avoid discussion of most of them in this report for several reasons. First and foremost, it remains a struggle within primary care to attract health professionals of all types who have ample opportunities for more lucrative specialty roles in the health care system. Most of the recommended actions in the committee's implementation plan focus on solving the problems common to all of the professions engaged in primary care with the goal of building more effective teams and addressing patients' needs. Second, in most cases, patients need teams of health professionals able to address the widest spectrum of conditions and issues presented anywhere in the health care system and to do so in a comprehensive, sustained way. In these teams, each health professional brings important capacities and competencies that should not be constrained by laws or policy if they are able to contribute to good care. Third, given the diversity of communities and the general struggle to equitably serve them all, primary care cannot be delivered through a single model, and laws or policies should be enabling of serving every community and meeting their particular needs. While the committee freely acknowledges that disagreements around scope of practice are real and related to structural, professional inequities, they are not unique to primary care and the committee felt that it was outside the scope of its Statement of Task to say how they should be resolved.

STUDY CONTEXT

Two earlier reports—*Defining Primary Care: An Interim Report* (IOM, 1994) and *Primary Care: America's Health in a New Era* (IOM, 1996)—were foundational and influential works that represented an ambitious plan to strengthen primary care in the United States. These reports defined primary care as "the provision of integrated, accessible health care services by clinicians who are accountable for addressing a large majority of personal health care needs, developing a sustained partnership with patients, and practicing in the context of family and community" (IOM, 1994, p. 15, 1996, p. 1).

The authoring committees emphasized in their reports that the term "primary" indicated that such care is first and fundamentally *care*, and primary care is not a specialty or a discipline but an essential, generalist function to which everyone in the population should have access. The inclusion of the words "integrated," "sustained partnership," and "context of family and community" reflected a responsibility to connect with other actors in the health system and a prominent population health perspective. It is the current committee's position that primary care's essential contribution to population health makes it a common good requiring investment and both societal and political support. While the 1996 definition[4] of primary care is still highly relevant, this study committee felt that it did not fully capture what high-quality primary care means today, and the committee offers an updated definition in Chapter 2.

Of the comprehensive recommendations in the 1996 report, most were never implemented but remain relevant today. That inaction can be attributed to a number of contextual factors and barriers, several of which are described below. The committee developed this report and its recommendations and implementation strategy with these barriers in mind.

A 2012 report, *Primary Care and Public Health: Exploring Integration to Improve Population Health* (IOM, 2012b), offered ways to expand the potency of primary care in partnership with public health. Broad recommendations included the need for interagency collaboration regarding maternal and child health, cardiovascular disease prevention, and colorectal cancer screening to address the broader social determinants of health (SDOH) and the comprehensive and interrelated aspects of physical, mental, and social health and well-being (Bielaszka-DuVernay, 2011; Bodenheimer et al., 2014; Landon et al., 2012; Love et al., 2019; Phillips and Bazemore, 2010; Starfield et al., 2005). The 2012 report's recommendations also remain largely unapplied, suggesting major barriers to implementing more robust primary care systems in partnership with public health.

This report revisits many of the outstanding issues these reports raised but through an updated, more expansive view of primary care. This committee also asserts that *primary care is a common good*—that every person in the United States should have access to high-quality primary care at all times in their lives; it should not be an optional service only available to certain age groups or classes of people. This report is not, however, an exhaustive review of the evidence supporting the importance of primary care writ large—that evidence is well documented (Basu et al., 2019; Levine et al., 2019; Macinko et al., 2003; Shi, 2012) and is an underlying assumption in the chapters that follow. Rather, this report focuses on implementing innovative solutions to improve the nation's ability to realize the full potential for primary care and addresses the systemic barriers that prevent attaining robust high-quality primary care for all U.S. populations.

Why the 1996 Recommendations Failed to Gain Traction

The committee began by evaluating the status and relevance of the 31 recommendations in *Primary Care: America's Health in a New Era* (IOM,

---

[4] Note that the IOM definition of primary care provided in *Primary Care: America's Health in a New Era* (IOM, 1996) first appeared in *Defining Primary Care: An Interim Report* (IOM, 1994). This report refers to this as "the 1996 IOM definition."

1996) (see Box 1-3 for a summary of the recommendations; see Appendix B for the complete text of the recommendations). As noted, many of the recommendations have not been implemented, which may be partly attributable to the presentation of many of the recommendations as aspirational goals, without identifying specific actors that would be accountable for following through. Systemic barriers to their implementation also existed, many of which persist today.

Lack of Centralized Accountability

Recommendation 9.1 from the 1996 report called for establishing a public–private consortium to oversee implementing the remaining recommendations. That study committee recognized the lack of an umbrella organizing body for the field of primary care and acknowledged that, without one, there was little chance for meaningful change. Today, there remains no singular, centralized body, professional society, or government agency, meaning that systemic change must occur by way of a number of independent stakeholders and actors, many of which may not be aligned, coordinated, or given shared accountability. In 2020, however, seven of the physician professional societies and boards did come together to propose sweeping changes in primary care policy, many of which align with the themes of this report (AAFP et al., 2020), suggesting that the field recognizes a need to be better aligned in purpose and mission.

Given that this committee's charge was to develop an implementation plan to improve primary care, the committee acknowledged the difficulty of developing specific strategies that would depend on a wide array of independent or poorly coordinated stakeholders and organizations and strongly agrees with the 1996 committee's idea that such an organization would help facilitate needed changes. Building on the 1996 recommendation, this committee proposes a more targeted, specific approach to ensuring that improvement efforts are coordinated and that stakeholders in the field are held accountable (see Chapter 12).

Demise of Health Care Reform

The demise of the federal effort to reform health care in 1994 also contributed to the limited impact of the 1996 recommendations. In 1993, at the beginning of the 1996 study process, the Clinton administration's proposal to comprehensively reform health care and guarantee universal health insurance coverage had widespread political and popular support and seemed likely to succeed (Skocpol, 1995). The plan contained a number of provisions that would have strengthened primary care and provided access to those previously uninsured, but political forces led to the ultimate

BOX 1-3
Primary Care: America's Health in a New Era
(IOM, 1996) Summary of Recommendations

- 2.1: Adopt committee's definition of primary care
- 9.1: Form a public–private, nonprofit primary care consortium

Care Delivery
- 5.1: Make primary care available to all Americans
- 5.2: Provide health care coverage for all Americans
- 5.3: Adopt payment methods that support primary care
- 5.4: Upgrade payments for primary care in fee-for-service
- 5.5: Use interdisciplinary teams
- 5.6: Include primary care in programs for underserved and special needs populations
- 5.7: Coordinate activities of health care plans and public health agencies
- 5.8: Better integrate primary care and mental health services
- 5.9: Better integrate primary care and long-term care
- 5.10: Adopt uniform performance measures of systems and individual clinicians
- 5.11: Accept primary care as a core mission of academic health centers, and provide leadership in teaching, research, and service delivery

Workforce
- 6.1: Continue efforts to increase supply of primary care clinicians
- 6.2: Monitor supply of and requirements for primary care clinicians
- 6.3: Explore how to alleviate geographic maldistribution
- 6.4: Amend scope of practice limitations for nurse practitioners and physician assistants

failure of the proposed Health Security Act.[5] Had health care reform passed in 1995, the health care community and the actors within it might have been more empowered to take up and implement many of the recommendations put forth by the 1996 report, including for universal access and coverage. The Patient Protection and Affordable Care Act[6] passed in 2010 enabled many previously uninsured Americans to obtain health insurance and did strengthen primary care in many ways (Davis et al., 2011), but it still fell short of the original 1996 recommendation for universal coverage. While reform that provides universal coverage and access would further strengthen primary care and the health of the nation considerably, the current committee considered the historical context of health care reform and

---

[5] Health Security Act, § 1757, 103rd Congress (1993–1994).
[6] Patient Protection and Affordable Care Act, Public Law 111-148 (March 23, 2010).

Education and Training
- 7.1: Train all medical students in primary care settings
- 7.2: Define core competencies
- 7.3: Support teaching of core competencies through accreditation and certification
- 7.4: Emphasize communication skills and cultural sensitivity
- 7.5: Develop an all-payer system to support professional education and training
- 7.6: Reallocate a portion of GME funds to cover costs of training in non-hospital settings
- 7.7: Include training in interdisciplinary team care
- 7.8: Determine best approaches for interdisciplinary teaching of collaborative care
- 7.9: Include core competencies in retraining programs; test and certify clinicians who have undergone retraining for primary care

Research
- 8.1: Identify and fund a lead agency for primary care research
- 8.2: Survey the nation's health care needs; include a uniform primary care data set
- 8.3: Support practice-based primary care research networks
- 8.4: Develop standards for data collection
- 8.5: Research the extent to which primary care is delivered by specialists, including
  - the impact on primary care workforce requirements and
  - the impact on costs and quality of and access to health care

strategies to facilitate universal access to high-quality primary care within the realities of the current health insurance landscape in the United States.

Limited Implementation of Newer Models of Care Delivery

New models of care have been developed since 1996, and one in particular, the patient-centered medical home (PCMH), was advanced as a solution to implementing many of the goals of the 1996 report. The PCMH model combines the essence of primary care with innovations to better align care processes with patient needs. The core principles include improved access, continuity of care, comprehensive team-based care, care coordination, quality and safety, and a reimbursement structure that supports the functions of primary care. A key component of the model is that everyone, both adults and children, maintains an ongoing relationship with a team at the practice level, led by a personal primary care clinician that collectively takes responsibility for ongoing care. While the model has been endorsed by many medical specialty groups and health care organizations, challenges inhibiting its widespread adoption include incompatible payment systems, significant upfront investment, and pervasive incentives to maintain current practice models, among other barriers (Arend et al., 2012; Basu et al., 2016, 2017; Fleming et al., 2017; Kizer, 2016; Reynolds et al., 2015) (see Chapter 9 on payment models). The PCMH model also falls short of community-oriented and people-centered primary care (WHO, 2016) and the integration with public health called for in prior IOM reports (1983, 2012a).

Lack of Collaboration to Improve Education and Training

The 1996 report made nine recommendations concerning education and training for primary care, but mental health, public health, primary care, and other clinical disciplines involved in primary care have not yet formed a collaboration to advance essential competencies. Despite calls to reform the basic organization and financing of clinician training (IOM, 2014), little progress has been made. In fact, despite repeated recommendations to realign graduate medical education (GME) funding and accountability to focus on primary care and population health (COGME, 2010; IOM, 1989, 2014), there have been no major reforms to GME that might shift the balance toward the future workforce that is needed.

The policy of hospitals being central to financing clinical medical education limits the extent to which training can take place in the settings where primary care actually occurs (COGME, 2007; IOM, 1989). Between 2006 and 2008, only about 25 percent of those from the medical education pipeline entered primary care and around 5 percent practiced in rural settings (Chen et al., 2013), an output insufficient to maintain the current proportion of primary care physicians in the overall physician workforce. While training models and environments do demonstrate higher primary care and rural outputs, these are not priorities for most major teaching hospitals (Phillips et al., 2009, 2013; Raffoul et al., 2019; Rosenthal, 2000). Remarkably little funding also goes to support postgraduate training of other health professionals to prepare for clinical practice in primary care. Chapter 6 discusses options to improve the education and training of the primary care workforce.

A series of IOM reports in the early 2000s showed that interprofessional teams and collaborative practices improve health outcomes (IOM, 2001, 2007), yet despite the evidence and the many calls to better integrate training across professions, its clinicians remain largely professionally siloed, and so the availability of joint learning experiences remains a challenge (Cuff et al., 2014; Lipstein et al., 2016; Ritchie et al., 2016; The Josiah Macy Jr. Foundation, 2010). Progress is needed on educational tools to enhance the communication and teamwork of clinicians in primary care and also for education on how specialists and primary care clinicians can improve care coordination and understanding of each other's roles. See Chapter 5 for more on the evidence behind team-based care, effective models, and resource needs.

Erosion of the Primary Care Workforce

The 1996 report made several recommendations to help strengthen the primary care workforce, but a shortage remains, particularly in rural areas. Increasing the density of primary care physicians[7] by adding 10 more per 100,000 people is associated with an increase in life expectancy of more than 51 days (Basu et al., 2019). That study also found that the U.S. primary care physician workforce had declined by 5.2 physicians per 100,000 population overall and 7.0 physicians per 100,000 population in rural counties between 2005 and 2015, the exact opposite of what is needed. This erosion of workforce capacity is associated with a loss of 85 lives per day overall and about 16 per day in rural counties, which is the equivalent of a 200-person airplane crashing every 2–3 days (see Appendix C for the committee's calculations). The failure of current primary care physician production and policies to make primary care a more viable career, especially in rural areas, has important implications for health outcomes and inequities.

Lack of a Primary Care Research Agenda

PCR is a distinct and unique area of scientific inquiry. It includes novel approaches to acute, chronic, and preventive care in the context of whole-person care; developing and improving systems of care; disseminating and implementing evidence-based care; addressing behavioral health and SDOH as part of care; using technology for care; and uniquely blending individual care and population health. While the past 25 years have shown rapid advances in technology and science that could improve the delivery and outcomes of primary care, no federal agency has embraced and funded PCR, and no dedicated research funding is available (Mendel et al., 2020). Specifically, no single entity is responsible for developing and advancing a robust program of research on primary care despite it being the largest

---

[7] Throughout the report, the committee's use of the word "physician" refers to both allopathic and osteopathic physicians.

platform for health care delivery and often the only source of health care for nearly half of people seeking care each year (Petterson et al., 2018).

The 1996 report recommended that the U.S. Department of Health and Human Services "identify a lead agency for primary care research and ... the Congress of the United States [should] appropriate funds for this agency in an amount adequate to build both the infrastructure required to conduct primary care research and fund high-priority research projects" (IOM, 1996, p. 11). Today, the Agency for Healthcare Research and Quality (AHRQ) is the only federal agency with a mandate for PCR, but its National Center for Excellence in Primary Care has no dedicated research funding, limiting its ability to meaningfully contribute to the field (CAFM, 2019). AHRQ's entire funding is $500 million per year compared to the $50 billion annual budget of the National Institutes of Health (NIH), and just 0.2 percent of NIH funding supports family medicine research (Cameron et al., 2016). See Chapter 10 for more on PCR needs.

Misaligned Payment Models

Since the 1996 report, the disconnection between fee-for-service (FFS) payment and high-quality primary care has become even more clear. Payment tied to individual services without the ability to either focus on whole-person care or support interprofessional teams that deliver flexible services tailored to patient and community needs has stalled progress and held the entire enterprise back. The growing misalignment between revenue and the expense of supporting the delivery of high-quality primary care has also challenged the advancement of primary care. For example, many practices discovered that the financial investments involved with practice transformation or meeting specific PCMH requirements far exceeded the added compensation for PCMH certification (Basu et al., 2017; Fleming et al., 2017; Halladay et al., 2016; Martsolf et al., 2016; Nutting et al., 2012; Patel et al., 2013). Similarly, the costs for adopting and implementing electronic health records were more than the Meaningful Use payments (see Chapter 8). While other segments of the health care system were able to rapidly increase charges and reimbursement rates to compensate for the high cost of labor (Papanicolas et al., 2018), primary care encountered similar hikes in administrative and personnel costs without comparable increases in payment rates. This left little or no choice for many small, independent primary care practices other than purchase by larger, for-profit health systems, which enabled them to increase rates for delivering essentially the same services (Mostashari, 2016; Scheffler et al., 2018). Yet, people cared for by smaller, independent practices are significantly more likely to have lower costs and comparable outcomes (Casalino et al., 2014; Mostashari, 2016).

The increasing popularity of high-deductible health insurance plans (KFF, 2019; Wilde Mathews, 2018) and shifting of costs to consumers to maintain insurance companies' profit margins (Altman and Mechanic, 2018) has disproportionately impacted primary care. It is a relatively low-cost service in comparison to others within the health care system, so many people must pay the entire bill for non-preventive services because the amount is below their deductible. Paradoxically, this phenomenon deters people from seeking primary care, arguably the most cost-effective type of care that could prevent much higher health care costs (Ganguli et al., 2020).

Fragmentation of the U.S. Health Care System

Isolated examples provide evidence of progress toward the 1996 report's nine recommendations regarding interdisciplinary education and training for primary care, and several good examples of integrated health systems exist today. However, care organization remains largely fragmented in most settings, perpetuating a less efficient, less effective, less equitable, and more expensive system of care (Stange, 2009). Attempts to correct this have been plentiful and valiant, if isolated; some exemplars are presented throughout this report. Ultimately, a degree of tribalism between professions and subspecialties and an emphasis on disease-specific care within the health care system exist at the expense of the long-term vision of integration that would benefit whole-person health. See Chapter 5 for more on integrated delivery.

The COVID-19 Pandemic and Calls for Social Justice

The COVID-19 pandemic began in the early stages of this committee's work; it revealed many vulnerabilities in how primary care is delivered today and further highlighted deep fissures in health equity resulting from racism and social injustice for individuals and families with undocumented immigration status or living in poverty (Dorn et al., 2020; Smith, 2020). If COVID-19 was a stress test of how well our country has supported its primary care infrastructure, the results have not been encouraging. Perhaps most notably, it has clearly demonstrated that large segments of our population do not have reliable access to primary care.

The pandemic also demonstrated that building a primary care system largely dependent on FFS payments is highly precarious. Such arrangements, which are the predominant payment method, have jeopardized the very existence of many primary care practices because the volume of visits declined rapidly as the pandemic took hold (Basu et al., 2020; Phillips et al., 2020). It is disappointing that the U.S. government hardly considered the role of primary care—our nation's largest and most distributed platform for health care—in its national epidemic planning (HHS, 2017; Holloway et al., 2014). This neglect is more marked considering that primary care is the frontline of COVID-19 triaging, testing, managing, and ultimately immunizing (Goodnough, 2021; Lewis et al., 2020). Congress also did not specifically consider primary care in its first four relief packages (Slavitt and Mostashari, 2020). By the time this report is published, the impacts of the pandemic may reveal more, particularly as care, testing, and vaccine administration for COVID-19 shift to primary care and patients reemerge, as cities and states begin to reopen, and make their way back to their primary care clinicians. A fundamental question will be whether primary care practices survive the economic crisis. Throughout this report, COVID-19 provides a useful lens on primary care problems, responses, and recommendations while also highlighting the gross inequalities and social injustices within society that are reflected in primary care practice.

In the midst of the COVID-19 pandemic, the United States also experienced a massive call for social justice, led by the Black Lives Matter movement, unlike anything experienced since the civil rights era of the 1960s. The nationwide discontent with the structural and institutional discrimination was further fueled by the disproportionate impact of the pandemic on the most disadvantaged and underserved populations, especially Black, Indigenous, and Hispanic groups (Tai et al., 2020). This is only the latest and perhaps most graphic illustration of racial and ethnic disparities in care and health outcomes that have been well documented and, along with growing economic inequities, are likely contributing to the decline in U.S. life expectancy in recent years (IOM, 2003; Woolf and Schoomaker, 2019).

The combination of events directly speaks to the committee's Statement of Task, particularly in terms of achieving health equity and population health goals and improving access, especially for underserved populations. While it is true that many of the same issues tackled in the 1996 report remain relevant, the United States of 2021 has radically changed due to the growth of the Internet, globalization, COVID-19, and the collective awakening to the impact of racism, all of which influence how people, families, and communities view and experience primary care. The implementation plan called for in the committee's Statement of Task attempts to address the barriers that thwarted the 1996 report's success, particularly in naming specific actors and actions that could secure this important foundation of health care and health. However, the committee considers other ideas and solutions that aim to achieve similar ends. COVID-19 and issues of equity are discussed throughout this report.

ORGANIZATION OF THE REPORT

The committee divided the report into 12 chapters. The remainder of this report lays out the committee's analysis of the current U.S. primary care system, which served as the basis for its recommendations and implementation plan. Chapter 2 provides a new definition of primary care, one that reflects the committee's vision for what it should be in the 21st century, and Chapter 3 presents the current state of U.S. primary care. Chapter 4 discusses the reasons primary care should be person centered, family centered, and community oriented, and Chapter 5 discusses how integrated primary care delivery is a foundational strategy for how health care organizations can support a culture of high-quality, person-centered, family-centered, and community-oriented primary care. Chapter 6 covers how the nation can build the workforce needed to enable primary care and interprofessional teams capable of supporting the whole person. Chapter 7 details why high-functioning digital technologies are an essential component of creating a high-quality primary care system that helps coordinate care and reduce clinician burnout, and Chapter 8 explains the importance of accountability and how the ability to monitor quality with metrics designed specifically for primary care will support implementing high-quality primary care. Chapter 9 discusses the critical role that revamping the current payment system can play in creating a system that can support independent primary care practices and the emerging array of new primary care delivery models. Chapter 10 makes the case for why the nation needs to invest specifically in PCR rather than relying on research in subspecialty care, hospitals, or single-disease cohorts. Chapter 11 describes the implementation, accountability, and public policy-making frameworks the committee used to develop its recommended implantation plan, presented in Chapter 12. Because many of the committee's recommended actions that comprise its implementation plan draw from information presented in more than one chapter, the specific actions of the implementation plan are included only in Chapter 12 and the Summary.

In addition to the core content, there are five appendixes. Appendix A presents the biographies of the committee members, fellows, and staff. Appendix B lists the full slate of the recommendations from the 1996 IOM report *Primary Care: America's Health in a New Era*. Appendix C includes the committee's calculations to determine the loss of life associated with decreased density of the primary care physician workforce presented earlier in this chapter. Appendix D maps the committee's recommended actions to different actors. Appendix E puts forth a scorecard for measuring the health of the U.S. primary care system.

REFERENCES

AAFP, AAP, ABFM, ABIM, ABP, ACP, and SGIM (American Academy of Family Physicians, American Academy of Pediatrics, American Board of Family Medicine, American Board of Internal Medicine, American Board of Pediatrics, American College of Physicians, and Society of General Internal Medicine). 2020. *A new primary care paradigm.* https://www.newprimarycareparadigm.org (accessed December 23, 2020).

Altman, S., and R. Mechanic. 2018. Health care cost control: Where do we go from here? *Health Affairs Blog.* https://www.healthaffairs.org/do/10.1377/hblog20180705.24704/full (accessed July 13, 2020).

Arend, J., J. Tsang-Quinn, C. Levine, and D. Thomas. 2012. The patient-centered medical home: History, components, and review of the evidence. *Mount Sinai Journal of Medicine* 79(4):433–450.

Baillieu, R., M. Kidd, R. Phillips, M. Roland, M. Mueller, D. Morgan, B. Landon, J. DeVoe, V. Martinez-Bianchi, H. Wang, R. Etz, C. Koller, N. Sachdev, H. Jackson, Y. Jabbarpour, and A. Bazemore. 2019. The primary care spend model: A systems approach to measuring investment in primary care. *BMJ Global Health* 4(4):e001601.

Basu, S., R. S. Phillips, Z. Song, B. E. Landon, and A. Bitton. 2016. Effects of new funding models for patient-centered medical homes on primary care practice finances and services: Results of a microsimulation model. *Annals of Family Medicine* 14(5):404–414.

Basu, S., R. Phillips, Z. Song, A. Bitton, and B. Landon. 2017. High levels of capitation payments needed to shift primary care toward proactive team and nonvisit care. *Health Affairs* 36:1599–1605.

Basu, S., S. A. Berkowitz, R. L. Phillips, A. Bitton, B. E. Landon, and R. S. Phillips. 2019. Association of primary care physician supply with population mortality in the United States, 2005–2015. *JAMA Internal Medicine* 179(4):506–514.

Basu, S., R. S. Phillips, R. Phillips, L. E. Peterson, and B. E. Landon. 2020. Primary care practice finances in the United States amid the COVID-19 pandemic. *Health Affairs* 39(9):1605–1614.

Bielaszka-DuVernay, C. 2011. Vermont's blueprint for medical homes, community health teams, and better health at lower cost. *Health Affairs* 30(3):383–386.

Bodenheimer, T., and C. Sinsky. 2014. From triple to quadruple aim: Care of the patient requires care of the provider. *Annals of Family Medicine* 12(6):573–576.

Bodenheimer, T., A. Ghorob, R. Willard-Grace, and K. Grumbach. 2014. The 10 building blocks of high-performing primary care. *Annals of Family Medicine* 12(2):166–171.

CAFM (Council of Academic Family Medicine). 2019. *Fund AHRQ's primary care research center.* Washington, DC: Council of Academic Family Medicine.

Cameron, B. J., A. W. Bazemore, and C. P. Morley. 2016. Lost in translation: NIH funding for family medicine research remains limited. *Journal of the American Board of Family Practice* 29(5):528–530.

Casalino, L. P., M. F. Pesko, A. M. Ryan, J. L. Mendelsohn, K. R. Copeland, P. P. Ramsay, X. Sun, D. R. Rittenhouse, and S. M. Shortell. 2014. Small primary care physician practices have low rates of preventable hospital admissions. *Health Affairs* 33(9):1680–1688.

CDC (Centers for Disease Control and Prevention). 2019. *Summary Health Statistics Tables: National Health Interview Survey, 2018 (Table A-16).* Atlanta, GA: Centers for Disease Control and Prevention.

Chen, C., S. Petterson, R. L. Phillips, F. Mullan, A. Bazemore, and S. D. O'Donnell. 2013. Towards graduate medical education (GME) accountability: Measuring the outcomes of GME institutions. *Academic Medicine* 88(9):1267–1280.

Christakis, D. A., L. Mell, T. D. Koepsell, F. J. Zimmerman, and F. A. Connell. 2001. Association of lower continuity of care with greater risk of emergency department use and hospitalization in children. *Pediatrics* 107(3):524–529.

Christian, E., V. Krall, S. Hulkower, and S. Stigleman. 2018. Primary care behavioral health integration: Promoting the quadruple aim. *North Carolina Medical Journal* 79(4):250–255.

COGME (Council on Graduate Medical Education). 2007. *New paradigms for physician training for improving access to health care.* Washington, DC: Council on Graduate Medical Education.

COGME. 2010. *Advancing primary care.* Rockville, MD: Council on Graduate Medical Education.

Coker, T. R., T. Thomas, and P. J. Chung. 2013. Does well-child care have a future in pediatrics? *Pediatrics* 131(Suppl 2):S149–S159.

Cooley, W. C., J. W. McAllister, K. Sherrieb, and K. Kuhlthau. 2009. Improved outcomes associated with medical home implementation in pediatric primary care. *Pediatrics* 124(1):358–364.

Coutinho, A. J., Z. Levin, S. Petterson, R. L. Phillips, Jr., and L. E. Peterson. 2019. Residency program characteristics and individual physician practice characteristics associated with family physician scope of practice. *Academic Medicine* 94(10):1561–1566.

Cuff, P., M. Schmitt, B. Zierler, M. Cox, J. De Maeseneer, L. L. Maine, S. Reeves, H. C. Spencer, and G. E. Thibault. 2014. Interprofessional education for collaborative practice: Views from a global forum workshop. *Journal of Interprofessional Care* 28(1):2–4.

Davis, K., M. Abrams, and K. Stremikis. 2011. How the Affordable Care Act will strengthen the nation's primary care foundation. *Journal of General Internal Medicine* 26(10):1201–1203.

Dorn, A. V., R. E. Cooney, and M. L. Sabin. 2020. COVID-19 exacerbating inequalities in the US. *The Lancet* 395(10232):1243–1244.

Fleming, N. S., B. da Graca, G. O. Ogola, S. D. Culler, J. Austin, P. McConnell, R. McCorkle, P. Aponte, M. Massey, and C. Fullerton. 2017. Costs of transforming established primary care practices to patient-centered medical homes (PCMHs). *Journal of the American Board of Family Medicine* 30(4):460–471.

Ganguli, I., T. H. Lee, and A. Mehrotra. 2019. Evidence and implications behind a national decline in primary care visits. *Journal of General Internal Medicine* 34(10):2260–2263.

Ganguli, I., Z. Shi, E. J. Orav, A. Rao, K. N. Ray, and A. Mehrotra. 2020. Declining use of primary care among commercially insured adults in the United States, 2008–2016. *Annals of Internal Medicine* 172(4):240–247.

Goodnough, A. 2021. In quest for herd immunity, giant vaccination sites proliferate. *The New York Times.* https://www.nytimes.com/2021/02/28/health/covid-vaccine-sites.html (accessed March 1, 2021).

Green, L. A., G. E. Fryer, Jr., B. P. Yawn, D. Lanier, and S. M. Dovey. 2001. The ecology of medical care revisited. *New England Journal of Medicine* 344(26):2021–2025.

Halladay, J. R., K. Mottus, K. Reiter, C. M. Mitchell, K. E. Donahue, W. M. Gabbard, and K. Gush. 2016. The cost to successfully apply for level 3 medical home recognition. *Journal of the American Board of Family Practice* 29(1):69–77.

HHS (U.S. Department of Health and Human Services). 2017. *Pandemic influenza plan: 2017 update.* Washington, DC: U.S. Department of Health and Human Services.

Holloway, R., S. A. Rasmussen, S. Zaza, N. J. Cox, and D. B. Jernigan. 2014. *Updated preparedness and response framework for influenza pandemics.* Washington, DC: Centers for Disease Control and Prevention.

HRSA (Health Resources and Services Administration). 2020a. *Behavioral health and primary care integration.* https://bphc.hrsa.gov/qualityimprovement/clinicalquality/behavioralhealth/index.html (accessed March 2, 2021).

HRSA. 2020b. *Oral health and primary care integration.* https://bphc.hrsa.gov/qualityimprovement/clinicalquality/oralhealth/index.html (accessed March 2, 2021).

International Conference on Primary Health Care. 1978. *Declaration of Alma-Ata.* Alma-Ata, USSR: World Health Organization.

IOM (Institute of Medicine). 1983. *Community oriented primary care: New directions for health services delivery.* Washington, DC: National Academy Press.

IOM. 1989. *Primary care physicians: Financing their graduate medical education in ambulatory settings.* Washington, DC: National Academy Press.

IOM. 1994. *Defining primary care: An interim report.* Washington, DC: National Academy Press.

IOM. 1996. *Primary care: America's health in a new era.* Washington, DC: National Academy Press.

IOM. 2001. *Crossing the quality chasm: A new health system for the 21st century.* Washington, DC: National Academy Press.

IOM. 2003. *Unequal treatment: Confronting racial and ethnic disparities in health care.* Washington, DC: The National Academies Press.

IOM. 2007. *Preventing medication errors.* Washington, DC: The National Academies Press.

IOM. 2011a. *Advancing oral health in America.* Washington, DC: The National Academies Press.

IOM. 2011b. *The future of nursing: Leading change, advancing health.* Washington, DC: The National Academies Press.

IOM. 2012a. *For the public's health: Investing in a healthier future.* Washington, DC: The National Academies Press.

IOM. 2012b. *Primary care and public health: Exploring integration to improve population health.* Washington, DC: The National Academies Press.

IOM. 2014. *Graduate medical education that meets the nation's health needs.* Washington, DC: The National Academies Press.

Johansen, M. E., S. M. Kircher, and T. R. Huerta. 2016. Reexamining the ecology of medical care. *New England Journal of Medicine* 374(5):495–496.

Kempski, A., and A. Greiner. 2020. *Primary care spending: High stakes, low investment.* Washington, DC: Primary Care Collaborative.

KFF (Kaiser Family Foundation). 2019. *Employer health benefits: 2019 annual survey.* San Francisco, CA: Kaiser Family Foundation.

Kizer, K. W. 2016. Understanding the costs of patient-centered medical homes. *Journal of General Internal Medicine* 31(7):705–706.

Koller, C. F., and D. Khullar. 2017. Primary care spending rate—a lever for encouraging investment in primary care. *New England Journal of Medicine* 377(18):1709–1711.

Kringos, D. S., W. Boerma, J. van der Zee, and P. Groenewegen. 2013. Europe's strong primary care systems are linked to better population health but also to higher health spending. *Health Affairs* 32(4):686–694.

Landon, B. E., K. Grumbach, and P. J. Wallace. 2012. Integrating public health and primary care systems: Potential strategies from an IOM report. *JAMA* 308(5):461–462.

Levine, D. M., B. E. Landon, and J. A. Linder. 2019. Quality and experience of outpatient care in the United States for adults with or without primary care. *JAMA Internal Medicine* 179(3):363–372.

Lewis, C., S. Seervai, T. Shah, M. K. Abrams, and L. Zephyrin. 2020. *Primary care and the COVID-19 pandemic.* https://www.commonwealthfund.org/blog/2020/primary-care-and-covid-19-pandemic (accessed July 1, 2020).

Liaw, W. R., A. Jetty, S. M. Petterson, L. E. Peterson, and A. W. Bazemore. 2016. Solo and small practices: A vital, diverse part of primary care. *Annals of Family Medicine* 14(1):8–15.

Lipstein, S. H., A. L. Kellermann, B. Berkowitz, R. Phillips, D. Sklar, G. D. Steele, and G. E. Thibault. 2016. *Workforce for 21st century health and health care: A vital direction for health and health care.* Washington, DC: National Academy of Medicine.

Long, W. E., H. Bauchner, R. D. Sege, H. J. Cabral, and A. Garg. 2012. The value of the medical home for children without special health care needs. *Pediatrics* 129(1):87–98.

Love, H. E., J. Schlitt, S. Soleimanpour, N. Panchal, and C. Behr. 2019. Twenty years of school-based health care growth and expansion. *Health Affairs* 38(5):755–764.

Macinko, J., B. Starfield, and L. Shi. 2003. The contribution of primary care systems to health outcomes within Organization for Economic Cooperation and Development (OECD) countries, 1970–1998. *Health Services Research* 38(3):831–865.

Martin, S., R. L. Phillips, Jr., S. Petterson, Z. Levin, and A. W. Bazemore. 2020. Primary care spending in the United States, 2002–2016. *JAMA Internal Medicine* 180(7):1019–1020.

Martsolf, G. R., R. Kandrack, R. A. Gabbay, and M. W. Friedberg. 2016. Cost of transformation among primary care practices participating in a medical home pilot. *Journal of General Internal Medicine* 31(7):723–731.

MedPAC (Medicare Payment Advisory Commission). 2008. *Report to the Congress: Reforming the delivery system.* Washington, DC: Medicare Payment Advisory Commission.

MedPAC. 2014. *Report to the Congress: Medicare and the health care delivery system.* Washington, DC: Medicare Payment Advisory Commission.

Mendel, P., C. A. Gidengil, A. Tomoaia-Cotisel, S. Mann, A. J. Rose, K. J. Leuschner, N. S. Qureshi, V. Kareddy, J. L. Sousa, and D. Kim. 2020. *Health services and primary care research study: Comprehensive report.* Santa Monica, CA: RAND Corporation.

Mostashari, F. 2016. The paradox of size: How small, independent practices can thrive in value-based care. *Annals of Family Medicine* 14(1):5–7.

NASEM (National Academies of Sciences, Engineering, and Medicine). 2016. *Assessing progress on the Institute of Medicine report* The Future of Nursing. Washington, DC: The National Academies Press.

NRC (National Research Council) and IOM. 2013. *U.S. health in international perspective: Shorter lives, poorer health.* Washington, DC: The National Academies Press.

Nutting, P. A., B. F. Crabtree, and R. R. McDaniel. 2012. Small primary care practices face four hurdles—including a physician-centric mind-set—in becoming medical homes. *Health Affairs* 31(11):2417–2422.

OECD (Organisation for Economic Co-operation and Development). 2019. *Deriving preliminary estimates of primary care spending under the SHA 2011 framework.* Paris, France: Organisation for Economic Co-operation and Development.

Papanicolas, I., L. R. Woskie, and A. K. Jha. 2018. Health care spending in the United States and other high-income countries. *JAMA* 319(10):1024–1039.

Park, B., S. B. Gold, A. Bazemore, and W. Liaw. 2018. How evolving United States payment models influence primary care and its impact on the quadruple aim. *Journal of the American Board of Family Medicine* 31(4):588–604.

Patel, M. S., M. J. Arron, T. A. Sinsky, E. H. Green, D. W. Baker, J. L. Bowen, and S. Day. 2013. Estimating the staffing infrastructure for a patient-centered medical home. *American Journal of Managed Care* 19(6):509–516.

Petterson, S., R. McNellis, K. Klink, D. Meyers, and A. Bazemore. 2018. *The state of primary care in the United States: A chartbook of facts and statistics.* Washington, DC: Robert Graham Center.

Phillips, R. L., Jr., and A. W. Bazemore. 2010. Primary care and why it matters for U.S. health system reform. *Health Affairs* 29(5):806–810.

Phillips, R. L., Jr., M. Dodoo, S. Petterson, I. Xierali, A. Bazemore, B. Teevan, K. Bennett, C. Legagneur, J. Rudd, and J. Phillips. 2009. *Specialty and geographic distribution of the physician workforce: What influences medical student and resident choices?* Washington, DC: Robert Graham Center.

Phillips, R. L., Jr., S. Petterson, and A. Bazemore. 2013. Do residents who train in safety net settings return for practice? *Academic Medicine* 88(12):1934–1940.

Phillips, R. L., Jr., A. Bazemore, and A. Baum. 2020. The COVID-19 tsunami: The tide goes out before it comes in. *Health Affairs Blog.* https://www.healthaffairs.org/do/10.1377/hblog20200415.293535/full (accessed December 18, 2020).

Raffoul, M., G. Bartlett-Esquilant, and R. L. Phillips, Jr. 2019. Recruiting and training a health professions workforce to meet the needs of tomorrow's health care system. *Academic Medicine* 94(5):651–655.

Ray, K. N., Z. Shi, I. Ganguli, A. Rao, E. J. Orav, and A. Mehrotra. 2020. Trends in pediatric primary care visits among commercially insured U.S. children, 2008–2016. *JAMA Pediatrics* 174(4):350–357.

Reid, R., C. Damberg, and M. W. Friedberg. 2019. Primary care spending in the fee-for-service medicare population. *JAMA Internal Medicine* 179(7):977–980.

Reiff, J., N. Brennan, and J. Fuglesten Biniek. 2019. Primary care spending in the commercially insured population. *JAMA* 322(22):2244–2245.

Reynolds, P. P., K. Klink, S. Gilman, L. A. Green, R. S. Phillips, S. Shipman, D. Keahey, K. Rugen, and M. Davis. 2015. The patient-centered medical home: Preparation of the workforce, more questions than answers. *Journal of General Internal Medicine* 30(7):1013–1017.

Ritchie, C., R. Andersen, J. Eng, S. K. Garrigues, G. Intinarelli, H. Kao, S. Kawahara, K. Patel, L. Sapiro, A. Thibault, E. Tunick, and D. E. Barnes. 2016. Implementation of an interdisciplinary, team-based complex care support health care model at an academic medical center: Impact on health care utilization and quality of life. *PLOS ONE* 11(2):e0148096.

Rittenhouse, D. R., J. A. Wiley, L. E. Peterson, L. P. Casalino, and R. L. Phillips. 2020. Meaningful use and medical home functionality in primary care practice. *Health Affairs* 39(11):1977–1983.

Rosenthal, T. C. 2000. Outcomes of rural training tracks: A review. *Journal of Rural Health* 16(3):213–216.

Rui, P., and T. Okeyode. 2016. *National Ambulatory Medical Care Survey: 2016 national summary tables.* Atlanta, GA: Centers for Disease Control and Prevention.

Scheffler, R. M., D. R. Arnold, and C. M. Whaley. 2018. Consolidation trends in California's health care system: Impacts on ACA premiums and outpatient visit prices. *Health Affairs* 37(9):1409–1416.

Shi, L. 2012. The impact of primary care: A focused review. *Scientifica* 2012:432892.

Skocpol, T. 1995. The rise and resounding demise of the Clinton plan. *Health Affairs* 14(1):66–85.

Slavitt, A., and F. Mostashari. 2020. Covid-19 is battering independent physician practices. They need help now. *STAT.* https://www.statnews.com/2020/05/28/covid-19-battering-independent-physician-practices (accessed December 1, 2020).

Smith, D. B. 2020. The pandemic challenge: End separate and unequal healthcare. *The American Journal of the Medical Sciences* 360(2):109–111.

Stange, K. C. 2009. The problem of fragmentation and the need for integrative solutions. *Annals of Family Medicine* 7(2):100–103.

Starfield, B., L. Shi, and J. Macinko. 2005. Contribution of primary care to health systems and health. *Milbank Quarterly* 83(3):457–502.

Tai, D. B. G., A. Shah, C. A. Doubeni, I. G. Sia, and M. L. Wieland. 2020. The disproportionate impact of COVID-19 on racial and ethnic minorities in the united states. *Clinical Infectious Diseases* ciaa815.

The Josiah Macy Jr. Foundation. 2010. *Educating nurses and physicians: Toward new horizons conference summary.* Palo Alto, CA: The Josiah Macy Jr. Foundation, The Carnegie Foundation for the Advancement of Teaching.

The Larry A. Green Center, and PCC (Primary Care Collaborative). 2020. *Quick COVID-19 primary care survey: Clinician series 9 fielded May 8–11, 2020.* https://www.green-center.org/covid-survey (accessed January 21, 2021).

White, K. L., T. F. Williams, and B. G. Greenberg. 1961. The ecology of medical care. *New England Journal of Medicine* 265:885–892.

WHO (World Health Organization). 2016. *Framework on integrated, people-centered health services.* Geneva, Switzerland: World Health Organization.

Wilde Mathews, A. 2018. Behind your rising health-care bills: Secret hospital deals that squelch competition. *The Wall Street Journal.* https://www.wsj.com/articles/behind-your-rising-health-care-bills-secret-hospital-deals-that-squelch-competition-1537281963 (accessed January 8, 2020).

Woolf, S. H., and H. Schoomaker. 2019. Life expectancy and mortality rates in the United States, 1959–2017. *JAMA* 322(20):1996–2016.

2

Defining High-Quality
Primary Care Today

The report *Primary Care: America's Health in a New Era* (IOM, 1996) presented the following definition of primary care:

Primary care is the provision of integrated, accessible health care services by clinicians who are accountable for addressing a large majority of personal health care needs, developing a sustained partnership with patients, and practicing in the context of family and community.

This definition advanced several important ideas about primary care that are still relevant today. First, and perhaps most significant to the current committee, is the idea that the relationship (referred to as a "sustained partnership" in the definition) is foundational to primary care. While the definition describes a relationship between patients and clinicians, this committee's view is that this foundational relationship is sustained through interactions between patients, their families, and any member (or members) of the primary care team (IOM, 1996). While the primary care team will change over time, primary care relationships are important throughout a person's life, beginning at childhood and into adolescence, adulthood, and old age. Second, primary care is not provided in a vacuum but rather occurs within the context of the patient's family and community. Third, primary care is best delivered in an integrated and accessible system. While these ideas were widely embraced as ideal (Halfon and Hochstein, 2002; IOM, 2012; Starfield et al., 2005), progress has been markedly limited in making them a reality for most primary care practices (Frey, 2018; Larson et al., 2005; Levene et al., 2018). Other notions, such as comprehensively addressing a large majority of a person's health care needs, were not new at the time, but nonetheless highlighted an important core function of primary care that continues today.

AN UPDATED DEFINITION OF PRIMARY CARE

While the committee agreed that the essence of the 1996 Institute of Medicine (IOM) definition was still highly relevant, it felt that the definition did not fully capture certain important shifts in primary care since 1996. Specifically, the committee felt an accurate, contemporary definition should

- shift the emphasis from the provision of health care *services* to integrated, whole-person health;
- emphasize the foundational sustained relationships at the core of high-quality primary care;
- recognize the importance of communities and their critical roles in the provision of primary care;
- highlight the need for primary care to be equitable;
- recognize the interprofessional care teams that deliver primary care; and
- acknowledge the diversity of settings (and modalities used) in which primary care occurs.

Recognizing these six key shifts,[1] this committee offers an updated definition of high-quality primary care, largely based on the 1996 IOM definition but with several meaningful changes that, in its view, more accurately reflects what *high-quality* means today:

> **High-quality primary care is the provision of whole-person, integrated, accessible, and equitable health care by interprofessional teams that are accountable for addressing the majority of an individual's health and wellness needs across settings and through sustained relationships with patients, families, and communities.**

Like the 1996 definition, this updated definition is in many ways aspirational—that is, it describes what high-quality primary care *should be*. In reality, what most people have access to in the United States today does not fully realize the vision presented in this definition. Additionally, it presents an ideal that will require additional financial investment in many settings (see Chapter 9 for more on paying for primary care). This definition

---

[1] These topics are discussed in greater detail later in the chapter.

articulates the committee's vision and represents what this report's recommendations and implementation strategy broadly seek to achieve.

Figure 2-1 visualizes what high-quality primary care can look like for a family in the United States, showing how it is based on strong relationships between the interprofessional primary care team and the individual,

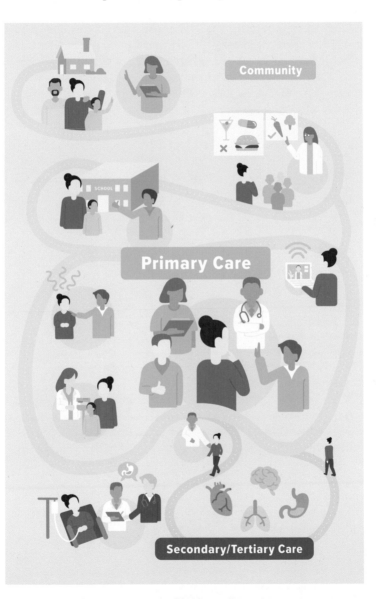

FIGURE 2-1 A visual representation of high-quality primary care.

family, and community and is delivered in a variety of settings. The person receiving care is in orange, physicians are in white, other team members are in blue, and family members are in olive. The top third of the illustration encompasses the many ways in which primary care can mesh with the community, while the bottom third represents connections that primary care should have with secondary and tertiary care. The figure also illustrates the unique roles of different members of the interprofessional primary care team in each of these settings.

If this definition is realized, primary care will better deliver both societal and individual benefits. In that sense, it is like public education—a common good to be assured, not a personal service to be delivered. Primary care's documented salutary effects for population outcomes and equity (and

---

BOX 2-1
Primary Care as a Common Good

The committee's position is that high-quality primary care, distinct from most other health care services, is a common good, delivering benefits for society and to individuals. Fundamentally, the committee holds that primary care is essential to the American values of "life, liberty and the pursuit of happiness" and merits status as a common good.

The economic definition[a] of a common good is a good or service that is both *rivalrous* (the resource is limited, so more for one person means less for another) and *non-excludable* (users cannot be prevented from accessing it, regardless of whether they have paid). While one might argue that morality and even U.S. public policy[b] dictate that all health care is a common good, primary care is to be particularly prioritized among health care services as a common good because of both its societal value (i.e., beneficial effect on population health for resources consumed) and its precarious status.

Responsible public policy requires that a common good—be it public education, grazing grounds for farm animals, or the capacity of primary care to meet the needs of a population—merits some degree of public policy for oversight and monitoring. In the absence of that, the good is depleted and not available when the need for it increases. Such has been the case for primary care during the COVID-19 pandemic.

Primary care does not, however, currently have the public policy support that reflects its importance as a common good. As Isaacs (2001) explains, for a health-based public good[c] to successfully take hold in a society and receive the public policy support it needs to succeed, a confluence of factors must be present:

1. **Highly credible scientific evidence** that can withstand critique from stakeholders whose interests may be threatened

contribution to inequity when missing or inadequate) within the United States, and the considerable evidence of its contribution to relative improvement in health outcomes in other developed countries, support this goal of making it a public benefit rather than a health service (Basu et al., 2019; Franks and Fiscella, 1998; Gong et al., 2019; Hansen et al., 2015; Starfield, 2009, 2012; Starfield et al., 2005; WHO and UNICEF, 2018). Doing so creates a public interest in high-quality, accessible primary care and the collective benefit it delivers, both of which are demonstrably greater than exists for other health care and clinical services. Given the challenges facing primary care cited throughout this report, this benefit undergirds the sense of urgency that this committee wishes to convey. (See Box 2-1 for more on primary care as a public good.)

2. **Strong advocacy** to make the issue visible
3. **Public awareness** driven by a partnership between the advocates and the media
4. **Laws and regulations** to codify the needed changes (Isaacs, 2001)

The evidence supporting the importance of primary care relative to other health care services is strong and convincing (Basu et al., 2019; Levine et al., 2019; Macinko et al., 2003; Shi, 2012). The committee acknowledges the absence of strong advocacy or even organized leadership for the field of primary care—this is discussed in greater detail in Chapter 3. Similarly, the media today offers little conversation on the importance of primary care, though stronger advocacy or leadership from the field of primary care and greater political support could position primary care more prominently in the media.

The implementation strategy outlined in Chapter 11 of this report accounts for the public policy-making process, through which consensus is achieved on the nature and priority of competing common goods through laws and regulations. Ignoring that process or explicitly relying on market-based mechanisms for allocating individually consumed private goods and services, in which primary care competes for its rightful share of the health care pie, have created the weakened condition that this report attempts to address.

---

[a] See http://wealthofthecommons.org/essay/why-distinguish-common-goods-public-goods (accessed February 14, 2021).

[b] For example, the federal Emergency Medical Treatment and Labor Act requires that no one be turned away from an emergency room.

[c] Though similar, a public good and common good are not identical. A common good can be overused and can disappear absent regulation, while a public good can be consumed or used by everyone simultaneously without affecting anyone else's ability to consume or use it. Isaacs refers specifically to a public good.

Embracing Integrated, Whole-Person Health

The current U.S. health care system focuses on delivering specific, reimbursable services centered around a disease process; this has resulted in increased health care spending, widening disparities, and inequitable health outcomes (Shi, 2012; Stange, 2009). While treating, diagnosing, and managing acute and chronic conditions are core functions of primary care, providing whole-person care requires a comprehensive person-centered, integrated approach based on relationships that account for mental, physical, emotional, and spiritual health and the social determinants of health in the context of community experiences (Ellner and Phillips, 2017; Feuerstein et al., 2016; Ring and Mahadevan, 2017; Sia et al., 2004). The whole-person approach considers health to be about the well-being of the person, not just the absence of disease (Thomas et al., 2018).

Integrated primary care facilitates care across different professionals, facilities, and support systems and is continuous over time and tailored to individual and family needs, values, and preferences (Singer et al., 2011). This care facilitation should occur within the immediate primary care team and with groups and services outside of that team, including community-based services and the health system overall, as seamlessly as possible. This supports whole health, ensuring that physical health, behavioral health, social needs, and oral health are comprehensively addressed (Ellner and Phillips, 2017) (see Chapter 5 for more on integrated delivery).

The Importance of Sustained, Foundational Relationships

While the 1996 definition does refer to "sustained partnerships," this committee felt it was important to frame this partnership as a relationship and to emphasize that these relationships are not just between patients and clinicians but between individuals, families, and the interprofessional care team more broadly who work together in achieving personal health care needs and whole-person health.

Fundamentally, primary care supports the health of a person in the context of their life and community. Care should be contextualized to each person's situation and evolve as needs change over time. To meet a person's needs most effectively, clinicians, the individual, and other partners (including family members, informal caregivers, and extended interprofessional team members) need to come to shared understandings of the context of the individual's life. This activity is inherently a relational one, requiring trust and respect between the individual and their care team and others involved in their lives and their communities. A relationship implies that individuals and their families seeking primary care have identified one or more clinicians in the practice who accepts accountability for their care, health, and wellness and whom they trust and prefer to see. Thus, delivering primary care is a social and local activity in which relationships and interdependencies need to be carefully cultivated and supported (Buckley et al., 2013; Colwill et al., 2016; Ellner and Phillips, 2017; Flieger, 2017; Frey, 2010; Gottlieb, 2013; Green and Puffer, 2016; Kravitz and Feldman, 2017).

The evidence for the important role of relationships, often captured as continuity of care and self-reported outcomes, is some of the strongest for primary care's beneficial effect (see Chapter 8 for more on primary care measures). Building this relationship and trust to make primary care centered on people, their families, and communities includes ensuring that primary care is accessible, convenient, and desirable, which requires flexibility and variation in the way in which care occurs across and within communities.

Primary care means different things across different age groups, settings, and health statuses. For example, to a healthy 25-year-old, it may be an occasional sick visit at a retail clinic with a nurse practitioner. This type of care is symptom specific and may include very little interaction or relationship building but may be adequate for that person at that moment in their life. An individual with multiple chronic comorbidities or a disability, however, may depend more on a primary care team to coordinate care across multiple specialists and locations, and, more importantly, to help define priorities and health goals that will guide choices across the set of subspecialty services. Similarly, a mother with a healthy infant may depend on her primary care team to help her navigate preventive care and developmental needs and address the family's social needs that may impact her infant's health and well-being. For these individuals and all others, regardless of need or complexity, a strong relationship with a care team will help ensure that personal values and needs are honored and met. See Chapter 4 for more on primary care relationships.

The Role of the Community

For decades now, community involvement in delivering primary care has been recognized as critical to help achieve whole-person health goals. Focusing on the community was one of the features of the Declaration of Alma-Ata in 1978[2] (International Conference on Primary Health Care, 1978), and adding community-oriented primary care to the new conceptualization

---

[2] The Declaration of Alma-Ata was adopted at the International Conference on Primary Health Care in what was then known as Alma-Ata in the Soviet Socialist Republic (today, it is known as Almaty, Kazakhstan). The conference and declaration called for national and international action to strengthen primary health care throughout the world (International Conference on Primary Health Care, 1978).

addresses the individual's and family's culture and social context as they are embedded within a medical and social neighborhood, rather than from a solely delivery-centric model (Braddock et al., 2013; Buchmueller and Carpenter, 2010; Chokshi and Cohen, 2018; Davis et al., 2005; DeVoe et al., 2009; Driscoll et al., 2013; Edgoose and Edgoose, 2017; Enard and Ganelin, 2013; Etz, 2016; Finkelstein et al., 2020; IOM, 1983; Kramer et al., 2018; Landon et al., 2012; McNall et al., 2010; Possemato et al., 2018; Starfield, 2011; Yoon et al., 2018).

In community-oriented care, families and other informal caregivers are integrated with formal care to better support older adults (Miller and Weissert, 2000) or keep children and adults with special needs healthy. Increasing access to community- and school-based health centers and telephone visits would pull the gravitational center of health care toward the individual being treated. Community health workers (CHWs) can also play a particularly important role in this regard. In addition, community-oriented primary care facilitates coordination between public health approaches and primary care delivery, opening the door for primary care to play a central role in improving the health of the community (Eng et al., 1992), particularly those with disadvantaged populations (Cyril et al., 2015; Derose et al., 2019; Shukor et al., 2018). See Chapter 4 for more on the role of the community in primary care.

Primary Care's Role in Improving Health Equity

Health inequity costs the U.S. health care system billions of dollars per year (LaVeist et al., 2011), and the COVID-19 pandemic has exposed how that system does not serve all Americans equally (Tai et al., 2020; Webb Hooper et al., 2020). Since 1996, there has been increased focus on the critical role that primary care can play in improving equity (Shi, 2012; Starfield, 2009, 2012; Starfield et al., 2005) and in reducing, and ultimately eliminating, disparities in health and its determinants, including social determinants. Health equity involves striving for whole-person care that meets the highest possible standard of health that is available to everyone, which speaks to equal access, but should also aim to improve health outcomes specifically for disadvantaged populations, reduce disparities in clinical care, and address the social determinants of health (Braveman, 2014). Using interprofessional primary care teams that reflect the communities they serve, within an integrated system that supports building and developing relationships with individuals, families, and communities, is integral to achieving health equity.

According to a 2017 report by the Robert Wood Johnson Foundation, achieving health equity "requires removing obstacles to health such as poverty, discrimination, and their consequences, including powerlessness and lack of access to good jobs with fair pay, quality education and housing, safe environments, and health care" (Braveman et al., 2017, p. 2). While primary care alone cannot remove all of these obstacles, this report will examine the role primary care can play in making health care more equitable. Much like the World Health Organization Declaration of Alma-Ata stating that health is not merely the absence of disease but complete physical, mental, and social well-being, health equity is about not merely equal access to care or addressing inequalities but rather justice and fairness in attaining equal opportunities to achieve complete physical, mental, and social well-being (International Conference on Primary Health Care, 1978).

The Role of Interprofessional Teams in Primary Care

An optimal team to deliver high-quality primary care includes a variety of clinical and nonclinical team members who can effectively and efficiently deliver whole-person care that meets the needs of the community or population they serve. This team may look different across settings, communities, and populations and should ideally reflect the diversity of its community. Interprofessional team-based delivery, however, does not abdicate individual accountability, especially for the primary care clinician (or clinicians) on the team—individual team members are responsible for their assigned roles and responsibilities. In many instances, non-clinician team members, such as health coaches and CHWs, can fill a critical role as the main point of contact for primary care and even may be the most effective keepers of the relationship between the individual and the care team, even if they are not accountable for delivering the actual care (Bodenheimer, 2019; Bodenheimer and Smith, 2013; Brownstein et al., 2011; Grumbach et al., 2012; Kangovi et al., 2018; Margolius et al., 2012) (see Chapter 6 for more information about primary care teams).

Furthermore, interprofessional care teams should ideally be highly engaged in promoting population health in the communities in which they are practicing and addressing community needs that impact health. The COVID-19 pandemic has demonstrated that primary care and public health cannot exist in silos and that the primary care and public health workforces need to work together in improving population health (IOM, 2012) and to be accountable for the health of the populations they serve.[3] See Chapter 6 for more on interprofessional primary care teams.

---

[3] This committee adopts the definition of population health as the health outcomes of a group of individuals, including the distribution of those outcomes, from Kindig and Stoddart (2003). Groups are most often determined by geography but may also be employees of the same organization, share an ethnic group, or be cared for within a system (e.g., veterans who seek care through the U.S. Department of Veterans Affairs).

The Wide Variety of Settings and Modalities Providing Primary Care

Compared to 1996, people today obtain primary care in a variety of ways—beyond traditional face-to-face visits in clinician offices—that did not exist at all or were very limited in their application 25 years ago, including retail clinics, virtual encounters via telehealth, community settings, such as schools and workplaces, direct messaging via patient portals and smartphone applications, and other modalities that were inconceivable in 1996. In some settings, primary care is provided through integration into specialty practices (Sandberg et al., 2016). In many ways, an individual chooses a setting to receive primary care based on their health needs at that point in their life. For example, as discussed in Chapter 3, young adults, who are less likely to have complex health needs, are more likely to use retail clinics than older adults. Older adults in nursing homes or assisted living facilities may receive most of their primary care in those settings.

In communities with few physical health care facilities or local clinicians, virtual visits may be the optimal way to make care accessible to those who do not require a face-to-face consultation to receive the majority of their care, via telehealth visits with a clinician, communication on mobile applications or patient portals, or asynchronous consultation with a care team that is not physically present. Ideally, these technologies are used to strengthen, not replace, the relationship between people and the interprofessional care team (Weiner and Biondich, 2006). The COVID-19 pandemic rapidly expanded information technology–enabled care, and both patients and clinicians hope that it will remain a routine option (Bashshur et al., 2020; Hollander and Carr, 2020). Using technology, however, requires ensuring that people have equal access to it. For those that do not or cannot obtain access, or for the many who do require face-to-face consultation, alternate access points need to be made available.

FACILITATORS OF HIGH-QUALITY PRIMARY CARE

The committee identified seven facilitators that can help develop and sustain the updated definition of high-quality primary care and support primary care teams in achieving the vision of accessible high-quality primary care for all. The first five (payment models, accountability and improving quality, digital health care, interprofessional care teams, and research) have dedicated chapters in this report. The others (leadership and policy, laws, and regulations) are considered throughout the chapters that follow. See Box 2-2 for a summary of all the facilitators.

BOX 2-2
Facilitators of High-Quality Primary Care

1. **Payment Models.** Payment models that support integrated, interprofessional teams working in sustained relationships with patients will ensure that high-quality primary care is possible to implement and sustain.
2. **Accountability and Improving Quality.** Effective measurement that is not onerous and holds primary care accountable for its high-value function will facilitate improvement over time.
3. **Digital Health Care.** An equitable use of technology can make care more accessible and make the primary care experience more efficient, higher quality, and convenient for people and the interprofessional care team.
4. **Interprofessional Care Teams.** Care provided by teams of clinicians and other professionals fit to the needs of communities, working to the top of their skills, and in coordination leads to better health.
5. **Research.** Building the empirical evidence on the epidemiology, organization, and provision of primary care will facilitate continuous improvement within the field.
6. **Leadership.** Coordination among primary care leaders will provide a unified voice on critical issues that will guide decisions of health care organizations and government while increasing accountability.
7. **Policy, Laws, and Regulations.** Federal and state policy, laws, and regulations that are compatible with locally tailored care can enable primary care stakeholders to implement needed changes.

Payment Models

Payment for primary care is currently insufficient relative to the value and amount of care provided. As discussed in Chapter 1, the sector that provides more than one-third of all care, and that can help govern downstream health care costs, receives about 5 percent of total spending (Jabbarpour et al., 2019; Johansen et al., 2016; Martin et al., 2020; Reid et al., 2019). To ensure the United States can implement the committee's vision, payment models for primary care need to be able to support it. Currently, most primary care (and health care in general) relies on a fee-for-service (FFS) model, which pays clinicians for billable services provided, regardless of the quality of those services or their outcomes. This payment model does not support flexible, interprofessional team-based care that uses a variety of health care professionals to build and maintain lasting meaningful relationships with patients. It also often does not cover less traditional delivery modalities (e.g., telehealth or patient portal communications) that can improve access to care, facilitate relationship building, and make care delivery and workflow more efficient.

In response to the COVID-19 pandemic, the Centers for Medicare & Medicaid Services (CMS) relaxed some payment rules to make most telehealth visits reimbursable at the same rate as in-person visits (CMS, 2020a), and several states' Medicaid programs and many private insurers did the same (Bodenheimer and Laing, 2020). However, these changes were slow, incomplete, and only some have been made permanent. COVID-19 also showed that FFS payment does not facilitate rapid and flexible changes in delivering primary care to meet communities' needs and cannot sustain primary care when a crisis significantly reduces visit volume (Scott, 2020; Slavitt and Mostashari, 2020). In addition, current common payment models may not cover care provided by some team members at all (e.g., CHWs or health coaches) (Basu et al., 2016, 2017; Hudak et al., 2017; Kangovi, 2020; Katkin et al., 2017; Smith et al., 2018).[4]

However, even in a capitated payment model, high-quality primary care remains elusive when payment inadequately covers the expenses necessary to support integrated, team-based care. Current capitated arrangements cannot sustain primary care when individuals and families have medical and social complexity that requires more care services and a wider interprofessional team (Hudak et al., 2017). Health care practices and systems will need financial support to transition toward a more integrated, team-based primary care delivery model (primary care payment is discussed further in Chapter 9).

Accountability and Improving Quality

Since the 1996 IOM report, there has been a movement toward improved health care quality and measurement to hold the health care system accountable to its stated goals (IOM, 2001). The delivery of primary care is distinctly different from specialized care and ideally occurs in integrated settings that are adaptable to the unique needs of individuals and communities. Therefore, many of the quality measures used in other sectors of health care are not directly transferable (Chen et al., 2012; Johnston et al., 2015; Kronenberg et al., 2017). Furthermore, it is critically necessary to be thoughtful about the measures that will identify accountability within primary care and facilitate improvement in settings of care where primary care teams and delivery modalities will differ from each other. Currently, primary care is measured mostly by its parts, relying on hundreds of disease

---

[4] The Center for Medicare & Medicaid Innovation does allow states to file plans to reimburse for services delivered by CHWs (https://www.cdc.gov/dhdsp/programs/spha/docs/1305_ta_guide_chws.pdf [accessed October 8, 2020]). In addition, the American Medical Association approved new billing codes for health coaches that went into effect in 2020 (https://blog.gethealthie.com/2019/12/11/guide-to-new-health-coach-cpt-codes [accessed February 19, 2021]).

and process measures that present an incomplete assessment of quality and drive care away from patient values, relationships, and effective management of health (Mutter et al., 2018; Shuemaker et al., 2020). As discussed in Chapter 8, better measures of the high-value functions of primary care could better align the intrinsic and extrinsic motivations to improve care, improve population health, and reduce burnout (Etz et al., 2017, 2019; Phillips et al., 2019; Stange et al., 2014).

Digital Health Care

Today, digital technologies touch every aspect of care. In fact, no other aspect of patient care delivery has changed as dramatically since the 1996 IOM report. Digital health care applications and technologies can be used to facilitate the relationship building between the care team and the individual and improve access while sustaining those relationships (Meskó et al., 2017). However, while digital tools, such as patient portals and telehealth, can improve access to care for some (IQVIA Institute, 2017), patient populations have differing levels of access, capacity, and familiarity with them (Estacio et al., 2019), and clinicians need to be flexible and able to use the tools that their patients have access to and can use. Within the care team, digital health tools should enable team members to seamlessly communicate with each other, share patient data, effectively monitor patient populations, and do their jobs more efficiently without contributing to professional burnout.

Digital health data can provide valuable metrics on care delivery and patient outcomes, and digital health technologies have promise for use in changing and shaping health behaviors, helping with patient- and family-level prevention and care management, and incorporating health-related data across sectors outside of health, such as education and community (Nittas et al., 2019; Vassiliou et al., 2020). Ultimately, the information in these data systems needs to be interoperable and accessible to improve care delivery to individuals and communities. Ideally, the transfer of information across systems should be seamless, to enable efficient coordination and reduce administrative burden associated with manual entry of patient data (NASEM, 2019).

Digital health care tools also expand the scope of primary care and may shift diagnostic and therapeutic capacity from subspecialty care back to the primary care setting (Damhorst et al., 2019; Howick et al., 2014; Young and Nesbitt, 2017). Point-of-care ultrasound, for example, has been able to replace X-rays and magnetic resonance imaging in some applications and may enhance the quality of some procedures. Given the rapid and transformative technological and digital changes in health care in the past two decades, the committee considered the importance of digital advances throughout this report and discusses it in detail in Chapter 7.

Interprofessional Teams

Compared to 1996, primary care today is more of an interprofessional team effort. The breadth of skills that a well-functioning team of diverse clinical and non-clinical professions offers can more comprehensively support the whole-person health goals of primary care than any individual clinician is capable of doing.

Primary care teams today need preparation to function in integrated systems with multiple types of health care workers and others in the community supporting the goals of primary care. Challenges include determining the size of the workforce that is needed; the types of team members needed in different communities; the necessary competencies of team members to function in an integrated, interprofessional manner; the funding and payment needed to ensure an adequate workforce and team composition; and the ways that the workforce can integrate and coordinate care with public health. Most recent evidence suggests that the primary care workforce is eroding generally, but this particularly true in rural areas (Basu et al., 2019) (see Chapter 6 for more on primary care team members).

Research

A better understanding of best practices in the delivery of primary care will also lead to further improvement, new discoveries, and cutting-edge innovation. While research is commonly conducted within primary care settings, it is primarily focused on a disease or condition and seldom designed to examine the science of effective models of providing or organizing primary care itself. The Agency for Healthcare Research and Quality is home to the National Center for Excellence in Primary Care Research, but the center has never had regular funding and currently has none (NIH and NIRSQ, 2020). The National Institutes of Health funds research that occurs in primary care, but it is routinely less than 0.4 percent of its budget (Cameron et al., 2016; Lucan et al., 2008). About 30 percent of the most recent funding from the Patient-Centered Outcomes Research Institute (PCORI) was directed to primary care research (PCR), most of it limited to comparative effectiveness research (Balster et al., 2019). While PCORI has become the mainstay for PCR funding and also funds essential infrastructure, it alone does not sufficiently meet the needs for PCR. Furthermore, this organization could change its focus and move away from primary care topics and/or fail to be reauthorized by Congress and disappear completely.

Primary care is one of the largest sectors of care yet remains unexplored territory for the origins and prevalence of disease, treatment outcomes, and care improvement. A dedicated home for research funding, sustained funding for PCR infrastructure, and funding mechanisms to study how to improve the care delivery are all needed to help inform, guide, and improve primary care learning health systems. Research is needed to improve the quality, experience, and cost of primary care and the experience of the primary care team. Research testing novel approaches, comparing various approaches, and studying the implementation of primary care would all be equally important. Research using primary care–specific metrics could also lead to creating a primary care learning health system.

Leadership

Primary care lacks a focal voice for its own advocacy, which may be the most important reason why the IOM's 1996 recommendations were not implemented. It lacks organization at local, state, and national levels. Despite several primary care professional societies, each of which is very active in professional and patient advocacy, there is no conjoint mechanism for them to come together on common issues of great import. The very interprofessional nature of primary care demands that the focal voice be able to speak across disciplinary boundaries. Within government, leadership is needed to better coordinate the many primary care activities across agencies. For this report to succeed in launching an effective implementation plan, and with that, increased accountability of primary care for implementing changes, more coordination of primary care's voice across organizations, disciplines, and government is required. Regardless, primary care will face increased accountabilities without sufficient resources. For example, it spends more time reporting quality measures than any other health care sector (Casalino et al., 2016) and is increasingly held responsible for point-of-care collection of social determinants and management of related issues without sufficient preparation or support (DeVoe et al., 2016; Solberg, 2016). Addressing the powerful combined forces of systemic discrimination and structural racism in education, housing, finance, social services, and the health care system is also likely to fall first to primary care, as it is where most people interact with health care. Collaboration across primary care professional associations will require leaders to embrace the generalist model of high-quality primary care put forth in this report.

Policy, Laws, and Regulations

A patchwork of federal and state policy, laws, and regulations directly and indirectly influence the scope, quality, availability, and accessibility of health care, including primary care. Law helps determine how primary care is delivered, who is able to deliver it, whether care will be accessible, where and how it is paid for, and the types of technology that can be used in its delivery. Additionally, law can have a large impact on innovation—both as a mechanism that can enable positive change as well as a means of limiting progress. As noted by Shin and colleagues (2010, p. 1):

> Law, as embodied in federal or state statutes, regulations, executive orders, administrative agency decisions, and court decisions, plays a profound role in shaping life circumstances, particularly as it relates to access, financing, and quality of individual health care.

The Patient Protection and Affordable Care Act (ACA)[5] in 2010 offers an example of how changes in federal law can facilitate improved access to health care generally (e.g., by making health insurance more affordable for millions of previously uninsured Americans) and primary care specifically (e.g., by financing the expansion of the Health Resources and Services Administration–funded health center program).

On the other hand, many current federal and state policies, laws, and regulations may deter or actually serve to undermine the growth of high-quality primary care and prevent primary care from attaining the common good status it deserves. For example, federal Medicare law[6] grants the U.S. Department of Health and Human Services (HHS) Secretary broad powers to determine Medicare payment rates and adjust the program's physician fee schedule to reflect payment for specific types of care. The Medicare fee schedule plays a role far beyond Medicare itself, since it is used as a payment benchmark by private insurers and employer health plans and thus largely determines the range of primary care procedures that will be compensated along with their payment levels, as well as the classes of health professionals who are qualified to directly bill the program and receive payment in their own right (Clemens et al., 2015). As discussed in Chapter 9, the fee schedule is a key driver of the undervaluation of primary care services and activities and this effectively is built into both broader financing schemes such as the capitation payments made by insurers and employer plans to large-scale integrated delivery systems in their networks or the fees insurers and plans pay to individual participating physicians (Trish et al., 2017). Several states, however, have passed laws to help correct this imbalance by requiring private insurers to increase the share of spending that goes to primary care (Delaware DOI, 2020; Jabbarpour et al., 2019;

---

[5] Patient Protection and Affordable Care Act, Public Law 111-148 (March 23, 2010).
[6] 42 U.S.C. § 1395w-4.

Koller et al., 2010). See Chapter 9 for a detailed discussion on primary care payment, including the policy, laws, and regulations that shape it.

Federal and state laws also play a significant role in codifying the training and practice requirements and programs that govern the health care workforce. As discussed in Chapter 6, trainees of many primary care professions are ineligible for the largest source of federal funding support, which comes through Medicare's graduate medical education payment system (IOM, 2014). The funds are also primarily distributed to teaching hospitals, not community-based settings where most primary care is delivered. By amending the ACA, Congress has, however, taken steps to fund training in non-hospital settings through the Teaching Health Center Graduate Medical Education program (HRSA, 2021; Mach and Kinzer, 2018). Similarly, while funding support through Title VII and Title VIII health professions training programs is open to more professions in community settings, actual annual appropriations levels remain low, limiting their impact on strengthening the workforce and improving access for the underserved (Palmer et al., 2008; Phillips and Turner, 2012).

Regarding the underlying scope of practice itself, despite national frameworks for education, training, and paying for health care, states retain the power to determine who may lawfully practice health care, to what extent, and under what conditions. State health professions practice acts, implementing regulations, and a web of legal rulings establish licensure competency requirements and the range of health care services each health profession may provide and under what conditions. This power has the effect of exposing health care practice itself to the political decisions of individual states, rather than ensuring that decisions regarding the regulation of health care practice are based on education and training competencies and evidence (IOM, 2011). See Chapter 3 for more on state-by-state scope of practice variation.

In a nation (and health care system) as varied and complex as the United States, there is no one-size-fits-all solution for the regulation of and payment for primary care. But that does not mean that laws do not evolve. Federal law can encourage innovation by promoting broad standards for coverage and payment of primary care, up to the limits of state-sanctioned licensure standards. As we have seen in recent federal action to broaden the classes of health professionals who may administer vaccines during a public health emergency, law can even preempt narrow state restrictions that impede access to lifesaving treatment (HHS, 2021). States can, of course, learn from one another regarding health professions regulatory innovation and encourage the growth of primary care models that are more person centered, integrated, and community oriented. This can be achieved, in part, through policies, laws, and regulations that allow for local adaptations of care delivery to enable primary care teams the flexibility to meet the needs of the populations they serve. Altering primary care payment policy is one major change that can help catalyze innovation at the practice level and allow the needed flexibility for practices to deliver primary care that aligns with the committee's definition. Changes in laws, policies, and regulations can also strengthen incentives for trainees to enter the primary care workforce and eventually work in federally designated shortage areas. Additionally, states can further enable high-quality, team-based care by altering their health professions regulatory standards to allow all health care professionals to work at the top of their license. Making permanent the policy and regulatory changes introduced during the COVID-19 pandemic (as CMS did for some, but not all, of the 2020 Physician Fee Schedule and telehealth expansion changes) will strengthen the delivery of and payment for services such as telehealth (CMS, 2020b; Verma, 2020).

The 2018 Declaration of Astana,[7] endorsed by the world's health ministers and HHS, affirms primary health care within a framework of universal health care and acknowledges that the fruits of effective primary health care can only be realized if everyone has access to it (WHO, 2018). The U.S. delegation had a different perspective on assuring access but nonetheless agreed that it was necessary. Policy solutions that solve the problem of inequity will also require addressing the underlying social, economic, political, justice, educational, *and* health systems that individually contribute to systemic, structural racism (Hardeman et al., 2020). Fully addressing the policies, laws, and regulations that enable and perpetuate societal inequalities and inequitable health care is beyond the scope of this report; however, legal, regulatory, and policy changes can improve equitable access to high-quality primary care regardless of insurance status, facilitate improvements to the care delivered, and enable the integration of that care with the broader health care system.

The impact of law (including federal and state statutes, policies, and regulations) is a major and overarching consideration for the delivery of and payment for all of health care. Various aspects of the law as they apply specifically to primary care are discussed throughout this report. An extensive examination of the interaction between law and health care delivery, including all of the barrier-creating and barrier-removing elements, is beyond the scope of this report. However, the important broader context of this relationship warrants follow-up examination and discussion as the recommendations within this report are implemented.

---

[7] In 2018, governments, nongovernmental organizations, professional organizations, and other stakeholder groups met at the Global Conference on Primary Health Care in Astana, Kazakhstan, to endorse a new declaration that reaffirmed a commitment to improving primary health care around the world.

REFERENCES

Balster, A., S. Mazur, A. Bazemore, and D. J. Merenstein. 2019. How well does the Patient-Centered Outcomes Research Institute fund primary care and comparative effectiveness research? *Journal of General Internal Medicine* 34(9):1680–1681.

Bashshur, R., C. R. Doarn, J. M. Frenk, J. C. Kvedar, and J. O. Woolliscroft. 2020. Telemedicine and the COVID-19 pandemic, lessons for the future. *Telemedicine and e-Health* 26(5):571–573.

Basu, S., R. S. Phillips, Z. Song, B. E. Landon, and A. Bitton. 2016. Effects of new funding models for patient-centered medical homes on primary care practice finances and services: Results of a microsimulation model. *Annals of Family Medicine* 14(5):404–414.

Basu, S., R. Phillips, Z. Song, A. Bitton, and B. Landon. 2017. High levels of capitation payments needed to shift primary care toward proactive team and nonvisit care. *Health Affairs* 36:1599–1605.

Basu, S., S. A. Berkowitz, R. L. Phillips, A. Bitton, B. E. Landon, and R. S. Phillips. 2019. Association of primary care physician supply with population mortality in the United States, 2005–2015. *JAMA Internal Medicine* 179(4):506–514.

Bodenheimer, T. 2019. Building powerful primary care teams. *Mayo Clinic Proceedings* 94(7):1135–1137.

Bodenheimer, T., and B. Y. Laing. 2020. *After COVID-19: How to rejuvenate primary care for the future.* https://www.healthaffairs.org/do/10.1377/hblog20200515.372874/full (accessed May 21, 2020).

Bodenheimer, T. S., and M. D. Smith. 2013. Primary care: Proposed solutions to the physician shortage without training more physicians. *Health Affairs* 32(11):1881–1886.

Braddock, C. H., 3rd, L. Snyder, R. L. Neubauer, G. S. Fischer, American College of Physicians Ethics, Professionalism and Human Rights Committee, and The Society of General Internal Medicine Ethics Committee. 2013. The patient-centered medical home: An ethical analysis of principles and practice. *Journal of General Internal Medicine* 28(1):141–146.

Braveman, P. 2014. What are health disparities and health equity? We need to be clear. *Public Health Reports* 129(Suppl 2):5–8.

Braveman, P., E. Arkin, T. Orleans, D. Proctor, and A. Plough. 2017. *What is health equity? And what difference does a definition make?* Princeton, NJ: Robert Wood Johnson Foundation.

Brownstein, J. N., G. R. Hirsch, E. L. Rosenthal, and C. H. Rush. 2011. Community health workers "101" for primary care providers and other stakeholders in health care systems. *Journal of Ambulatory Care Management* 34(3):210–220.

Buchmueller, T., and C. S. Carpenter. 2010. Disparities in health insurance coverage, access, and outcomes for individuals in same-sex versus different-sex relationships, 2000–2007. *American Journal of Public Health* 100(3):489–495.

Buckley, D. I., P. McGinnis, L. J. Fagnan, R. Mardon, J. Johnson, Maurice, and C. Dymek. 2013. *Clinical-community relationships evaluation roadmap.* Rockville, MD: Agency for Healthcare Research and Quality.

Cameron, B. J., A. W. Bazemore, and C. P. Morley. 2016. Lost in translation: NIH funding for family medicine research remains limited. *Journal of the American Board of Family Practice* 29(5):528–530.

Casalino, L. P., D. Gans, R. Weber, M. Cea, A. Tuchovsky, T. F. Bishop, Y. Miranda, B. A. Frankel, K. B. Ziehler, M. M. Wong, and T. B. Evenson. 2016. U.S. physician practices spend more than $15.4 billion annually to report quality measures. *Health Affairs* 35(3):401–406.

Chen, A. Y., S. M. Schrager, and R. Mangione-Smith. 2012. Quality measures for primary care of complex pediatric patients. *Pediatrics* 129(3):433–445.

Chokshi, D. A., and L. Cohen. 2018. Progress in primary care—from Alma-Ata to Astana. *JAMA* 320(19):1965–1966.

Clemens, J., J. D. Gottlieb, and T. L. Molnár. 2015. *The anatomy of physician payment: Contracting subject to complexity.* Cambridge, MA: National Bureau of Economic Research.

CMS (Centers for Medicare & Medicaid Services). 2020a. *Medicare telemedicine health care provider fact sheet.* https://www.cms.gov/newsroom/fact-sheets/medicare-telemedicine-health-care-provider-fact-sheet (accessed May 21, 2020).

CMS. 2020b. *Trump administration finalizes permanent expansion of Medicare telehealth services and improved payment for time doctors spend with patients.* https://www.cms.gov/newsroom/press-releases/trump-administration-finalizes-permanent-expansion-medicare-telehealth-services-and-improved-payment (accessed January 27, 2021).

Colwill, J. M., J. J. Frey, M. A. Baird, J. W. Kirk, and W. W. Rosser. 2016. Patient relationships and the personal physician in tomorrow's health system: A perspective from the Keystone IV conference. *Journal of the American Board of Family Medicine* 29(Suppl 1):S54–S59.

Cyril, S., B. J. Smith, A. Possamai-Inesedy, and A. M. Renzaho. 2015. Exploring the role of community engagement in improving the health of disadvantaged populations: A systematic review. *Global Health Action* 8:29842.

Damhorst, G. L., E. A. Tyburski, O. Brand, G. S. Martin, and W. A. Lam. 2019. Diagnosis of acute serious illness: The role of point-of-care technologies. *Current Opinion in Biomedical Engineering* 11:22–34.

Davis, K., S. C. Schoenbaum, and A. M. Audet. 2005. A 2020 vision of patient-centered primary care. *Journal of General Internal Medicine* 20(10):953–957.

Delaware DOI (Department of Insurance). 2020. *Delaware health care affordability standards: An integrated approach to improve access, quality and value.* Dover, DE: Delaware Department of Insurance.

Derose, K. P., M. V. Williams, C. A. Branch, K. R. Flórez, J. Hawes-Dawson, M. A. Mata, C. W. Oden, and E. C. Wong. 2019. A community-partnered approach to developing church-based interventions to reduce health disparities among African-Americans and Latinos. *Journal of Racial and Ethnic Health Disparities* 6(2):254–264.

DeVoe, J. E., J. W. Saultz, L. Krois, and C. J. Tillotson. 2009. A medical home versus temporary housing: The importance of a stable usual source of care. *Pediatrics* 124(5):1363–1371.

DeVoe, J. E., A. W. Bazemore, E. K. Cottrell, S. Likumahuwa-Ackman, J. Grandmont, N. Spach, and R. Gold. 2016. Perspectives in primary care: A conceptual framework and path for integrating social determinants of health into primary care practice. *Annals of Family Medicine* 14(2):104–108.

Driscoll, D. L., V. Hiratsuka, J. M. Johnston, S. Norman, K. M. Reilly, J. Shaw, J. Smith, Q. N. Szafran, and D. Dillard. 2013. Process and outcomes of patient-centered medical care with Alaska Native people at Southcentral Foundation. *Annals of Family Medicine* 11(Suppl 1):S41–S49.

Edgoose, J. Y. C., and J. M. Edgoose. 2017. Finding hope in the face-to-face. *Annals of Family Medicine* 15(3):272–274.

Ellner, A. L., and R. S. Phillips. 2017. The coming primary care revolution. *Journal of General Internal Medicine* 32(4):380–386.

Enard, K. R., and D. M. Ganelin. 2013. Reducing preventable emergency department utilization and costs by using community health workers as patient navigators. *Journal of Healthcare Management* 58(6):412–427; discussion 428.

Eng, E., M. E. Salmon, and F. Mullan. 1992. Community empowerment: The critical base for primary health care. *Family & Community Health: The Journal of Health Promotion & Maintenance* 15(1):1–12.

Estacio, E. V., R. Whittle, and J. Protheroe. 2019. The digital divide: Examining socio-demographic factors associated with health literacy, access and use of Internet to seek health information. *Journal of Health Psychology* 24(12):1668–1675.

Etz, R. S. 2016. People are primary: A perspective from the Keystone IV conference. *Journal of the American Board of Family Practice* 29(Suppl 1):S40–S44.

Etz, R. S., M. M. Gonzalez, E. M. Brooks, and K. C. Stange. 2017. Less and more are needed to assess primary care. *Journal of the American Board of Family Practice* 30(1):13–15.

Etz, R. S., S. J. Zyzanski, M. M. Gonzalez, S. R. Reves, J. P. O'Neal, and K. C. Stange. 2019. A new comprehensive measure of high-value aspects of primary care. *Annals of Family Medicine* 17(3):221–230.

Feuerstein, J. D., V. Sheppard, A. S. Cheifetz, and K. Ariyabuddhiphongs. 2016. How to develop the medical neighborhood. *Journal of Medical Systems* 40(9):196.

Finkelstein, A., A. Zhou, S. Taubman, and J. Doyle. 2020. Health care hotspotting—a randomized, controlled trial. *New England Journal of Medicine* 382(2):152–162.

Flieger, S. P. 2017. Implementing the patient-centered medical home in complex adaptive systems: Becoming a relationship-centered patient-centered medical home. *Health Care Management Review* 42(2):112–121.

Franks, P., and K. Fiscella. 1998. Primary care physicians and specialists as personal physicians. Health care expenditures and mortality experience. *Journal of Family Practice* 47(2):105–109.

Frey, J. J., 3rd. 2010. In this issue: Relationships count for patients and doctors alike. *Annals of Family Medicine* 8(2):98–99.

Frey, J. J., 3rd. 2018. Colluding with the decline of continuity. *Annals of Family Medicine* 16(6):488–489.

Gong, G., S. G. Phillips, C. Hudson, D. Curti, and B. U. Philips. 2019. Higher U.S. rural mortality rates linked to socioeconomic status, physician shortages, and lack of health insurance. *Health Affairs* 38(12):2003–2010.

Gottlieb, K. 2013. The Nuka system of care: Improving health through ownership and relationships. *International Journal of Circumpolar Health* 72.

Green, L. A., and J. C. Puffer. 2016. Reimagining our relationships with patients: A perspective from the Keystone IV conference. *Journal of the American Board of Family Medicine* 29(Suppl 1):S1–S11.

Grumbach, K., E. Bainbridge, and T. Bodenheimer. 2012. Facilitating improvement in primary care: The promise of practice coaching. *Issue Brief (Commonwealth Fund)* 15:1–14.

Halfon, N., and M. Hochstein. 2002. Life course health development: An integrated framework for developing health, policy, and research. *Milbank Quarterly* 80(3):433–479.

Hansen, J., P. P. Groenewegen, W. G. Boerma, and D. S. Kringos. 2015. Living in a country with a strong primary care system is beneficial to people with chronic conditions. *Health Affairs* 34(9):1531–1537.

Hardeman, R. R., E. M. Medina, and R. W. Boyd. 2020. Stolen breaths. *New England Journal of Medicine* 383:197–199.

HHS (U.S. Department of Health and Human Services). 2021. Notice of amendment: Fifth amendment to declaration under the public readiness and emergency preparedness act for medical countermeasures against COVID-19. As published on February 2, 2021. *Federal Register* 8(20). https://www.govinfo.gov/content/pkg/FR-2021-02-02/pdf/2021-02174.pdf (accessed March 30, 2021).

Hollander, J. E., and B. G. Carr. 2020. Virtually perfect? Telemedicine for COVID-19. *New England Journal of Medicine* 382(18):1679–1681.

Howick, J., J. W. L. Cals, C. Jones, C. P. Price, A. Plüddemann, C. Heneghan, M. Y. Berger, F. Buntinx, J. Hickner, W. Pace, T. Badrick, A. Van den Bruel, C. Laurence, H. C. van Weert, E. van Severen, A. Parrella, and M. Thompson. 2014. Current and future use of point-of-care tests in primary care: An international survey in Australia, Belgium, the Netherlands, the UK and the USA. *BMJ Open* 4(8):e005611.

HRSA (Health Resources and Services Administration). 2021. *Teaching Health Center Graduate Medical Education (THCGME) program.* https://bhw.hrsa.gov/grants/medicine/thcgme (accessed March 30, 2021).

Hudak, M. L., M. E. Helm, and P. H. White. 2017. Principles of child health care financing. *Pediatrics* 140(3):e20172098.

International Conference on Primary Health Care. 1978. *Declaration of Alma-Ata.* Alma-Ata, USSR: World Health Organization.

IOM (Institute of Medicine). 1983. *Community oriented primary care: New directions for health services delivery.* Washington, DC: National Academy Press.

IOM. 1996. *Primary care: America's health in a new era.* Washington, DC: National Academy Press.

IOM. 2001. *Crossing the quality chasm: A new health system for the 21st century.* Washington, DC: National Academy Press.

IOM. 2011. *The future of nursing: Leading change, advancing health.* Washington, DC: The National Academies Press.

IOM. 2012. *Primary care and public health: Exploring integration to improve population health.* Washington, DC: The National Academies Press.

IOM. 2014. *Graduate medical education that meets the nation's health needs.* Washington, DC: The National Academies Press.

IQVIA Institute. 2017. *The growing value of digital health.* Parsippany, NJ: IQVIA Institute.

Isaacs, S. L. 2001. Where the public good prevailed: Lessons from success stories in health. *The American Prospect* 12(10):26.

Jabbarpour, Y., A. Greiner, A. Jetty, M. Coffman, C. Jose, S. Petterson, K. Pivaral, R. Phillips, A. Bazemore, and A. Neumann Kane. 2019. *Investing in primary care: A state-level analysis.* Washington, DC: Patient-Centered Primary Care Collaborative.

Johansen, M. E., S. M. Kircher, and T. R. Huerta. 2016. Reexamining the ecology of medical care. *New England Journal of Medicine* 374(5):495–496.

Johnston, S., C. Kendall, M. Hogel, M. McLaren, and C. Liddy. 2015. Measures of quality of care for people with HIV: A scoping review of performance indicators for primary care. *PLOS ONE* 10(9):e0136757.

Kangovi, S. 2020. *To protect public health during and after the pandemic, we need a new approach to financing community health workers.* https://www.healthaffairs.org/do/10.1377/hblog20200603.986107/full (accessed November 17, 2020).

Kangovi, S., N. Mitra, L. Norton, R. Harte, X. Zhao, T. Carter, D. Grande, and J. A. Long. 2018. Effect of community health worker support on clinical outcomes of low-income patients across primary care facilities: A randomized clinical trial. *JAMA Internal Medicine* 178(12):1635–1643.

Katkin, J. P., S. J. Kressly, A. R. Edwards, J. M. Perrin, C. A. Kraft, J. E. Richerson, J. S. Tieder, and L. Wall. 2017. Guiding principles for team-based pediatric care. *Pediatrics* 140(2):e20171489.

Kindig, D., and G. Stoddart. 2003. What is population health? *American Journal of Public Health* 93(3):380–383.

Koller, C. F., T. A. Brennan, and M. H. Bailit. 2010. Rhode Island's novel experiment to rebuild primary care from the insurance side. *Health Affairs* 29(5):941–947.

Kramer, B. J., B. Creekmur, M. N. Mitchell, and D. Saliba. 2018. Expanding home-based primary care to American Indian reservations and other rural communities: An observational study. *Journal of the American Geriatrics Society* 66(4):818–824.

Kravitz, R. L., and M. D. Feldman. 2017. Reinventing primary care: Embracing change, preserving relationships. *Journal of General Internal Medicine* 32(4):369–370.

Kronenberg, C., T. Doran, M. Goddard, T. Kendrick, S. Gilbody, C. R. Dare, L. Aylott, and R. Jacobs. 2017. Identifying primary care quality indicators for people with serious mental illness: A systematic review. *British Journal of General Practice* 67(661):e519–e530.

Landon, B. E., K. Grumbach, and P. J. Wallace. 2012. Integrating public health and primary care systems: Potential strategies from an IOM report. *JAMA* 308(5):461-462.

Larson, E. B., K. B. Roberts, and K. Grumbach. 2005. Primary care, generalism, public good: Déjà vu? Again! *Annals of Internal Medicine* 142(8):671–674.

LaVeist, T. A., D. Gaskin, and P. Richard. 2011. Estimating the economic burden of racial health inequalities in the united states. *International Journal of Health Services* 41(2):231–238.

Levene, L. S., R. Baker, N. Walker, C. Williams, A. Wilson, and J. Bankart. 2018. Predicting declines in perceived relationship continuity using practice deprivation scores: A longitudinal study in primary care. *British Journal of General Practice* 68(671):e420–e426.

Levine, D. M., B. E. Landon, and J. A. Linder. 2019. Quality and experience of outpatient care in the United States for adults with or without primary care. *JAMA Internal Medicine* 179(3):363–372.

Lucan, S. C., R. L. Phillips, Jr., and A. W. Bazemore. 2008. Off the roadmap? Family medicine's grant funding and committee representation at NIH. *Annals of Family Medicine* 6(6):534–542.

Mach, A. L., and J. Kinzer. 2018. *Legislative actions to modify the Affordable Care Act in the 111th-115th congresses.* Washington, DC: Congressional Research Service.

Macinko, J., B. Starfield, and L. Shi. 2003. The contribution of primary care systems to health outcomes within Organization for Economic Cooperation and Development (OECD) countries, 1970–1998. *Health Services Research* 38(3):831–865.

Margolius, D., J. Wong, M. L. Goldman, J. Rouse-Iniguez, and T. Bodenheimer. 2012. Delegating responsibility from clinicians to nonprofessional personnel: The example of hypertension control. *Journal of the American Board of Family Medicine* 25(2):209–215.

Martin, S., R. L. Phillips, Jr., S. Petterson, Z. Levin, and A. W. Bazemore. 2020. Primary care spending in the United States, 2002–2016. *JAMA Internal Medicine* 180(7):1019–1020.

McNall, M. A., L. F. Lichty, and B. Mavis. 2010. The impact of school-based health centers on the health outcomes of middle school and high school students. *American Journal of Public Health* 100(9):1604–1610.

Meskó, B., Z. Drobni, É. Bényei, B. Gergely, and Z. Győrffy. 2017. Digital health is a cultural transformation of traditional healthcare. *mHealth* 3:38.

Miller, E. A., and W. G. Weissert. 2000. Predicting elderly people's risk for nursing home placement, hospitalization, functional impairment, and mortality: A synthesis. *Medical Care Research and Review* 57(3):259–297.

Mutter, J. B., W. Liaw, M. A. Moore, R. S. Etz, A. Howe, and A. Bazemore. 2018. Core principles to improve primary care quality management. *Journal of the American Board of Family Medicine* 31(6):931–940.

NASEM (National Academies of Sciences, Engineering, and Medicine). 2019. *Taking action against clinician burnout: A systems approach to professional well-being.* Washington, DC: The National Academies Press.

NIH and NIRSQ (National Institutes of Health and National Institute for Research on Safety and Quality). 2020. *Major changes in the fiscal year 2021 president's budget request.* Washington, DC: National Institutes of Health and National Institute for Research on Safety and Quality.

Nittas, V., P. Lun, F. Ehrler, M. A. Puhan, and M. Mütsch. 2019. Electronic patient-generated health data to facilitate disease prevention and health promotion: Scoping review. *Journal of Medical Internet Research* 21(10):e13320.

Palmer, E. J., P. J. Carek, S. M. Carr-Johnson, and Association of Family Medicine Residency Directors. 2008. Title VII: Revisiting an opportunity. *Annals of Family Medicine* 6(2):180–181.

Phillips, R. L., Jr., and B. J. Turner. 2012. The next phase of Title VII funding for training primary care physicians for America's health care needs. *Annals of Family Medicine* 10(2):163–168.

Phillips, R. L., Jr., A. W. Bazemore, and W. P. Newton. 2019. Pursuing practical professionalism: Form follows function. *Annals of Family Medicine* 17(5):472–475.

Possemato, K., L. O. Wray, E. Johnson, B. Webster, and G. P. Beehler. 2018. Facilitators and barriers to seeking mental health care among primary care veterans with posttraumatic stress disorder. *Journal of Traumatic Stress* 31(5):742–752.

Reid, R., C. Damberg, and M. W. Friedberg. 2019. Primary care spending in the fee-for-service Medicare population. *JAMA Internal Medicine* 179(7):977–980.

Ring, M., and R. Mahadevan. 2017. Introduction to integrative medicine in the primary care setting. *Primary Care* 44(2):203–215.

Sandberg, S. F., S. A. Shipman, and C. Erikson. 2016. *Innovations at the interface of primary and specialty care*. Washington, DC: AAMC.

Scott, D. 2020. Coronavirus has created a crisis for primary care doctors and their patients. *Vox*. https://www.vox.com/2020/4/27/21231528/coronavirus-covid-19-primary-care-doctors-crisis (accessed June 1, 2020).

Shi, L. 2012. The impact of primary care: A focused review. *Scientifica* 2012:432892.

Shin, P., F. R. Byrne, E. Jones, J. Teitelbaum, L. Repasch, and S. Rosenbaum. 2010. *Medical-legal partnerships: Addressing the unmet legal needs of health center patients (Geiger Gibson/RCHN Community Health Foundation Research Collaborative policy research brief no. 18)*. Washington, DC: George Washington University, School of Public Health and Health Services, Department of Health Policy.

Shuemaker, J. C., R. L. Phillips, and W. P. Newton. 2020. Clinical quality measures in a post-pandemic world: Measuring what matters in family medicine (ABFM). *Annals of Family Medicine* 18(4):380–382.

Shukor, A. R., S. Edelman, D. Brown, and C. Rivard. 2018. Developing community-based primary health care for complex and vulnerable populations in the Vancouver coastal health region: Healthconnection clinic. *The Permanente Journal* 22:18-010.

Sia, C., T. F. Tonniges, E. Osterhus, and S. Taba. 2004. History of the medical home concept. *Pediatrics* 113(5):1473–1478.

Singer, S. J., J. Burgers, M. Friedberg, M. B. Rosenthal, L. Leape, and E. Schneider. 2011. Defining and measuring integrated patient care: Promoting the next frontier in health care delivery. *Medical Care Research and Review* 68(1):112–127.

Slavitt, A., and F. Mostashari. 2020. COVID-19 is battering independent physician practices. They need help now. *STAT*. https://www.statnews.com/2020/05/28/covid-19-battering-independent-physician-practices (accessed December 1, 2020).

Smith, C., C. Balatbat, S. Corbridge, A. Dopp, J. Fried, R. Harter, S. Landefeld, C. Martin, F. Opelka, L. Sandy, L. Sato, and C. Sinsky. 2018. Implementing optimal team-based care to reduce clinician burnout. *NAM Perspectives* 8.

Solberg, L. I. 2016. Theory vs practice: Should primary care practice take on social determinants of health now? No. *Annals of Family Medicine* 14(2):102–103.

Stange, K. C. 2009. The problem of fragmentation and the need for integrative solutions. *Annals of Family Medicine* 7(2):100–103.

Stange, K. C., R. S. Etz, H. Gullett, S. A. Sweeney, W. L. Miller, C. R. Jaen, B. F. Crabtree, P. A. Nutting, and R. E. Glasgow. 2014. Metrics for assessing improvements in primary health care. *Annual Review of Public Health* 35:423–442.

Starfield, B. 2009. Primary care and equity in health: The importance to effectiveness and equity of responsiveness to people's needs. *Humanity & Society* 33(1–2):56–73.

Starfield, B. 2011. Is patient-centered care the same as person-focused care? *The Permanente Journal* 15:63–69.

Starfield, B. 2012. Primary care: An increasingly important contributor to effectiveness, equity, and efficiency of health services. SESPAS report 2012. *Gaceta Sanitaria* 26(Suppl 1):20–26.

Starfield, B., L. Shi, and J. Macinko. 2005. Contribution of primary care to health systems and health. *Milbank Quarterly* 83(3):457–502.

Tai, D. B. G., A. Shah, C. A. Doubeni, I. G. Sia, and M. L. Wieland. 2020. The disproportionate impact of COVID-19 on racial and ethnic minorities in the United States. *Clinical Infectious Diseases* ciaa815.

Thomas, H., G. Mitchell, J. Rich, and M. Best. 2018. Definition of whole person care in general practice in the English language literature: A systematic review. *BMJ Open* 8(12):e023758.

Trish, E., P. Ginsburg, L. Gascue, and G. Joyce. 2017. Physician reimbursement in Medicare Advantage compared with traditional medicare and commercial health insurance. *JAMA Internal Medicine* 177(9):1287–1295.

Vassiliou, A. G., C. Georgakopoulou, A. Papageorgiou, S. Georgakopoulos, S. Goulas, T. Paschalis, P. Paterakis, P. Gallos, D. Kyriazis, and V. Plagianakos. 2020. Health in all policy making utilizing big data. *Acta Informatica Medica* 28(1):65–70.

Verma, S. 2020. Early impact of CMS expansion of Medicare telehealth during COVD-19. *Health Affairs Blog* (July 15). https://www.healthaffairs.org/do/10.1377/hblog 20200715.454789/full/ (accessed December 2, 2020).

Webb Hooper, M., A. M. Nápoles, and E. J. Pérez-Stable. 2020. COVID-19 and racial/ethnic disparities. *JAMA* 323(24):2466–2467.

Weiner, M., and P. Biondich. 2006. The influence of information technology on patient-physician relationships. *Journal of General Internal Medicine* 21:S35–S39.

WHO (World Health Organization). 2018. *Integrated primary health care-based service delivery in the global conference on primary health care, Astana, Kazakhstan.* https:// www.who.int/servicedeliverysafety/areas/people-centred-care/news/ipchs-astana/en (accessed October 23, 2020).

WHO and UNICEF (United Nations Children's Fund). 2018. *Declaration of Astana.* Astana, Kazakhstan: World Health Organization and United Nations Children's Fund.

Yoon, J., E. Chang, L. V. Rubenstein, A. Park, D. M. Zulman, S. Stockdale, M. K. Ong, D. Atkins, G. Schectman, and S. M. Asch. 2018. Impact of primary care intensive management on high-risk veterans' costs and utilization: A randomized quality improvement trial. *Annals of Internal Medicine* 168(12):846–854.

Young, H. M., and T. S. Nesbitt. 2017. Increasing the capacity of primary care through enabling technology. *Journal of General Internal Medicine* 32(4):398–403.

3

Primary Care in the United States: A Brief History and Current Trends

For the first two-thirds of the 20th century, the lone general practitioner served as the face of primary care in the United States. However, primary care was a shrinking presence with the rise of subspecialty care and urbanization following World War II (Stevens, 2001). Three commissioned reports on the challenges facing primary care—Millis (Citizens Commission on Graduate Medical Education, 1966), Folsom (National Commission on Community Health Services, 1967), and Willard (AMA et al., 1966)—were soon followed in 1969 by establishing family practice, the 20th medical specialty, as part of an effort to reverse the decline in primary care. General internal medicine, geriatric medicine, and general pediatrics also found their ways into academic medical centers in response to the needs of their patients and communities. The first neighborhood health centers focused on primary care, which became today's health centers,[1] were also established in the mid-1960s as part of President Lyndon Johnson's War on Poverty (CHroniCles, 2020), and the nurse practitioner (NP) certification project was started at the University of Colorado Medical School to "bridge the gap between health care needs of children and families' ability to access and afford primary health care" (Ford, 1979, p. 517). In the 1970s, the recognition of the number of aging veterans (and their impact on the

---

[1] Health centers, as defined by section 330 of the Public Health Service Act (42 U.S.C. § 254b), include outpatient clinics in federally designated underserved areas that qualify for specific reimbursement systems under Medicare and Medicaid. They include (but are not limited to) federally qualified health centers (FQHCs), FQHC look-alikes, rural health clinics, school-based health centers, and tribal and urban Indian health centers.

veteran's health care system) led the U.S. Department of Veterans Affairs to establish the first Geriatric Research, Education and Clinical Centers (GRECCs) (Morley, 2004). The GRECCs supported education and training in geriatrics, and developed interdisciplinary team training programs to provide care for the aging population.

In the early 1980s, most primary care practices were independent, small, and organized around relationships, patient loyalty, reputation, place, a "pay what you can" fee-for-service (FFS) model, professional duty, and personal and family care, with an emphasis on comprehensiveness, continuity, and access. Often, this period is seen through the lens of fond nostalgia, but general practice in those days was paternalistic, driven almost exclusively by physicians (who were nearly all male and white), and lacked transparency about the quality of care. These practices were also disconnected from each other and only connected to the larger health care system and local community through personal relationships and the more close-knit neighborhoods of the time. Information sharing with other parts of the larger health care system, such as specialty care, was limited or even nonexistent (Kim et al., 2015).

By the start of the 21st century, most primary care practices would be almost unrecognizable to past generations of primary care clinicians. Relative to decades ago, practices today are larger (Liebhaber and Grossman, 2007), often part of health care systems (Kane, 2019), and generally not organized around values, professionalism, and relationships. Instead, they exist within a new administrative and technological context, including National Committee for Quality Assurance recognition, accountable care organization requirements, the ubiquitous use of electronic health records, compensation based on relative value unit productivity, and pay-for-performance metrics. New models of care, such as patient-centered medical homes, developed originally as a pediatric care model, and Advanced Primary Care, addressed many of the concerns of the traditional care model because they aimed to be more collaborative and transparent, associated with various measures of quality, and more formally connected with each other and the health system. However, this new organization of primary care has come with rising moral distress and disturbingly high levels of burnout in clinicians, community and personal disconnections, and inordinate and surprising dissatisfaction all around (Kim et al., 2018; Shanafelt et al., 2012; Sinaiko et al., 2017).

Today, NPs, physicians, and physician assistants (PAs) provide most of the in-office, primary care services in the United States (IOM, 2011). Increasingly, though, they also work with an interprofessional team that may include community health workers (CHWs) or aides, promotores de salud, health coaches, informal caregivers, certified nurse-midwives (CNMs),[2] and behavioral health specialists, who can help primary care practices address the socioeconomic conditions and behaviors that research has shown are major determinants of health (Kangovi et al., 2020). Also, because informal caregivers, CHWs, and promotores de salud reflect the communities they serve, these team members can help shift the primary care workforce from its clinician-centric traditions to an approach that includes the people, families, and communities that it addresses (Chernoff and Cueva, 2017; Manchanda, 2015). In 2017, approximately 223,125 (31.9 percent) of all office-based, direct patient care physicians were primary care physicians (Petterson et al., 2018). Data from 2019 show that 25 percent of PAs work in primary care settings (NCCPA, 2020). The National Sample Survey of Registered Nurses estimates that 15 percent of registered nurses and 29 percent of advanced practice registered nurses (APRNs)[3] reported that they spend most of their patient-care time in primary care settings (HHS et al., 2020). While it is unclear precisely how many work in primary care settings (Sabo et al., 2017), the U.S. Bureau of Labor Statistics estimated nearly 59,000 CHWs in the United States, with approximately 5,100 in outpatient care centers, 4,720 in general medical and surgical hospitals, and 3,700 in physician offices (BLS, 2019).

It is surprisingly difficult, however, to describe the broader primary care workforce in detail, because national data neglect many professions, such as behavioral health specialists, pharmacists, health coaches, and others who make up interprofessional primary care teams (see Chapter 6 for more on the workforce). Better data on the professionals in such teams will be useful as primary care practice continues to become more team based and inclusive of non-clinician care team members.

While oral health is an essential component of the health of the whole person, dental care remains largely siloed in both payment and delivery from the rest of health care, including from primary care. While there are examples of oral health integration into models of primary care delivery (notably in health centers), oral health professionals are generally not included in most interprofessional primary care teams today and it is unclear how many are working in integrated settings.

While the numbers of NPs and PAs are steadily increasing, the proportion working in primary care settings has decreased (AANP, 2020; NASEM, 2016; NCCPA, 2020), as has the proportion of medical students and residents entering primary care in recent years (Naylor and Kurtzman, 2010;

---

[2] CNMs are licensed, independent health care clinicians with prescriptive authority in all 50 states, the District of Columbia, American Samoa, Guam, Puerto Rico, and the U.S. Virgin Islands. CNMs are defined as primary care clinicians under federal law (ACNM, 2019).

[3] APRNs include NPs, CNMs, nurse anesthetists, and clinical nurse specialists. This report focuses on NPs, who work most consistently in primary care, except where data reports at the APRN level only.

NRMP, 2020). The number of CHWs is increasing, though it is difficult to quantify exactly how many are working in primary care because they have more than 100 different job titles (Sabo et al., 2017).

The rapid growth of health care professionals other than physicians has increased their contributions to the primary care workforce, particularly in rural areas, but the nationwide distribution of all health care workers is uneven (AHRQ, 2012). One contributor to this result for NPs, PAs, and CHWs, for example, is variation in state scope of practice regulations, some of which still prohibit them from working independently from a supervising physician. As of 2021, only 23 states and the District of Columbia allow NPs to independently evaluate patients; diagnose, order, and interpret diagnostic tests; and initiate and manage treatments, including prescribing medications and controlled substances. Laws in another 16 states restrict at least one element of practice and require a career-long, regulated collaborative agreement with another health provider in order for the NP to provide patient care (AANP, 2021) (see Figure 3-1). For PAs, 37 states allow for the determination of scope of practice to be jointly established through a written agreement between the supervising physician and PA at the practice level (AAFP, 2019). As of 2016, 16 states had laws addressing scope of practice for CHWs (CDC, 2017), and each state had its own particular take on what it should be.

This regulatory variation can make it difficult to organize primary care teams effectively. Nearly a decade ago, more than 50 percent of family physicians worked with NPs, PAs, and CNMs, and the percentage was even higher in rural areas (Peterson et al., 2013). Responding to this finding, Jean Johnson, former dean of the School of Nursing at The George Washington University, said,

> Rather than NPs and FPs [family physicians] continuing to focus on issues of who is the captain of the team or who can have an independent practice, the overriding principle for continued dialogue should keep the patient at the center of our efforts. There is too much work to be done to meet the health care needs of the United States for nursing and medicine to be at odds. (Johnson, 2013, p. 242)

Relatedly, NPs and PAs do not have dedicated, public databases about the two workforces, making it difficult to discern how many from each profession are working in primary care settings versus those who were trained in that setting. As cited earlier in this chapter, the National Sample Survey of Registered Nurses offers estimates of those practicing in primary care (HHS et al., 2020) but does not provide a broader workforce enumeration and monitoring function the way that the American Medical Association Physician Masterfile[4] or the Health Resources and Services Administration

---

[4] See https://www.ama-assn.org/practice-management/masterfile/ama-physician-masterfile (accessed February 14, 2021).

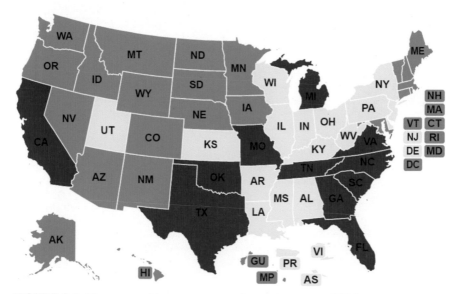

FIGURE 3-1 Nurse practitioner state practice environment, 2021.
NOTE: States in green allow full practice, states in yellow reduced practice, and states in red restricted practice.
SOURCE: AANP, 2021.

(HRSA) Area Health Resources File[5] does for physicians. Membership files for several PA organizations offer better insights and monitoring capacity (Orcutt, 2015), but a combined, cleaned file would give a clearer picture.

Primary Care Specialties

Another notable change from earlier generations of primary care is the growth of primary care specialties, including family medicine, general internal medicine, general pediatrics, adolescent medicine, and geriatric medicine, each with its own professional organizations and advocacy groups (Dalen et al., 2017). A growing number of primary care physicians are also moving into niche areas, such as sleep medicine, hospital-based care, and sports medicine, often seeking greater income and improved lifestyle (Cassel and Reuben, 2011). The primary care advanced practice professions also have their own professional organizations and accreditation bodies, adding to the complexity of the field. This continued fragmentation of practice has diminished the generalist role of primary care and the ability to focus on

---

[5] See https://data.hrsa.gov/topics/health-workforce/ahrf (accessed February 14, 2021).

BOX 3-1
The Value of the Generalist Role in Primary Care

A generalist is usually someone who possesses a wide breadth of skills rather than highly specific skills in a narrower area of expertise. Primary care is at its heart a generalist approach, designed to address undifferentiated symptoms and the majority of whole-person care needs and health concerns, which are often broad, as opposed to seeing only individuals with specific types of diagnoses or health issues. Recapturing this generalist function was the main call of the 1966 American Medical Association Graduate Medical Education report (commonly known as the "Millis Commission" report) that helped birth family medicine (Citizens Commission on Graduate Medical Education, 1966) and also of the 1978 Declaration of Alma-Ata, led by the World Health Organization and endorsed by the world's health ministers (International Conference on Primary Health Care, 1978). It is also a focus of the 2018 Declaration of Astana, 40 years after Alma-Ata, which put primary care into the broader context called "primary health care" (including public health and sanitation) (WHO and UNICEF, 2018). This report is partly a response to the Astana Declaration and how the United States could better fit the international commitment to primary care.

The committee believes strongly that there is real risk when primary care is considered just one among many "health service lines" rather than being seen as the general and most frequent basis for entry into health care and a critical link to the overall population health of a community. Generalism is increasingly recognized as a valuable societal good, but with the explosion of specialized health care, true generalism is a vanishing function (Epstein, 2019).

The generalist approach has several strengths, including serving to achieve the following:

- develop long-standing, continuous relationships focused on developing and promoting health and healing;
- address most acute and chronic care needs that do not require specialty care;
- act as filter between patients and high-technology care to avoid neglecting necessary care and delivering unnecessary care;
- care for people whose symptoms do not have or do not yet have a diagnosis;

the health of a community or population (see Box 3-1 for more information on the value of the generalist). Other care disciplines that contribute to primary care in some models include dental health, physical therapy, social work, occupational therapy, pharmacy, and behavioral health, each with its own professional organizations and description of the roles it plays in primary care.

- help people engage in health behaviors and change health-harming behaviors over time;
- meet population health goals for prevention and wellness; and
- work with community partners and public health to address community sources of health inequity (Ferrer et al., 2005).

Solving complex problems, as are often presented in primary care settings, requires practicing discernment across multiple levels, working with openness and humility, and focusing on observing, learning, refocusing, connecting, integrating, iterating between the parts and the whole—in short, the generalist approach epitomized in high-quality primary care that focuses on relationships with people over time (Gunn et al., 2008; Mercer and Howie, 2006; Palmer et al., 2007; Stange, 2009a).

However, the COVID-19 pandemic has revealed how chronic underinvestment in health care as a relationship and overinvestment in it as a commodity (Miller et al., 2003; Olaisen et al., 2020; Scott et al., 2008; Stange, 2018) cause illness by compromising ongoing health care (DeVoe, 2020) and exacerbating inequities (Souch and Cossman, 2020; Wang and Tang, 2020). Generalist knowledge is needed now to iteratively prioritize attention and combine different ways of knowing particulars to create an integrated whole (Stange, 2010; Stange et al., 2001). The fragmented, impersonal, often inaccessible response to the pandemic brings to light the need for primary care to contextualize acute, chronic, preventive, and mental health care by knowing the person in their family and community context (IOM, 1996).

High-quality primary care complements specialist expertise by starting with a focus on the whole person and their family, within the context of their community, and then iteratively identifying and working on the most important concern in that moment, while keeping the whole in view (McWhinney, 1989; O'Connor et al., 2017; Stange, 2002). That fundamental, essential, integrating, personalizing, and prioritizing role of the generalist is not widely understood and has largely been eliminated in the U.S. health care system (Loxterkamp, 1991, 2009; Montgomery et al., 2017; Stange, 2009b). With a rising proportion of the population in the United States experiencing multiple chronic conditions, patients have a series of specialists focused on specific diagnoses and often lack one primary care team whose focus is the combination of all of their diagnoses.

CURRENT PRIMARY CARE PRACTICE TYPES

As of 2014, some 56 percent of primary care physicians worked in practices in which they were full or partial owners, while 41 percent were employees, of either a physician-owned or non-physician-owned practice (see Figure 3-2). Of the 26 percent in non-physician-owned practices, 51.9 percent were in practices owned by insurers, health plans, health maintenance organizations, or other corporate entities, while 41.8 percent were

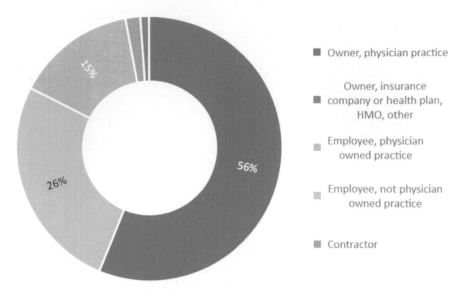

FIGURE 3-2 Primary care physicians by employment status, 2014.
NOTES: HMO = health maintenance organization. Contractor = 2%; Owner, insurance company or health plan, HMO, other = 1%.
SOURCE: Petterson et al., 2018.

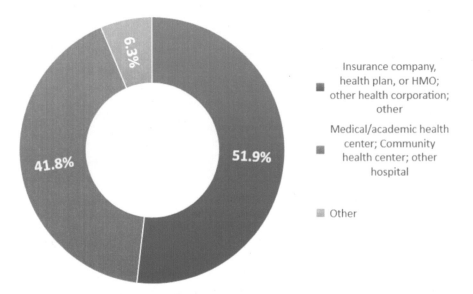

FIGURE 3-3 Distribution of primary care physicians in non-physician-owned practices, 2014.
NOTE: HMO = health maintenance organization.
SOURCE: Petterson et al., 2018.

in a medical or academic health center, community health center, or other hospital (Petterson et al., 2018) (see Figure 3-3).

Solo and small practices of fewer than five physicians have long been an important component of the U.S. primary care system. However, a combination of factors are changing the landscape of primary care practices and leading to consolidation and loss of independent practices. A 2017 study found that between 2010 and 2016, the percentage of primary care physicians working in a practice owned by a hospital or health system increased from 28 to 44, and the percentage of those working in an independently owned practice decreased by a similar amount (Fulton, 2017) (see Figure 3-4). More recently, a study by the Physicians Advocacy Institute and Avalere Health found that between 2016 and 2018, hospitals acquired some 8,000 medical practices and approximately 14,000 physicians left private practice to work in hospitals (PAI and Avalere Health, 2019). Another study found that while physicians of all specialties are moving from smaller to larger group practices, primary care practices are consolidating much faster than specialty practices (Muhlestein and Smith, 2016) (see Figure 3-5). The financial pressures that the COVID-19 pandemic wrought on independent primary care practices that rely largely on FFS payments (Basu et al., 2020) may accelerate this shift.

Research on the effects of consolidation on access to care and quality of care is scant, with most focusing on how it has contributed to the rising cost of care (Baker et al., 2014; Dunn and Shapiro, 2014). One study did

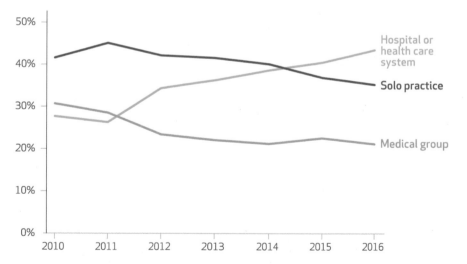

FIGURE 3-4 Primary care physicians are leaving independent practices and medical groups to work directly for hospitals or health care systems.
SOURCE: Fulton, 2017.

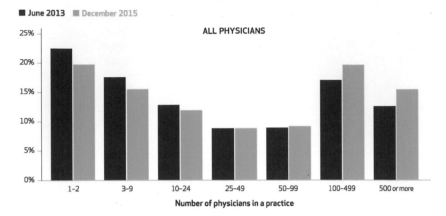

FIGURE 3-5 Percentages of U.S. primary care physicians in practice groups of various sizes.
SOURCE: Muhlestein and Smith, 2016.

find that clinician concentration was associated with relative improvements in Medicaid beneficiaries' access to care (Bond et al., 2017). Another study found that Medicare patients had worse health outcomes and higher health care expenditures when receiving treatment in areas where clinician concentration was highest (Koch et al., 2018).

Retail and Direct-to-Consumer Urgent Care Clinics

A relatively recent trend is the growth of retail or direct-to-consumer clinics, typically staffed by NPs and PAs. A 2014 market assessment estimated the size of the U.S. retail clinic market at $1.4 billion and projected an annual growth rate of 20 percent through 2025 (Grand View Research, 2017). While retail clinics have been promoted as a means of reducing emergency department visits and decreasing health care spending, research findings have been mixed as to whether those two claims are correct (Alexander et al., 2019a,b; RAND, 2016). In addition, policy makers are concerned that increased use of retail clinics will create missed opportunities for preventive care, make coordination and continuity of care more challenging, and pose a threat to the financial viability of primary care practices by treating the latter's most profitable cases (Weinick et al., 2011). Nevertheless, the number of retail clinics is expected to reach 3,000 in 2020 (up from close to 1,200 in 2000) (CCA, 2017). At the same time, health systems are opening a growing number of urgent care clinics that can compete with retail clinics. The Urgent Care Association notes that there were 9,279 urgent care centers as of June 2019 and that their number has been growing by 400 to 500 centers annually since 2014 (UCA, 2019).

Both retail and urgent care clinics typically serve younger adults who otherwise do not have a primary care clinician (RAND, 2016). Still, a 2015 survey asking individuals where they would go for treatment of a non-emergency or non-life-threatening situation found that a plurality of those in the 18–34 age group still preferred traditional primary care, delivered in an office setting, over all other options, and that a majority of consumers age 35 years and older preferred traditional primary care over other options (FAIR Health, 2015) (see Table 3-1).

While the growth of both retail and urgent care clinics are evidence that both settings will continue to deliver a substantial amount of problem-based care, it is important to note that the committee's definition of high-quality primary care (see Chapter 2) is largely incompatible with the retail clinic and urgent care delivery models. Of particular note, the episodic nature of the care delivered in these settings is not conducive to either whole-person health or individuals and their families building and maintaining relationships with their primary care team (it may instead be a PA or an NP who is different at every visit) (Reid et al., 2012). The increase in health systems starting urgent care clinics is a mechanism to link the person who visits an urgent care clinic when their primary care service is closed back to the larger primary care network.

TABLE 3-1 Settings Where Consumers Would Most Likely Go for Treatment for a Non-Emergency or Non-Life-Threatening Situation

Age	Primary Care in a Traditional Office Setting	Emergency Room	Urgent Care	Walk-in Clinic at a Pharmacy or Retail Center
18–34	43%	25%	21%	7%
35–44	54%	21%	19%	3%
45–54	64%	19%	8%	5%
55–64	62%	16%	13%	7%
65+	59%	22%	9%	4%
Total Population	55%	21%	15%	5%

SOURCE: FAIR Health, 2015.

ACCESS TO PRIMARY CARE

More than 80 million individuals live in a primary care Health Professional Shortage Area (HPSA) (HRSA, 2020) (see Figure 3-6).[6] These designations are often used by the HRSA to prioritize funding for health centers and by the Centers for Medicare & Medicaid Services (CMS) for reimbursement and payment incentives for primary care clinicians (CMS, 2019).

Since 2000, health centers' capacity to provide primary care has nearly tripled, and they now provide care to nearly 30 million people in the United States (Sharac et al., 2018). Despite this considerable investment in health centers and the National Health Service Corps,[7] rural and underserved areas continue to experience an inadequate primary care workforce, which is generally a source of health inequity (Basu et al., 2019; Gong et al., 2019). Nearly 20 percent of the U.S. population resides in a primary care HPSA, with HRSA designating nearly 40 percent of rural areas (counties) as such (HRSA, 2020). Although the supply of primary care clinicians is greater in urban than rural areas (Xue et al., 2019), predominantly Black, brown, and

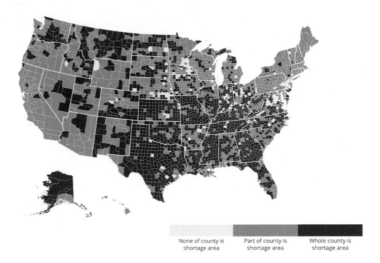

None of county is   Part of county is   Whole county is
shortage area   shortage area   shortage area

FIGURE 3-6 Primary care Health Professional Shortage Areas by county, 2019.
SOURCE: HRSA, 2020.

---

[6] A HPSA is an area HRSA designates if the supply of primary care physicians does not meet the needs of the local population based on the population-to-clinician threshold of 3,500:1.

[7] The National Health Service Corps is an HRSA scholarship and loan repayment program designed to incentivize primary care medical, dental, and mental and behavioral health professionals to work in HPSAs. See https://nhsc.hrsa.gov (accessed February 14, 2021) for more information.

Indigenous neighborhoods in urban areas are significantly more likely to have a shortage of primary care clinicians when compared to other neighborhoods (Brown et al., 2016; Huang and Finegold, 2013). Given the large population of urban counties, differences in the availability of primary care clinicians are only observed at the neighborhood level.

The number of U.S. primary care physicians per capita has declined in recent years (Basu et al., 2019). In 2016, HRSA estimated that by 2025, an additional 23,640 will be needed to meet the projected demand, with the southern region being hardest hit (HRSA and NCHWA, 2016). HRSA also estimated that the supply of primary care NPs and PAs will exceed demand by 2025 and that "with delivery system changes and full utilization of NP and PA services, the projected shortage of [primary care physicians] can be effectively mitigated" (HRSA and NCHWA, 2016, p. 4). (See Chapter 6 for a more detailed discussion of primary care workforce issues.) This assessment demonstrates a general lack of understanding regarding complementary or team-based care. The problem of scope convergence is not just an expansion for NPs and PAs but also a narrowing for physicians. Advanced, interprofessional primary care models do not presume that these clinicians have identical roles but rather that they offer a combined, broader scope of services that their unique training and experience support.

Factors other than clinician supply limit access to primary care, including lack of health insurance (Ayanian et al., 2000; Freeman et al., 2008; Hadley, 2003; Tolbert and Oregera, 2020), type of insurance (Alcalá et al., 2018; Hsiang et al., 2019), language-related barriers (Cheng et al., 2007; Ponce et al., 2006), disabilities (Krahn et al., 2006), inability to take time off work to attend appointments (Gleason and Kneipp, 2004; O'Malley et al., 2012), and geographic and transportation-related barriers (Douthit et al., 2015). Lack of insurance decreases the use of preventive and primary care services, which translates into poor health outcomes (Ayanian et al., 2000), an issue that is particularly acute for racial and ethnic minority populations (Brown et al., 2000). While the Patient Protection and Affordable Care Act (ACA)[8] led to historic gains in health insurance coverage—fewer than 26.7 million non-elderly Americans were uninsured in 2016, down from 46.5 million in 2010, before the ACA went into effect—the number of uninsured increased to 28.9 million in 2019 and the uninsured rate has increased steadily since 2017 as a result of changes made to the ACA (Tolbert and Orgera, 2020). Most of those without insurance are in low-income families with at least one worker in the family, with adults and people of color more likely to be uninsured than children or non-Hispanic white people.

The COVID-19 pandemic has also had notable implications for access

---

[8] Patient Protection and Affordable Care Act, Public Law 111-148 (March 23, 2010).

to primary care. In response, many practices eliminated nonessential in-person visits. In some cases, practices were able to provide access to care via telehealth. However, while the change in CMS and many private insurers' rules ensured that more types of visits could be delivered virtually, many practices did not have the infrastructure in place to make the shift quickly or at all. Furthermore, many people did not have access to the technology required (Nouri et al., 2020; Velasquez and Mehrotra, 2020). Many services that require in-person appointments, such as immunizations and other types of preventive care most commonly delivered in primary care settings, have been delayed during the pandemic (Czeisler et al., 2020).

PRIMARY CARE USAGE TRENDS

Despite the new research, reforms, and policy changes of the last two decades emphasizing the importance of primary care, the rate of in-office primary care visits has decreased (Chou et al., 2019; Ganguli et al., 2020). Total visits by commercially insured adults to primary care offices decreased by 24.2 percent between 2008 and 2016 (Ganguli et al., 2020). This reduction is driven by a decline in problem-based visits, down by 30.5 percent, whereas preventive care visits actually increased by 40.6 percent during this time (Ganguli et al., 2020). These changes in visit type and the avoidance of care may be related to rapid adoption of high deductible health insurance; it demonstrably reduces problem-based primary care services, which often require copays (wellness or preventive care visits often do not) (Rabin et al., 2017; Reddy et al., 2014). The changes in visit type may also be a reflection of people choosing convenient visits to urgent care and retail clinics for problem-based care, while maintaining yearly scheduled wellness or preventive care with primary care clinicians. A study of commercially insured children found similar patterns during this same period, although the overall decline in office visits was not as great (14.4 percent) (Ray et al., 2020). Despite this overall decline, primary care services from NPs and PAs continues to grow (Frost and Hargraves, 2018; Ganguli et al., 2020). Reflecting these trends, a 6 percent decline in spending on primary care office visits also occurred between 2012 and 2016, but spending on specialist visits increased by 31 percent (Frost et al., 2018).

Several possible explanations exist for the decrease in primary care visits. One theory is that primary care's efforts to emphasize the clinician–patient relationship, incorporate technology, and provide comprehensive care are working. While the number of visits overall is in decline, the appointments that do take place are typically longer, are more likely to be via Internet or telephone, and result in fewer follow-up appointments and fewer unneeded appointments (Ganguli et al., 2020; Rao et al., 2019). With greater attention to continuity and coordination of care, visits that do occur may be more efficient and productive and result in fewer face-to-face follow-up appointments (Ganguli et al., 2019). Lack of insurance or insurance with high deductibles may also explain the decline. Average out-of-pocket cost per problem-based primary care visits has increased steadily as well, rising more than $10 (from $29.7 to $39.1) between 2008 and 2016 (Ganguli et al., 2020).

Despite these potential explanations, systemic access problems persist and are a contributing factor to declining office visits. The insufficient supply of primary care clinicians and their uneven geographic dispersal leads to an inadequate supply of appointments, particularly for the often last-minute needs of problem-based visits (Ganguli et al., 2019). With emergency department usage rates increasing 12 percent between 2002 and 2015 (Chou et al., 2019), and people opting for other "convenient care" options, such as urgent care and retail clinics, many people likely prioritize access and immediacy for their acute care, especially outside of typical office hours (Chang et al., 2015; Kangovi et al., 2013; Rocovich and Patel, 2012). The decline in problem-based primary care visits is tellingly largest among low-income communities, which are more affected by increases to out-of-pocket expenses (Ganguli et al., 2020; Rabin et al., 2017).

Confronted by these barriers to care, people may simultaneously perceive diminished need for in-person primary care. The abundance of websites such as WebMD, symptom checkers, and online patient communities may replace formal care, particularly for low-acuity problems (Ganguli et al., 2019). Indeed, primary care offices saw fewer visits regarding easily researched conditions, such as conjunctivitis (Ganguli et al., 2020).

FINDINGS AND CONCLUSIONS

Primary care in the United States has changed dramatically in recent decades. The changes have eroded its generalist role and led to the consolidation and reduction in its scope and an erosion of its physician workforce, particularly in rural and underserved areas, coupled with the growth of NPs, PAs, CHWs, and other health care workers in primary care. Limited access to primary care in federally designated shortage areas covering much of the country and changes in primary care use all threaten the capacity of primary care to serve the needs of the U.S. population.

REFERENCES

AAFP (American Academy of Family Physicians). 2019. *Scope of practice—physicians assistants.* Leawood, KS: American Academy of Family Physicians.

AANP (American Association of Nurse Practitioners). 2020. *Historical timeline.* https://www.aanp.org/about/about-the-american-association-of-nurse-practitioners-aanp/historical-timeline (accessed October 29, 2020).

AANP. 2021. *2021 nurse practitioner state practice environment.* Arlington, VA: American Association of Nurse Practitioners.

ACNM (American College of Nurse-Midwives). 2019. *Essential facts about midwives.* Silver Spring, MD: American College of Nurse-Midwives.

AHRQ (Agency for Healthcare Research and Quality). 2012. *The distribution of the U.S. primary care workforce.* https://www.ahrq.gov/research/findings/factsheets/primary/pcwork3/index.html (accessed October 28, 2020).

Alcalá, H. E., D. H. Roby, D. T. Grande, R. M. McKenna, and A. N. Ortega. 2018. Insurance type and access to health care providers and appointments under the Affordable Care Act. *Medical Care* 56(2):186–192.

Alexander, D., J. Currie, and M. Schnell. 2019a. Check up before you check out: Retail clinics and emergency room use. *Journal of Public Economics* 178:104050.

Alexander, D., J. Currie, M. Schnell, and L. C. McKay. 2019b. *Check up before you check out.* Chicago, IL: Federal Reserve Bank of Chicago.

AMA (American Medical Association), Ad Hoc Committee on Education for Family Practice, and Council on Medical Education. 1966. *Meeting the challenge of family practice (also known as the "Willard Report").* Chicago, IL: American Medical Association.

Ayanian, J. Z., J. S. Weissman, E. C. Schneider, J. A. Ginsburg, and A. M. Zaslavsky. 2000. Unmet health needs of uninsured adults in the United States. *JAMA* 284(16):2061–2069.

Baker, L. C., M. K. Bundorf, and D. P. Kessler. 2014. Vertical integration: Hospital ownership of physician practices is associated with higher prices and spending. *Health Affairs* 33(5):756–763.

Basu, S., S. A. Berkowitz, R. L. Phillips, A. Bitton, B. E. Landon, and R. S. Phillips. 2019. Association of primary care physician supply with population mortality in the United States, 2005–2015. *JAMA Internal Medicine* 179(4):506–514.

Basu, S., R. S. Phillips, R. Phillips, L. E. Peterson, and B. E. Landon. 2020. Primary care practice finances in the United States amid the COVID-19 pandemic. *Health Affairs* 10.1377/hlthaff.2020.00794.

BLS (U.S. Bureau of Labor Statistics). 2019. *Occupational employment and wages, May 2019: 21-1094 community health workers.* https://www.bls.gov/oes/current/oes211094.htm (accessed November 24, 2020).

Bond, A., W. Pajerowski, D. Polsky, and M. R. Richards. 2017. Market environment and Medicaid acceptance: What influences the access gap? *Health Economics* 26(12):1759–1766.

Brown, E. J., D. Polsky, C. M. Barbu, J. W. Seymour, and D. Grande. 2016. Racial disparities in geographic access to primary care in Philadelphia. *Health Affairs* 35(8):1374–1381.

Brown, E. R., V. D. Ojeda, R. Wyn, and R. Levan. 2000. *Racial and ethnic disparities in access to health insurance and health care.* Los Angeles, CA: University of California, Los Angeles, Center for Health Policy Research, Henry J. Kaiser Family Foundation.

Cassel, C. K., and D. B. Reuben. 2011. Specialization, subspecialization, and subsubspecialization in internal medicine. *New England Journal of Medicine* 364(12):1169–1173.

CCA (Convenient Care Association). 2017. *Convenient care clinics: Increasing access.* Philadelphia, PA: Convenient Care Association.

CDC (Centers for Disease Control and Prevention). 2017. *What evidence supports state laws to establish community health worker scope of practice and certification?* Atlanta, GA: Centers for Disease Control and Prevention.

Chang, J. E., S. C. Brundage, and D. A. Chokshi. 2015. Convenient ambulatory care—promise, pitfalls, and policy. *New England Journal of Medicine* 373(4):382–388.

Cheng, E. M., A. Chen, and W. Cunningham. 2007. Primary language and receipt of recommended health care among Hispanics in the United States. *Journal of General Internal Medicine* 22(Suppl 2):283–288.

Chernoff, M., and K. Cueva. 2017. The role of Alaska's tribal health workers in supporting families. *Journal of Community Health* 42(5):1020–1026.

Chou, S.-C., A. K. Venkatesh, N. S. Trueger, and S. R. Pitts. 2019. Primary care office visits for acute care dropped sharply in 2002–15, while ED visits increased modestly. *Health Affairs* 38(2):268–275.

CHroniCles. 2020. *Health centers then & now.* https://www.chcchronicles.org/histories (accessed October 8, 2020).

Citizens Commission on Graduate Medical Education. 1966. *The graduate education of physicians.* Chicago, IL: American Medical Association.

CMS (Centers for Medicare & Medicaid Services). 2019. Chapter 13—rural health clinic (RHC) and federally qualified health center (FQHC) services. In *Medicare benefit policy manual.* Washington, DC: Centers for Medicare & Medicaid Services.

Czeisler, M., K. Marynak, K. E. N. Clarke, Z. Salah, I. Shakya, J. M. Thierry, N. Ali, H. McMillan, J. F. Wiley, M. D. Weaver, C. A. Czeisler, S. M. W. Rajaratnam, and M. E. Howard. 2020. Delay or avoidance of medical care because of COVID-19-related concerns—United States, June 2020. *Morbidity and Mortality Weekly Report* 69(36):1250–1257.

Dalen, J. E., K. J. Ryan, and J. S. Alpert. 2017. Where have the generalists gone? They became specialists, then subspecialists. *The American Journal of Medicine* 130(7):766–768.

DeVoe, J. E. 2020. Primary care is an essential ingredient to a successful population health improvement strategy. *Journal of the American Board of Family Medicine* 33(3):468–472.

Douthit, N., S. Kiv, T. Dwolatzky, and S. Biswas. 2015. Exposing some important barriers to health care access in the rural USA. *Public Health* 129(6):611–620.

Dunn, A., and A. H. Shapiro. 2014. Do physicians possess market power? *The Journal of Law & Economics* 57(1):159–193.

Epstein, D. 2019. *Range: Why generalists triumph in a specialized world.* New York: Macmillan Publishers.

FAIR Health. 2015. *FAIR health survey: Viewpoints about ER use for non-emergency care vary significantly by race, age, education and income.* New York: PRNewswire.

Ferrer, R. L., S. J. Hambidge, and R. C. Maly. 2005. The essential role of generalists in health care systems. *Annals of Internal Medicine* 142(8):691–699.

Ford, L. C. 1979. A nurse for all settings: The nurse practitioner. *Nursing Outlook* 27(8):516–521.

Freeman, J. D., S. Kadiyala, J. F. Bell, and D. P. Martin. 2008. The causal effect of health insurance on utilization and outcomes in adults: A systematic review of U.S. studies. *Medical Care* 46(10):1023–1032.

Frost, A., and J. Hargraves. 2018. *HCCI brief: Trends in primary care visits.* Washington, DC: Health Care Cost Institute.

Frost, A., J. Hargraves, and S. Rodriguez. 2018. *2016 health care cost and utilization report.* Washington, DC: Health Care Cost Institute.

Fulton, B. D. 2017. Health care market concentration trends in the United States: Evidence and policy responses. *Health Affairs* 36(9):1530–1538.

Ganguli, I., T. H. Lee, and A. Mehrotra. 2019. Evidence and implications behind a national decline in primary care visits. *Journal of General Internal Medicine* 34(10):2260–2263.

Ganguli, I., Z. Shi, E. J. Orav, A. Rao, K. N. Ray, and A. Mehrotra. 2020. Declining use of primary care among commercially insured adults in the United States, 2008–2016. *Annals of Internal Medicine* 172(4):240–247.

Gleason, R. P., and S. M. Kneipp. 2004. Employment-related constraints: Determinants of primary health care access? *Policy, Politics, & Nursing Practice* 5(2):73–83.

Gong, G., S. G. Phillips, C. Hudson, D. Curti, and B. U. Philips. 2019. Higher U.S. rural mortality rates linked to socioeconomic status, physician shortages, and lack of health insurance. *Health Affairs* 38(12):2003–2010.

Grand View Research. 2017. *U.S. Retail clinics market size, share & trends analysis report by ownership type (retail-owned, hospital-owned), competitive landscape, and segment forecasts, 2018–2025.* https://www.grandviewresearch.com/industry-analysis/us-retail-clinics-market (accessed October 29, 2020).

Gunn, J. M., V. J. Palmer, L. Naccarella, R. Kokanovic, C. J. Pope, J. Lathlean, and K. C. Stange. 2008. The promise and pitfalls of generalism in achieving the Alma-Ata vision of health for all. *The Medical Journal of Australia* 189(2):110–112.

Hadley, J. 2003. Sicker and poorer—the consequences of being uninsured: A review of the research on the relationship between health insurance, medical care use, health, work, and income. *Medical Care Research and Review* 60(Suppl 2):3S–75S; discussion 76S–112S.

HHS, HRSA, and NCHWA (U.S. Department of Health and Human Services, Health Resources and Services Administration, and National Center for Health Workforce Analysis). 2020. *Characteristics of the U.S. nursing workforce with patient care responsibilities: Resources for epidemic and pandemic response.* Rockville, MD: Health Resources and Services Administration.

HRSA. 2020. *Shortage areas.* https://data.hrsa.gov/topics/health-workforce/shortage-areas (accessed August 20, 2020).

HRSA and NCHWA. 2016. *National and regional projections of supply and demand for primary care practitioners: 2013–2025.* Rockville, MD: U.S. Department of Health and Human Services, Health Resources and Services Administration.

Hsiang, W. R., A. Lukasiewicz, M. Gentry, C. Y. Kim, M. P. Leslie, R. Pelker, H. P. Forman, and D. H. Wiznia. 2019. Medicaid patients have greater difficulty scheduling health care appointments compared with private insurance patients: A meta-analysis. *Inquiry: A Journal of Medical Care Organization, Provision and Financing* 56:46958019838118.

Huang, E. S., and K. Finegold. 2013. Seven million Americans live in areas where demand for primary care may exceed supply by more than 10 percent. *Health Affairs* 32(3):614–621.

International Conference on Primary Health Care. 1978. *Declaration of Alma-Ata.* Alma-Ata, USSR: World Health Organization.

IOM (Institute of Medicine). 1996. *Primary care: America's health in a new era.* Washington, DC: National Academy Press.

IOM. 2011. *The future of nursing: Leading change, advancing health.* Washington, DC: The National Academies Press.

Johnson, J. E. 2013. Working together in the best interest of patients. *Journal of the American Board of Family Practice* 26(3):241–243.

Kane, C. K. 2019. *Updated data on physician practice arrangements: For the first time, fewer physicians are owners than employees.* Chicago, IL: American Medical Association.

Kangovi, S., F. K. Barg, T. Carter, J. A. Long, R. Shannon, and D. Grande. 2013. Understanding why patients of low socioeconomic status prefer hospitals over ambulatory care. *Health Affairs* 32(7):1196–1203.

Kangovi, S., N. Mitra, D. Grande, J. A. Long, and D. A. Asch. 2020. Evidence-based community health worker program addresses unmet social needs and generates positive return on investment. *Health Affairs* 39(2):207–213.

Kim, B., M. A. Lucatorto, K. Hawthorne, J. Hersh, R. Myers, A. R. Elwy, and G. D. Graham. 2015. Care coordination between specialty care and primary care: A focus group study of provider perspectives on strong practices and improvement opportunities. *Journal of Multidisciplinary Healthcare* 8:47–58.

Kim, L. Y., D. E. Rose, L. M. Soban, S. E. Stockdale, L. S. Meredith, S. T. Edwards, C. D. Helfrich, and L. V. Rubenstein. 2018. Primary care tasks associated with provider burnout: Findings from a Veterans Health Administration survey. *Journal of General Internal Medicine* 33(1):50–56.

Koch, T., B. Wendling, and N. E. Wilson. 2018. Physician market structure, patient outcomes, and spending: An examination of Medicare beneficiaries. *Health Services Research* 53(5):3549–3568.

Krahn, G. L., L. Hammond, and A. Turner. 2006. A cascade of disparities: Health and health care access for people with intellectual disabilities. *Mental Retardation and Developmental Disabilities Research Reviews* 12(1):70–82.

Liebhaber, A., and J. M. Grossman. 2007. *Physicians moving to mid-sized, single-specialty practices.* Washington, DC: Center for Studying Health System Change.

Loxterkamp, D. 1991. Being there: On the place of the family physician. *Journal of the American Board of Family Practice* 4(5):354–360.

Loxterkamp, D. 2009. Doctors' work: Eulogy for my vocation. *Annals of Family Medicine* 7(3):267–268.

Manchanda, R. 2015. Practice and power: Community health workers and the promise of moving health care upstream. *Journal of Ambulatory Care Management* 38(3):219–224.

McWhinney, I. R. 1989. "An acquaintance with particulars..." *Family Medicine* 21(4):296–298.

Mercer, S. W., and J. G. Howie. 2006. CQI-2—a new measure of holistic interpersonal care in primary care consultations. *British Journal of General Practice* 56(525):262–268.

Miller, W. L., B. F. Crabtree, M. B. Duffy, R. M. Epstein, and K. C. Stange. 2003. Research guidelines for assessing the impact of healing relationships in clinical medicine. *Alternative Therapies in Health and Medicine* 9(3):A80–A95.

Montgomery, L., S. Loue, and K. C. Stange. 2017. Linking the heart and the head: Humanism and professionalism in medical education and practice. *Family Medicine* 49(5):378–383.

Morley, J. E. 2004. A brief history of geriatrics. *The Journals of Gerontology: Series A* 59(11):1132–1152.

Muhlestein, D. B., and N. J. Smith. 2016. Physician consolidation: Rapid movement from small to large group practices, 2013–15. *Health Affairs* 35(9):1638–1642.

NASEM (National Academies of Sciences, Engineering, and Medicine). 2016. *Assessing progress on the Institute of Medicine report* The Future of Nursing. Washington, DC: The National Academies Press.

National Commission on Community Health Services. 1967. *Health is a community affair: Report of the National Commission on Community Health Services.* Cambridge, MA: Harvard University Press.

Naylor, M. D., and E. T. Kurtzman. 2010. The role of nurse practitioners in reinventing primary care. *Health Affairs* 29(5):893–899.

NCCPA (National Commission on Certification of Physician Assistants). 2020. *2019 statistical profile of certified physician assistants.* Johns Creek, GA: National Commission on Certification of Physician Assistants.

Nouri, S., E. C. Khoong, C. R. Lyles, and L. Karliner. 2020. *Addressing equity in telemedicine for chronic disease management during the COVID-19 pandemic.* https://catalyst.nejm.org/doi/full/10.1056/CAT.20.0123 (accessed January 8, 2021).

NRMP (National Resident Matching Program). 2020. *Results and data: 2020 main residency match.* Washington, DC: National Resident Matching Program.

O'Connor, P. J., J. M. Sperl-Hillen, K. L. Margolis, and T. E. Kottke. 2017. Strategies to prioritize clinical options in primary care. *Annals of Family Medicine* 15(1):10–13.

Olaisen, R. H., M. D. Schluchter, S. A. Flocke, K. A. Smyth, S. M. Koroukian, and K. C. Stange. 2020. Assessing the longitudinal impact of physician-patient relationship on functional health. *Annals of Family Medicine* 18(5):422–429.

O'Malley, A. S., D. Samuel, A. M. Bond, and E. Carrier. 2012. After-hours care and its co-ordination with primary care in the U.S. *Journal of General Internal Medicine* 27(11): 1406–1415.

Orcutt, V. L. 2015. Exploring physician assistant data sources. *Journal of the American Academy of Physician Assistants* 28(8):49–50, 52–56.

PAI (Physicians Advocacy Institute) and Avalere Health. 2019. *Updated physician practice acquisition study: National and regional changes in physician employment 2012–2018.* Austin, TX: Physicians Advocacy Institute.

Palmer, V. J., L. Naccarella, and J. M. Gunn. 2007. Are you my generalist or the specialist of my care? *The New Zealand Family Physician* 34(6).

Peterson, L. E., R. L. Phillips, J. C. Puffer, A. Bazemore, and S. Petterson. 2013. Most family physicians work routinely with nurse practitioners, physician assistants, or certified nurse midwives. *Journal of the American Board of Family Medicine* 26(3):244–245.

Petterson, S., R. McNellis, K. Klink, D. Meyers, and A. Bazemore. 2018. *The state of primary care in the United States: A chartbook of facts and statistics.* Washington, DC: Robert Graham Center.

Ponce, N. A., R. D. Hays, and W. E. Cunningham. 2006. Linguistic disparities in health care access and health status among older adults. *Journal of General Internal Medicine* 21(7):786–791.

Rabin, D. L., A. Jetty, S. Petterson, Z. Saqr, and A. Froehlich. 2017. Among low-income re-spondents with diabetes, high-deductible versus no-deductible insurance sharply reduces medical service use. *Diabetes Care* 40(2):239–245.

RAND. 2016. *The evolving role of retail clinics.* Santa Monica, CA: RAND Corporation.

Rao, A., Z. Shi, K. N. Ray, A. Mehrotra, and I. Ganguli. 2019. National trends in primary care visit use and practice capabilities, 2008–2015. *Annals of Family Medicine* 17(6):538–544.

Ray, K. N., Z. Shi, I. Ganguli, A. Rao, E. J. Orav, and A. Mehrotra. 2020. Trends in pedi-atric primary care visits among commercially insured U.S. children, 2008–2016. *JAMA Pediatrics* 174(4):350–357.

Reddy, S. R., D. Ross-Degnan, A. M. Zaslavsky, S. B. Soumerai, and J. F. Wharam. 2014. Impact of a high-deductible health plan on outpatient visits and associated diagnostic tests. *Medical Care* 52(1):86–92.

Reid, R. O., J. S. Ashwood, M. W. Friedberg, E. S. Weber, C. M. Setodji, and A. Mehrotra. 2012. Retail clinic visits and receipt of primary care. *Journal of General Internal Medicine* 28(4):504–512.

Rocovich, C., and T. Patel. 2012. Emergency department visits: Why adults choose the emergency room over a primary care physician visit during regular office hours? *World Journal of Emergency Medicine* 3(2):91–97.

Sabo, S., C. G. Allen, K. Sutkowi, and A. Wennerstrom. 2017. Community health workers in the United States: Challenges in identifying, surveying, and supporting the workforce. *American Journal of Public Health* 107(12):1964–1969.

Scott, J. G., D. Cohen, B. Dicicco-Bloom, W. L. Miller, K. C. Stange, and B. F. Crabtree. 2008. Understanding healing relationships in primary care. *Annals of Family Medicine* 6(4):315–322.

Shanafelt, T. D., S. Boone, L. Tan, L. N. Dyrbye, W. Sotile, D. Satele, C. P. West, J. Sloan, and M. R. Oreskovich. 2012. Burnout and satisfaction with work-life balance among U.S. physicians relative to the general U.S. population. *Archives of Internal Medicine* 172(18):1377–1385.

Sharac, J., P. Shin, R. Gunsalus, and S. Rosenbaum. 2018. *Community health centers con-tinued to expand patient and service capacity in 2017.* Washington, DC: Geiger Gibson Program in Community Health Policy, RCHN Community Health Foundation.

Sinaiko, A. D., M. B. Landrum, D. J. Meyers, S. Alidina, D. D. Maeng, M. W. Friedberg, L. M. Kern, A. M. Edwards, S. P. Flieger, P. R. Houck, P. Peele, R. J. Reid, K. McGraves-Lloyd, K. Finison, and M. B. Rosenthal. 2017. Synthesis of research on patient-centered medical homes brings systematic differences into relief. *Health Affairs* 36(3):500–508.

Souch, J. M., and J. S. Cossman. 2020. A commentary on rural-urban disparities in COVID-19 testing rates per 100,000 and risk factors. *Journal of Rural Health* 37(1):188–190.

Stange, K. C. 2002. The paradox of the parts and the whole in understanding and improving general practice. *International Journal for Quality in Health Care* 14(4):267–268.

Stange, K. C. 2009a. The generalist approach. *Annals of Family Medicine* 7(3):198–203.

Stange, K. C. 2009b. A science of connectedness. *Annals of Family Medicine* 7(5):387–395.

Stange, K. C. 2010. Ways of knowing, learning, and developing. *Annals of Family Medicine* 8(1):4–10.

Stange, K. C. 2018. In this issue: Continuity, relationships, and the illusion of a steady state. *Annals of Family Medicine* 16(6):486–487.

Stange, K. C., W. L. Miller, and I. McWhinney. 2001. Developing the knowledge base of family practice. *Family Medicine* 33(4):286–297.

Stevens, R. A. 2001. The Americanization of family medicine: Contradictions, challenges, and change, 1969–2000. *Family Medicine* 33(4):232–243.

Tolbert, J., and K. Orgera. 2020. *Key fact about the uninsured population.* https://www.kff.org/uninsured/issue-brief/key-facts-about-the-uninsured-population (accessed January 19, 2021).

UCA (Urgent Care Association). 2019. *Urgent care industry white paper: The essential role of the urgent care center in population health.* Warrenville, IL: Urgent Care Association.

Velasquez, D., and A. Mehrotra. 2020. Ensuring the growth of telehealth during COVID-19 does not exacerbate disparities in care. *Health Affairs Blog* (May 8). https://www.healthaffairs.org/do/10.1377/hblog20200505.591306/full (accessed January 8, 2021).

Wang, Z., and K. Tang. 2020. Combating COVID-19: Health equity matters. *Nature Medicine* 26(4):458.

Weinick, R. M., C. E. Pollack, M. P. Fisher, E. M. Gillen, and A. Mehrotra. 2011. Policy implications of the use of retail clinics. *RAND Health Quarterly* 1(3):9.

WHO and UNICEF (World Health Organization and United Nations Children's Fund). 2018. *Declaration of Astana.* Astana, Kazakhstan: World Health Organization and United Nations Children's Fund.

Xue, Y., J. A. Smith, and J. Spetz. 2019. Primary care nurse practitioners and physicians in low-income and rural areas, 2010–2016. *JAMA* 321(1):102–105.

4

Person-Centered, Family-Centered, and Community-Oriented Primary Care

Primary care does not exist within a vacuum. Rather, it is a reflection of societal norms and values. Many primary care settings today are structured in a way that prevents the team from understanding and addressing the context in which a patient lives. An approach to care limited in this way perpetuates disadvantage and health inequity. Institutional inequalities, including structural racism, sexism, and classism, that are present throughout American society also exist within primary care today (Feagin and Bennefield, 2014; NASEM, 2017). Over time, these influences have led to a dominant paradigm in primary care that is clinician centric and paternalistic, mirroring the broader U.S. health care system. The need to shift that paradigm has become even more clear given the unequal impact that the COVID-19 pandemic has had on disadvantaged communities and the current acceleration and amplification of long-standing calls for social justice and the dismantling of structural inequities, including racism, that are woven deeply within the fabric of society (Morse et al., 2020).

Fortunately, primary care has seized on opportunities to shift toward an approach that is more grounded in tenets of care that are crucial to high-quality primary care: *relationships* with the people, their families, and the communities being served; and *equity*, which acknowledges and empowers those people, families, and communities. These two tenets represent an important transition in how primary care needs to move forward in the twenty-first century. While it will require a shift in the dominant paradigm to accelerate this forward progress, it is important to acknowledge the long history and many successful models (current and historical) based on this approach (Geiger, 2002; IOM, 1983; Kark and Kark, 1999; National

Commission on Community Health Services, 1967; Rosen, 1971; The Folsom Group, 2012). Box 4-1 summarizes the history and outcomes of one of these models, the patient-centered medical home. (See Chapter 9 for more on this model's financing and outcomes.)

Crossing the Quality Chasm: A New Health System for the 21st Century (IOM, 2001) helped highlight the need to shift the paradigm, proposing the concept of patient-centered care and describing it as "respectful of and responsive to individual patient preferences, needs and values, and ensuring that patient values guide all clinical decisions" (p. 40). Since then, momentum has been growing to realize the ideal vision for primary care—moving further toward care that is person centered, family centered, and community oriented (a model developed in the 1940s [Kark and Kark, 1999; Kark and Riche, 1944]) rather than clinic oriented (Health centres of tomorrow, 1947; Susser et al., 1955). This conceptualization focuses on the entire individual over the course of their lifetime and in the context of their family and community, not solely on a specific health issue and a specific

---

BOX 4-1
The Patient-Centered Medical Home

The patient-centered medical home (PCMH) is one model of care built on the principles of person- and family-centeredness. First introduced by the American Academy of Pediatrics in the late 1960s to improve care for children with special needs, the PCMH is an organizing concept that is now seen as a model of care that can further the goals of disease prevention and management, population health improvement, and care coordination (Peikes et al., 2015). Today, several accrediting organizations recognize PCMHs, with the National Committee for Quality Assurance (NCQA) being the major accreditor (Philip et al., 2019). In 2017, more than 13,000 primary care practices, with some 67,000 clinicians, have achieved NCQA PCMH recognition (NCQA, 2020).

There is no one formula for a successful PCMH, but the characteristics they share include management of patient populations, interprofessional care teams to improve care coordination, and care safety, efficiency, and quality. By becoming a recognized PCMH, practices may receive private or public incentive payments. Passage of the Patient Protection and Affordable Care Act, which offers enhanced federal funding to states for health homes serving Medicaid beneficiaries, catalyzed increased interest in becoming a PCMH (Adamson, 2011). (See Chapter 9 for a discussion of payment models and incentives.)

A key feature of PCMH models is that individuals are aligned with a care coordinator, who can be a registered nurse, physician assistant, or social worker, whose main function is to manage the person's health throughout the care spectrum, simplifying access to care, facilitating improved compliance with treatment recommendations and preventive measures, and improving care (Adamson, 2011; Fortuna et al., 2020). Individuals who receive care in a PCMH report higher satisfaction with

clinical visit. It also emphasizes prevention and well-being, or well care rather than sick care. In addition, this conceptualization recognizes that knowledge accumulated over time—about the person, the family, and the community in which they live—creates a better foundation for recognizing health problems and the delivery of care that is appropriate in the context of other needs individuals might have (Starfield, 2011).

This chapter describes what the committee heard about what individuals seeking care, families, and communities want from primary care and then presents the evidence for why a person-centered, family-centered, and community-oriented approach can deliver on those wants, and in doing so, will benefit all parties involved. The chapter also discusses how primary care can overcome the historical barriers to fully operationalize these concepts, as well as two tenets of person-centered, family-centered, and community-oriented primary care: the primacy of relationships and health equity.

their care (Reid et al., 2010; Sarinopoulos et al., 2017). For clinicians, becoming a PCMH includes reporting on progress toward measurable outcomes that can result in the practice receiving incentives and bonus payments. The PCMH model is also associated with improved staff satisfaction (Reid et al., 2010), with one study finding that staff who reported they were "extremely satisfied" with their workplace increasing from 38.5 to 42.2 percent and burnout rates decreasing from 32.7 to 25.8 percent (AHRQ, 2017). A study of the U.S. Department of Veterans Affairs primary care personnel also found that working in adequately staffed PCMH settings was associated with lower rates of burnout than working in inadequately staffed settings (Helfrich et al., 2014). For health plans, PCMHs can reduce spending over time, improve health outcomes by better managing chronic conditions (Liss et al., 2013; van den Berk-Clark et al., 2018), increase member satisfaction and retention, and improve care collaboration (Adamson, 2011).

While the PCMH model has many advantages, it is not perfect. A small practice or solo practitioner may not have the resources available to meet the management and administrative demands and have to hire additional staff. Geographic limitations may also pose a challenge, as rural practices without adequate local specialists, non-physician primary care team members, or community resources may find it difficult to meet collaborative care standards. Implementing the digital health systems required for PCMH recognition is expensive and complicated and can be beyond the skills and financial capabilities of many practices. One study of 32 PCMH practices in Pennsylvania found that benefits may be limited to high-risk populations (Friedberg et al., 2014; Schwenk, 2014). Another study found that misalignment between current payment systems and PCMH goals was common, largely because primary care clinicians were unable to spend the extra time and effort needed to establish an engaging and well-integrated medical home with specialized and coordinated care for every patient (Alexander et al., 2013).

LISTENING TO INDIVIDUAL, FAMILY,
AND COMMUNITY VOICES

In a survey that asked people about their personal definitions of health, answers included "not being sick" but also being happy, calm and relaxed, and able to live independently (AAFP, 2018). Separately, community health workers (CHWs) in Philadelphia asked approximately 10,000 people "what do you need to improve your health?" Their answers were not limited to care focused on disease but also included psychosocial support, health behavior coaching, health-promoting resources, health system navigation, and clinical care (NASEM, 2019b). They expressed a desire to eliminate the racism and systematic injustice that permeates their daily lives and influences their experiences with health care, their health outcomes, and their life expectancy (Kangovi et al., 2014a; Williams et al., 2019a,b). These drivers of health mirror epidemiologic studies suggesting that socioeconomic and behavioral factors influence health outcomes more than health care or genetics do (Artiga and Hinton, 2018; Braveman and Gottlieb, 2014; McGinnis et al., 2002). While primary care teams have known this for a long time, primary care has encountered significant barriers—most notably incompatible payment models—that prevent it from moving away from a biomedical, disease-focused model to one that addresses people's expressed needs and preferences, includes individuals and families more in their care, and responds to the multitude of factors that impact health, including the context of the community (Puffer et al., 2015).

Early in its deliberations, the committee sought input from individuals and families on their experiences with primary care. On June 2, 2020, the committee hosted a webinar titled Patient Perspectives on Primary Care.[1] Representatives from AARP, Family Voices, the Migrant Clinicians Network, the National Patient Advocate Foundation, the National Health Council, the University of North Carolina Family Support Program, and the U.S. Department of Veterans Affairs (VA) participated in the webinar and presented on the following topics:

- What does primary care mean to the people, families, and communities your organization represents?
- What can primary care do to better serve them?

Separately, the committee also sought to hear from people directly about their experiences with primary care. Through an online form posted on the project website, people shared their stories, ideas, and experiences

---

[1] The webinar agenda, speaker bios, and archived presentations can be found at https://www.nationalacademies.org/event/06-02-2020/patient-perspectives-on-primary-care-a-webinar (accessed February 14, 2021).

with primary care. Anonymous submissions from this exercise and excerpts from conversations in the webinar appear below to illustrate the importance of relationships and equity in primary care and reinforce the importance of organizing primary care in a way that honors and responds to individual and family preferences, needs, values, and goals (Greene et al., 2012).

Continuity of Relationships

A defining aspect of the committee's vision of primary care is the trusting relationship between the interprofessional care team and the person seeking care. Patients and advocacy groups provided multiple descriptions of the importance of relationship building. One woman from New York views her primary care clinician as a whole-person health expert and not just someone that completes an annual exam. Others reported that if it were not for primary care, no one would know—or care about—their overall health. The primacy of this relationship was described by a 33-year-old woman from rural Iowa:

> I live in a rural community, and my primary physician is truly a "one-stop shop" for all of my health care questions. Not that all services and supports are provided by my physician, but there is always a way to ask a question and be referred to what I need.

Part of this trusting relationship involves an element of partnership and inclusivity. People felt positive about feeling heard and negative when their care remained unaligned with their personal preferences and priorities. The following two submissions are, respectively, from a 52-year-old in Ohio who illustrates the importance of being heard and a 77-year-old woman in Massachusetts who remarks on a breach of trust that compelled her to seek care elsewhere:

> I like that my doctor and I have a long history together. He listens to my suggestions if I have a medical issue and tries to address them based on my symptoms or issues.

> I have been living in a nursing home for 18 1/2 years. A medical director was my primary care physician here for many years. Then, one year, I read my medical record and saw that I was on nine unnecessary medications— either for medical conditions I did not have or for which treatment wasn't needed. This physician did not have the expertise I needed, so I now go outpatient for primary care. He never apologized either.

Gwen Darien with the National Patient Advocate Foundation spoke to the primacy of relationships and said, "it's very fair to say ... that health care relationships used to just be doctors and patients, but we have certainly gone well beyond doctors and patients in our health care." She went on to describe the importance of the relationship with the person who coordinates a patient's care and of a trusting relationship that patients can depend on, particularly those with multiple health conditions. She also questioned why, when people get into the U.S. specialist system, there is no transition back into primary care, which should be about follow-up and continued relationships.

Marc Boutin, chief executive officer of the National Health Council, stressed that taking time to understand people's circumstances and personal goals is the basis of relationship building. With this knowledge, the care team should design care that can help the person and their family achieve the goal that was most important to them. Integrating these two processes would dramatically change how health is viewed and help us get the outcomes that matter for the person and family.

Jennifer Purdy from the VA illustrated important components of the clinician–patient relationship and how the VA health system solicits feedback to better understand that relationship. The VA asks for the patient's perspective on what it was like before the visit and how the patient felt they needed to prepare for it. They also listen to the patient's perspective of the experience of arriving at a facility or clinic to receive care or even clicking the telehealth button to start an appointment. They ask questions about what it was like to have care in the exam itself. Veterans have reported that they want to feel heard and to be able to trust their clinician without explaining themselves over and over again. They want to know what comes next and understand their role in their whole health care. The VA also inquires about what happens after the visit and when the person returned home, including how fast they would see test results that mattered to them and their role in receiving the next parts of their care.

Amy Liebman from the Migrant Clinician Network also talked about building relationships when a person's residence is not fixed. She stated that health systems need to be redesigned to ensure that the relationship can be maintained even with challenges of migrant populations. The ultimate goal, she said, is not to interrupt the health care relationship. The COVID-19 pandemic has provided an illustration of how telehealth has enabled primary care relationships to be maintained and even flourish when office visits are not possible.

Family Focus

While "family" in the 21st century can mean different things to different people (and many people may not have anyone in their lives that they consider to be part of their family), the patient advocacy webinar panelists and individuals from the community presented many illustrations of the importance of the family in the delivery of primary care. That same 33-year-old woman from Iowa with the "one-stop shop" physician followed up to write that:

> My other experience with primary care that I would like to share, is the immense value when my doctor has knowledge of my family health. I was pregnant at 19 years old, and one great gift was that my daughter and I received care from the same doctor. We could attend appointments together (and did for many years) which reduced my burden of travel and time. The doctors could respond to our combined needs—the [e]ffect the health of another family member has on your health could be addressed, etc. In my dream for the future, primary care could be provided knowing the full context of the families experience and therefore be able to connect and respond to the needs and supports beyond just the individual in the office chair.

But others see the role of primary care through different lenses. Another individual from California submitted this:

> Since I'm a fairly healthy adult, I only use primary care episodically for minor acute issues. My perspective about primary care has more to do with helping my mother manage her care. There's much to be desired in terms of how involved the provider really wants to be in her overall care. It's not clear that the provider wants to go above the basics.

Allysa Ware from Family Voices spoke about her organization being a network of families with diverse experiences that share on-the-ground information on what is happening in primary care visits. In focus groups, Family Voices listened to families who felt doctors were just going through a checklist without a meaningful relationship. One family member said the doctor was checking off things on a paper but not personalizing it to their child and did not take environmental factors into account. The doctor did not offer suggestions for helping, seem to take her concerns seriously, or say anything to lessen those concerns. Family Voices often heard that visits are fast and families do not feel like partners. One theme was that the primary care team took a wait-and-see approach, instead of really listening to the parents. The fragile relationship was illustrated by families reporting fear that if they raised concerns or disagreed with their clinician, it would impact the care their child received.

Barbara Leach, a special projects coordinator in the University of North Carolina School of Social Work, reinforced the importance of primary care and family support with children and youth with special needs. Parents start out looking to their primary care physician, their family doctor, to make sure their child gets what they need and serve as the gatekeepers of information about their child. She also pointed out the important role of primary care in coordinating care with different specialists. Parents expect primary care clinicians to provide education and information about their child's challenging conditions and referrals to specialists and connect the family to community resources and supports. She described the role of primary care clinicians as comprehensive and conducted in partnership with the family, understanding the problems families face and helping them to learn and support their child's well-being.

Community Resources

The panel discussed at length the important role that primary care plays in connecting people with community resources and addressing issues related to the community. These resources (e.g., social services, nutrition assistance programs) are fundamental to whole-person health but are generally considered to be separate from traditional, disease-focused medical care. Ware described that families often do not know which way to go and that social determinants of health (SDOH) play a major role in the ability to navigate the community. The panelists gave examples of clinicians not always being sufficiently knowledgeable about the community to connect someone to resources that could help them, and people submitting their primary care experiences online also expressed the need for strong connections between primary care and additional health and community resources. One individual, a 31-year-old, non-binary woman from Massachusetts, experienced a rotating door of clinicians—six since 2017—and found that the majority avoided care related to mental health and eating disorders and were usually unable to create a safe care environment.

> Seeking primary care is difficult because I do not trust that doctors want me to have a healthier body, just a smaller one. I am queer and transgender, so safety comes to mind as well as [whether] the office will be respectful of my pronouns, my body, or my family. I have mental health needs, and many doctors do not want to touch or talk about that beyond the small survey at the end of visits. And it is clear despite the many and serious effects that eating disorders can have on the body, that PCPs are not trained in how to work with patients in ED recovery.

ACHIEVING PERSON-CENTERED CARE

The terms "patient-centered" and "person-centered" are often used interchangeably but are conceptually different. Moving from patient-centered to person-centered care represents an evolution of primary care to focus on individual people in the context of their lived experiences, family, social worlds, and community (Starfield, 2011; van Weel, 2011) (see Table 4-1).

The World Health Organization (WHO) defines people-centered care[2] as

> focused and organized around the health needs and expectations of people and communities rather than on diseases. People-centered care extends the concept of patient-centered care to individuals, families, communities and society. Whereas patient-centered care is commonly understood as focusing on the individual seeking care—the patient—people-centered care encompasses these clinical encounters and also includes attention to the health of people in their communities and their crucial role in shaping health policy and health services. (2020b, p. 12)

According to WHO's *Framework on Integrated People-Centered Health Services* (WHO, 2016), a people-centered approach is needed to ensure the following:

TABLE 4-1 The Differences Between Patient-Centered Care and Person-Centered Care

Patient-Centered Care	Person-Centered Care[a]
Generally refers to interactions in visits	Refers to interrelationships over time
May be episode oriented	Considers episodes as part of life-course experiences with health
Generally centers around the management of diseases	Views diseases as interrelated phenomena
Generally views comorbidity as number of chronic diseases	Often considers morbidity as combinations of types of illnesses (multimorbidity)
Generally views body systems as distinct	Views body systems as interrelated
Uses coding systems that reflect professionally defined conditions	Uses coding systems that also allow for specification of people's health concerns
Is concerned primarily with the evolution of patients' diseases	Is concerned with the evolution of people's experienced health problems as well as with their diseases

[a] Starfield (2011) uses "person-focused" rather than the committee's preferred term, "person-centered."
SOURCE: Starfield, 2011.

---

[2] WHO uses "people-centered care" instead of "person-centered care," but both terms represent the same concept.

- **Equity:** For everyone, everywhere to access the quality health services they need, when and where they need them. (See section below for more on this subject.)
- **Quality:** Safe, effective, and timely care that responds to people's comprehensive needs and is of the highest possible standards.
- **Responsiveness and participation:** Care that is coordinated around people's needs, respects their preferences, and allows for their participation in health affairs.
- **Efficiency:** The assurance that services are provided in the most cost-effective setting with the right balance between health promotion, prevention, and in-and-out care, avoiding duplication and waste of resources.
- **Resilience:** Strengthened capacity of health actors, institutions, and populations to prepare for, and effectively respond to, public health crises.

The essence of person-centered care is that it extends beyond any one clinical encounter and involves continuous and holistic knowledge of patients as people, their families, their social world, and the communities in which they live and work. This knowledge accrues over time and is not specific to disease-oriented episodes. Furthermore, this knowledge, and the time spent attaining it, strengthens the relationships between the primary care team and the people seeking care. Compared to patient-centered care, person-centered care has been shown to lead to agreement on care plans, better health outcomes, and higher patient satisfaction (Ekman et al., 2011). The WHO Astana Declaration in 2018 reiterated and refreshed commitments made by the world's governments to primary *health care* (WHO and UNICEF, 2018), which is the integration of primary care and public health, with the collective goal of caring for populations. This puts the goals of this report squarely in line with the Astana Declaration and the commitments of the U.S. government as one of its cosigners.

The Role of the Individual

Activating and empowering individuals to be a part of their own care team should function cyclically and iteratively—as people become more knowledgeable and confident in their own health care and continue to experience success, they may take on increasingly sustained and eventually proactive roles. While empowerment has become a highly visible initiative in public health and policy reforms in the past decade (e.g., some provisions of the Patient Protection and Affordable Care Act [ACA][3] encourage engaging

---

[3] Patient Protection and Affordable Care Act, Public Law 111-148 (March 23, 2010).

care-seekers in this way), the methods of reaching person-centered care can and should look different depending on context (Chen et al., 2016). One foundational tenet, though, is respecting people as experts in their own lives (Kennedy, 2003). The Chronic Care Model explicitly recognizes that "informed, activated patients" are needed to improve health outcomes for individuals with chronic diseases. One of the six components of that model is self-management support (Bodenheimer et al., 2002). Apart from engaging individuals in their own care, understanding the individual's goals for their care, particularly as they age, can be especially important. Naik and colleagues (2018) noted that "eliciting and documenting the personal values of older, multimorbid adults is uncommon in routine care, despite playing a central role in person-centered care." Models for capturing the goals, values, and preferences of older adults in the primary care setting have been shown to be feasible (Blaum et al., 2018; Naik et al., 2018).

The Role of Family and Informal Caregivers

Family members and other informal caregivers may not be licensed to provide care, but their voice and presence is an important component of person-centered primary care and can improve health outcomes, health care quality, and the overall care experience for people and their families. Primary care that includes family members or companions is associated with improved self-management, satisfaction, communication, and understanding (Cené et al., 2015; Rosland et al., 2011). In fact, an individual's most important health care resource may be their family or informal supports (if they have them) (Cole-Kelly and Seaburn, 1999). Research shows that most individuals prefer clinicians to involve their families and other informal caregivers in their health care (Andrades et al., 2013; Botelho et al., 1996). Family members play a supportive role in most consultations with clinicians (Andrades et al., 2013; Sayers et al., 2006), as well as helping their loved one to navigate the increasing complexity of health care systems, including making and keeping appointments and following up on referrals (Andrades et al., 2013; Botelho et al., 1996; Igel and Lerner, 2016; IOM, 2008). In addition, a family member or other informal caregiver can be a valuable source of health information and insights about the home and community environments that clinicians may not get from the person seeking care.

Family members can take many roles aside from providing companionship and comfort when they accompany a loved one to an office visit (Brown et al., 1998; Clayman et al., 2005; Cornelius et al., 2018; Schilling et al., 2002). As an advocate, they can communicate the person's needs and concerns and may translate or interpret in situations with a language gap, especially in emergencies (Rimmer, 2020). They can also act as an additional set of ears to ensure the person understands their disease, medications, procedures, and treatments, which may result in better outcomes (Whitehead et al., 2018). Family members can help someone make decisions that are aligned with their personal and cultural beliefs. For chronic illnesses, family members may come to see themselves as the primary care team's partner in providing care. It is important in such cases for communication to continue to include the individual, particularly when they are capable of making decisions about their care.

Research has identified core facilitators of family-centered care models that benefit the individual while protecting the health and well-being of family members (Kokorelias et al., 2019): (1) development and implementation of care plans that include the family; (2) collaboration between family members and health care clinicians in the delivery of care; (3) education for patients, families, and clinicians; and (4) dedicated policies and procedures that address inclusion of family members (Kokorelias et al., 2019). When implemented, family-centered primary care can reduce admissions, readmissions, and length of hospital stay; increase patient, family, and clinician satisfaction; and improve relationships (Kuhlthau et al., 2011; Park et al., 2018). However, despite the benefits of such inclusive care, family and informal caregivers often need additional support, including more consistent and explicit inclusion in the care team, training, respite, and financial security (IOM, 2008).

Examples from Medical Disciplines

Centering care around the family was a major driver in creating the medical specialty of family medicine in 1969 (Green and Puffer, 2010; Stephens, 2010). In the early years of this emerging new medical and academic discipline, family medicine adapted care based on the biopsychosocial model of care and incorporated unique training elements to strengthen the expertise of primary care teams to think of individuals within the context of their families and their communities (Borrell-Carrió et al., 2004; Engel, 2012; Martin et al., 2004). Today, family medicine teams often care for several members of the same family and have developed advanced skills to incorporate families into care plans and seamlessly care for multiple family members of various ages at one clinic visit or during one hospitalization (Beasley et al., 2004; Flocke et al., 1998). Other primary care medical disciplines not focused on all ages, such as pediatrics (Clay and Parsh, 2016; Jolley and Shields, 2009; Pettoello-Mantovani et al., 2009) and geriatrics, have also embraced family-centered care concepts and practices. Pediatric clinicians who adopt family-centered practices recognize the importance of including family members in evaluating, planning, and delivering treatment and incorporate that ideology into policies, programs, facility design, and day-to-day interactions (Committee on Hospital Care, 2003; Committee on Hospital Care and IPFCC, 2012).

Similarly, geriatricians understand that families can provide information that plays an important role in clinical decision making. Geriatrics care tends to focus on assessing function and cognition and emphasizes the goals of care. Involving the family in assessing and caring for older adults is both important and challenging, particularly for the many who have multiple chronic disorders (American Geriatrics Society Expert Panel on the Care of Older Adults with Multimorbidity, 2012; Boyd et al., 2005; Tinetti et al., 2012). The changes in sensory, cognitive, and physical functions that come with aging may prompt some older adults to need or want to involve family members or close friends in managing their health (IOM, 2008; Wolff and Roter, 2011). A 2015 survey of older adults and their preferences for care found that while nearly 70 percent of older adults manage their own care, they prefer family members, in addition to their clinicians, to be involved in making health care decisions (Wolff and Boyd, 2015).

The Role of Community and Community-Oriented Care

The importance of recognizing community needs in primary care has been described for decades. *Community-Oriented Primary Care: New Directions for Health Services Delivery* (IOM, 1983, p. 70) defined community-oriented primary care as

> an approach to medical practice that undertakes responsibility for the health of a defined population, by combining epidemiologic study and social intervention with the clinical care of individuals, so that the primary care practice itself becomes a community medicine program. Both the individual and the community or population are the focus of diagnosis, treatment, and ongoing surveillance.

People-centered and community-oriented care overlap considerably and link strongly to the goals of WHO and the World Health Assembly in the 2018 Declaration of Astana and subsequent commitments.

Adding community-oriented care to the new conceptualization of primary care addresses the individual's and family's cultural and social context as they are embedded within a medical and social neighborhood, rather than from a solely delivery-centric model (Braddock et al., 2013; Buchmueller and Carpenter, 2010; Chokshi and Cohen, 2018; Davis et al., 2005; DeVoe et al., 2009; Driscoll et al., 2013; Edgoose and Edgoose, 2017; Enard and Ganelin, 2013; Etz, 2016; Finkelstein et al., 2020; Kramer et al., 2018; Landon et al., 2012; Possemato et al., 2018; Starfield, 2011; Yoon et al., 2018). In addition, community-oriented care facilitates coordination between public health approaches and primary care delivery, opening the door for primary care to play a central role in improving community health (Eng et al., 1992), particularly for communities with disadvantaged populations (Cyril et al., 2015; Derose et al., 2019; Shukor et al., 2018).

Benefits of Community-Oriented Care

Community-oriented care improves outcomes in many areas and for different populations, including well-child care (Jones et al., 2018); maternal, neonatal, and child health (Black et al., 2017); and for people with depression (Izquierdo et al., 2018; Ong et al., 2017), obesity (Derose et al., 2019), hypertension (Epstein et al., 2002), and opioid use disorder (Wells et al., 2018). It can also play an important role in reducing health disparities (Derose et al., 2019), decreasing unnecessary use of the emergency department, and increasing the ability for older adults to live independently (Institute for Clinical Systems Improvement, 2014).

Despite the strong evidence that partnering with the community will benefit person- and family-centered care, studies have found that models involving shared decision making, such as integrating the community into primary care, can be challenging to the health care enterprise on practical, structural, and systematic levels. For example, some clinicians have difficulty recognizing the power dynamics between them and other care team members or people seeking care: specifically, the power that inherently comes with the position of health care clinician (Nimmon and Stenfors-Hayes, 2016; Singer, 1989).

Clinicians and systems may see community-oriented approaches as a means to bolster medical care but not necessarily whole-person health (Garfield and Kangovi, 2019). In addition, most challenges are exacerbated by fee-for-service (FFS) payment that incentivizes diagnosing and treating diseases, performing procedures, prescribing medications, and providing care based on traditional biomedical models. For example, a 2018 study found that primary care clinicians felt pressure to focus on diagnosis and treatment and had a hard time imagining how evidence-based, community-partnered programs for disease self-management and prevention could contribute to either of those primary functions (Leppin et al., 2018). The study authors concluded that "primary care and community-based programs exist in disconnected worlds. Without urgent and intentional efforts to bridge well-care and sick-care, interventions that support people's efforts to be and stay well in their communities will remain outside of—if not at odds with—health care" (p. 1). These words echo those of primary care clinicians nearly a century ago (Burnham, 1920; Susser et al., 1955; Wald, 1911). Such long-standing challenges can be overcome when payment is reformed to better align incentives to support community-oriented care

(Gofin et al., 2015; IOM, 1983; Lloyd et al., 2020). See Chapter 9 for more about primary care payment.

The Role of the Interprofessional Care Team

Ideally, person-centered care is delivered via interprofessional teams who establish long-term relationships with care-seeking individuals and their families. Achieving this aim requires a team structure that places individuals in the driver's seat of care that aligns with their needs and preferences. Well-designed teams can support nurturing, longitudinal, person-centered care (Mitchell et al., 2012; Sullivan and Ellner, 2015). A commonly used definition of team-based care is "the provision of health services to individuals, families, [and] their communities by at least two health providers who work collaboratively with patients and their caregivers—to the extent preferred by each patient—to accomplish shared goals within and across settings to achieve coordinated, high-quality care" (Mitchell et al., 2012, p. 5; Okun et al., 2014, p. 46) (see Chapter 6 for more on primary care teams).

The Role of Relationships in Primary Care

Primary care settings continue to expand beyond traditional health care settings and move beyond the walls of clinics and hospitals to community-based settings, such as schools, employment sites, and housing complexes. In addition, primary care is increasingly using technology-enabled care delivery modalities, including telehealth and smartphone apps. As a result, the personal relationship between the person seeking care and the care team providing that care as a foundation for consistency is more important than ever. The person–care team relationship is the "bedrock of value in primary care" and symbiotically related to other components of high-quality care, including whole-person care and coordination (Ellner and Phillips, 2017), and continuity of care (Andres et al., 2016; Rhodes et al., 2014). Evidence of the benefits of a strong relationship to both the individual and care team is well documented; a relationship built on respect and acceptance can lead to patient satisfaction and empowerment, improved outcomes and safety, increased adherence, prolonged engagement, and decreased burnout for care team members (Bogart et al., 2016; Brown et al., 2015; Chaudhri et al., 2019; Pollack, 2019).

Relationships can be healing in their own right, outside of any health services, and personal connections with care staff other than the immediate primary care team, such as front office staff, subspecialists, consultants, and care extenders, also contribute a vital dimension to the patient experience (Kravitz and Feldman, 2017). Over time, relationships encourage the care-seeker to feel understood, hopeful about the future, and comfortable with the care team or in a health environment (Scott et al., 2008). Comfort and trust are crucial for beginning to reduce health inequities and improve access for marginalized care-seekers, including formerly incarcerated individuals, those who are not U.S. citizens, people with disabilities, veterans, people who are homeless, and communities of color. Trauma-informed care and anti-racism curricula in training, in addition to diversified hiring practices for these teams, improve team members' abilities to connect with patients, foster a relationship of understanding and trust, and ultimately begin to improve disparities in health access and outcomes (Alsan et al., 2019, 2020; Chaudhri et al., 2019; Garcia et al., 2019; Saha et al., 1999; Shen et al., 2018). Relationships are a function of time, trust, and respect, measures of continuity and longitudinality, and patient-reported outcomes, described in Chapter 8, are an effort to assess relationships systematically as high-value measures of primary care.

Few primary care team members would likely disagree with the importance of relationships, and some evidence suggests that medical school graduates who go into primary care may choose it at least in part for its relationship aspect (Osborn et al., 2017). The reality, however, is less than the ideal, and care teams struggle with time constraints, reimbursement barriers, and administrative hurdles that get in the way of relationship building. While some suggest simply reprioritizing and freeing up time to work on relationships, other more novel options have been conceived including changes to the electronic medical record system, building communication skills, reconfiguring the primary care team, and overhauling payment models so they are compatible with the time and effort needed to build and sustain relationships with people seeking care (AHRQ, 2018; Montague and Asan, 2014; Pollack, 2019).

The patient–care team relationship is all the more important in times of crisis and uncertainty, such as during the COVID-19 pandemic. A survey found that even in the midst of the pandemic, the majority of primary care patients continue to value a relationship with their care clinician, citing desires for being known as individuals, help understanding current events, and a safe environment for asking questions; 83 percent expressed distress at the thought of losing that relationship (The Larry A. Green Center and PCC, 2020). In another wave of that survey, two-thirds of patients most preferred speaking with a member of their primary care team about potential exposure to COVID-19, as opposed to public health officials, hospital workers, or trained community members.[4] Additional research found doz-

---

[4] These data come from the third wave of the Green Center's COVID-19 survey, but were not published in the executive summary. The national aggregate data are available upon request from the project public access file. To request, follow the link on the project webpage (www.nationalacademies.org/primarycare [accessed February 14, 2021]) for contacting the Public Access Records Office.

ens of ways to improve relationships, even during telehealth visits, casting the pandemic as an opportunity to reinvent primary care's investment in relationships (Bergman et al., 2020).

Even though primary care's emphasis on relationships is not consistently realized, isolated exemplars do exist. For example, Southcentral Foundation's (SCF's) Nuka[5] System of Care built relationships into the core of its operational principles and responsibilities. The Alaska Native–owned, nonprofit health care organization also focuses on responding to the wide range of opportunities for feedback from patients, whom SCF refers to as "customer-owners." SCF succeeds in part as a result of the bespoke tailoring of its system for the people, families, and communities it serves. From the beginning, the entire health system was based on Alaska Native values and needs. This was possible thanks to federal legislation[6] that allows for self-governance and the foundation's reliance on customer-owner surveys and feedback (Gottlieb, 2013) (see Chapter 5 for a more detailed discussion of SCF's integrated system of care).

The Individualized Management for Patient-Centered Targets (IMPaCT) program is a community-based model founded on the notion that CHWs can improve outcomes by building relationships and providing person-centered support. CHWs provide personalized and holistic social support, advocacy, coaching, and health system navigation (Seervai, 2020), and the CHWs start by getting to know the person outside of their medical history and health complaints, initially addressing the social or behavioral needs that are obstacles to health care, such as loneliness or distrust of clinicians. The relationship, built on trust and understanding, is essential for this to happen, for it allows the CHWs to understand those in their care so that later in the relationship, they can guide them toward the health resources needed for whole-person care. IMPaCT has seen positive results across a wide variety of measures, including body mass index, hemoglobin and blood pressure levels, self-rated mental health, quality of care, total hospital days, and likelihood to complete a primary care follow-up appointment within 14 days of discharge from the hospital. The program yields a return on investment of $2.47 for every dollar invested by Medicaid and has been replicated across 20 states. Its success indicates that addressing socioeconomic and behavioral needs in a whole-person approach to care can improve access to and quality of primary care (Kangovi et al., 2014b, 2017).

---

[5] Nuka is an Alaska Native word used for strong, giant structures and living things.
[6] The Indian Self-Determination and Education Assistance Act, Public Law 93-638 (January 4, 1975).

HEALTH EQUITY AND THE ROLE OF PRIMARY CARE

Health equity is a guiding principle for many primary care teams. Primary care improves equity (Starfield, 2009, 2012; Starfield et al., 2005), and an ultimate goal for improving primary care is to reduce inequities as much as possible. Health disparities are the metrics used to measure progress toward achieving health equity (see Box 4-2). The United States has health disparities in terms of education, race, ethnicity, sex, sexual orientation, and place of residence (Adler et al., 2016). Greater equity is achieved by improving the health specifically of those who are economically or socially disadvantaged, and reductions in health disparities (both absolute and relative) are evidence of a move toward greater health equity. Achieving health equity means achieving social justice in health—no one is denied the possibility of a healthy life as a result of belonging to a population that has historically been disadvantaged (Braveman, 2014; Martinez-Bianchi et al., 2019). Health disparities and health care disparities are separate concepts and should not be confused. Ensuring equitable access to high-quality health care for all is not a guaranteed way to reduce health disparities and ensure health equity, given the many factors that have a much greater impact on health than health care does.

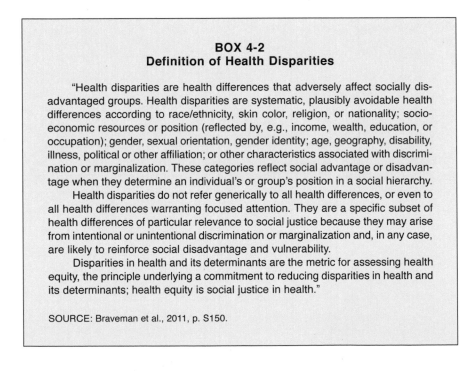

BOX 4-2
Definition of Health Disparities

"Health disparities are health differences that adversely affect socially disadvantaged groups. Health disparities are systematic, plausibly avoidable health differences according to race/ethnicity, skin color, religion, or nationality; socioeconomic resources or position (reflected by, e.g., income, wealth, education, or occupation); gender, sexual orientation, gender identity; age, geography, disability, illness, political or other affiliation; or other characteristics associated with discrimination or marginalization. These categories reflect social advantage or disadvantage when they determine an individual's or group's position in a social hierarchy.

Health disparities do not refer generically to all health differences, or even to all health differences warranting focused attention. They are a specific subset of health differences of particular relevance to social justice because they may arise from intentional or unintentional discrimination or marginalization and, in any case, are likely to reinforce social disadvantage and vulnerability.

Disparities in health and its determinants are the metric for assessing health equity, the principle underlying a commitment to reducing disparities in health and its determinants; health equity is social justice in health."

SOURCE: Braveman et al., 2011, p. S150.

Improving Primary Care Models to Address Inequities

A 2016 review comparing the standard medical model of primary care to community-oriented primary care found that the latter did a much better job of addressing sociocultural issues that act as barriers to care and SDOH that lead to health inequities among immigrant populations (Batista et al., 2018). The study's authors suggested that community-oriented primary care is better suited to address health equity in general.

A community-oriented approach to primary care is not the silver bullet to address inequities in health care—workforce solutions (Jackson and Gracia, 2014), digital health (Zhang et al., 2019), and policy measures (Holden et al., 2019) are also needed. However, it is an essential part of the solution. Over the past 40 years, practice-based research networks (PBRNs), each comprising at least 15 primary care clinicians or ambulatory practices that are linked closely with their communities, have been conducting research on how to improve primary care delivery, often with an explicit focus on health equity (Westfall et al., 2019). For example, the Southeast Regional Clinicians' Network PBRN, based out of the Morehouse School of Medicine and comprising 203 federally qualified health centers (FQHCs) across eight southeastern states (MSM, 2021), has studied equity-addressing interventions for improving cancer screening (Hunt and Hurlbert, 2016) and treatment of asthma (Rust et al., 1999), heart disease (Daniels et al., 2012), and mental health issues (Rust et al., 2005) for high-disparity, underserved populations.

Consistent with the concept of whole-person, equitable health care and the person-centered, family-centered, and community-oriented approaches described in this chapter, the need to address SDOH is a key feature of the committee's definition of high-quality primary care (see Chapter 2). In the past decade, consistent and compelling evidence concerning SDOH and their influence in shaping individual health have led the health care sector to reconsider its role in care. As discussed earlier in this chapter, a person's health is a culmination of factors and is not limited to the absence of disease. SDOH represent some of these factors and are defined as the "conditions in which people are born, grow, work, live, and age, and the wider set of forces and systems shaping the conditions of daily life" (WHO, 2020a). What these determinants mean for each individual can be different, though; they can enhance wellness for some yet embody barriers and social risk patterns that contribute to increased morbidity and mortality for others (NASEM, 2019a). Addressing SDOH is an essential component of whole-person health and can eliminate some of the factors that contribute to health inequities.

According to Healthy People 2020, these determinants come in five key areas that span spheres of influence on an individual: economic stability or socioeconomic status (SES), education, social and community context, health and health care, and neighborhood and built environment (ODPHP, 2020). Those with lower SES, and the resulting stress, shoulder a heavier burden of poor health than those with higher SES (Adler and Rehkopf, 2008; Bor et al., 2017). If SDOH inform social care and its integration into health care, clinicians can treat the upstream factors that so often become barriers to future health equity.

Integrating Social Care into the Delivery of Health Care to Improve the Nation's Health (NASEM, 2019a) looked at the current state of U.S. social care and recommended changes to health care and policy infrastructure that promote alignment across sectors in order to better inform care delivery for all people. This report details five areas where health care systems can work with people and communities to encourage better social care for all (NASEM, 2019a): promoting awareness, adjustment, assistance, alignment, and advocacy. All of these actions will ultimately benefit individuals seeking care. Adjustment and assistance focus on improving care delivery specifically for individuals based on information about their social needs, while alignment and advocacy focus more delivery activities that the health care sector can carry out through coordinated care.

Advocacy activities promote health equity for people who may not have a voice in the current value-based care system and can range from light-touch (e.g., referring people to social workers to obtain rental assistance) to high-touch (e.g., longer, more intensive interventions that seek to address social needs) assistance. One example of a successful advocacy program is the Boston Medical Center Medical-Legal Partnership, which involved a coordinated team of lawyers and clinicians who worked together to change utility shutdown regulation with the Massachusetts Department of Public Utilities, to ensure that high-risk people did not have their heat shut off during the winter (National Center for Medical-Legal Partnership, 2017). Activities such as these ensure that social needs and determinants are taken into account and those with more barriers are not necessarily relegated to worse health outcomes.

The Role of Empanelment

Empanelment, sometimes known internationally as "rostering," is the process of assigning all individuals in a given population to an interprofessional care team or team member that is then responsible for providing primary care. It is an approach that can help achieve equitable access to care for all and improved population health outcomes. Empanelment usually has delivery systems or care teams making the assignments, whereas attribution, covered further in Chapter 9, typically involves payers doing so (AIR, 2013). Approaches vary and can be based on geography, insurance, or patient preference (Joint Learning Network for Universal Health Coverage et al., 2019). Panel size is frequently predetermined to ensure sufficient resources for the target population. More sophisticated processes may also acknowledge population health profiles to more evenly distribute health needs among primary care teams and help team members better understand the needs of their panels (PHCPI, 2019).

Empanelment ensures that each individual in a given population has a consistent and reliable source of primary care. It can be a strong foundation for trusting, continuous team member–patient relationships and provides community members with the access to appointments when they need them (Bodenheimer et al., 2014; Wagner et al., 2012). For these reasons, empanelment is an important component of community-oriented and PCMH primary care models, which emphasize ease of access to care and sustained clinician–patient relationships (Brownlee and Van Borkulo, 2013). Ideally, empanelment can help primary care meet access and convenience needs that frequently drive people to retail clinics and emergency departments (Coster et al., 2017). However, empanelment is not a one-time fix; it requires proactive maintenance to ensure consistent, timely access and resource capacity for all panel members (Joint Learning Network for Universal Health Coverage et al., 2019). See Chapter 6 for more on empanelment, panel size, and building primary care teams to meet the needs of a population.

SHIFTING PRIMARY CARE TO BE
MORE COMMUNITY-ORIENTED

If one goal of person- and family-centered primary care is to move from a reactive to proactive approach, it is essential for teams to understand the health trends and demographic characteristics of the populations they serve (Hollander-Rodriguez and DeVoe, 2018). Multiple levers can help shift primary care toward community-oriented models, including data systems, workforce, care delivery settings, and partnerships between primary care, public health, and community-based organizations. All of these levers can be influenced by policy changes and innovative payment models (Bailey and Goodman-Bacon, 2015; Bitton et al., 2019; Cometto et al., 2018; Enard and Ganelin, 2013; Fertig et al., 2012; Gold et al., 2019; Hone et al., 2018; Krist et al., 2013; Ockene et al., 2007; SNOCAP-USA et al., 2014; Wiggins et al., 2013). The following sections discuss each lever in more detail.

Data Systems

Without data systems to understand the population being served, community-oriented primary care is not possible. Whereas the door-to-door data collection performed by the primary care leaders of the past century posed issues of representativeness and accuracy, today's data are often quite complete (Mullan and Epstein, 2002). Instead, care teams and their partners struggle with collecting and aggregating multiple data sources into a comprehensive, usable community-oriented system. Doing this will optimize tools such as patient registries, "community vital signs," and geographic information systems to take the pulse of a community, orienting local care teams to health and social needs, issues of access, and the intervention strategies and collaborations needed to address them (AMA, 2016; Hughes et al., 2016; Phillips et al., 2019; Rock et al., 2019). See Chapter 7 for more information regarding data tools in primary care's continued shift toward community-oriented care.

Workforce

In most settings, the primary care physician workforce does not reflect the people it serves and is disproportionately male and white compared to the U.S. population (Xierali and Nivet, 2018). Physicians also increasingly come from privileged backgrounds. One study showed that more than half of all first-year medical students came from households in the top income quintile, whereas fewer than 5 percent were from the bottom income quintile (Youngclaus and Roskovensky, 2018). Individuals and families may perceive this discordance as a barrier to care (Malat et al., 2009; Saha et al., 1999) and prefer to see racial-concordant physicians (Alsan et al., 2019; Cooper et al., 2003; Saha and Beach, 2020; Saha et al., 2000). Increasing workforce diversity is believed to be essential in "(1) advancing cultural competency, (2) increasing access to high-quality health care services, (3) strengthening the medical research agenda, and (4) ensuring optimal management of the health care system" (Cohen et al., 2002, p. 91) and can contribute to a more equitable system for all. Chapter 6 explores the factors influencing the composition of the primary care workforce and strategies to increase its number and diversity.

One critical strategy for aligning the primary care workforce with its community is to expand opportunities to integrate CHWs and promotores de salud into primary care teams. CHWs are trusted community members who share a common background with the people they serve and have often experienced obstacles to health care or other forms of injustice themselves. They reflect the diversity of disadvantaged Americans: 65 percent are Black or Hispanic, 23 percent are white, 10 percent are American Indian or Alaska Native, and 2 percent are Asian or Pacific Islander (Arizona Prevention Research Center, 2015).

A large body of evidence suggests that CHWs can engage people with underlying socioeconomic issues into primary care (Wang et al., 2012), improve preventive screening rates (O'Brien et al., 2010), and reduce costly hospitalizations (Campbell et al., 2015). The use of CHWs, however, should not deter the necessary efforts to diversify the overall primary care workforce across professions to create a local workforce that reflects the diversity of the community in which it is practicing. See Chapter 6 for more on the primary care workforce.

Delivery Setting

Primary care is often delivered in settings outside of the clinician's office and more integrated into community settings. Innovative models of community-oriented primary care further integrate care delivery in non-clinical settings, including the workplace, college campuses and schools, recreation centers, places of worship, retail shops (e.g., barbershops), homeless shelters, housing for older adults, and institutions (e.g., prisons and jails). This shift to primary care in non-clinical settings increases access to care, allows for greater community participation, and relies on settings that are contextualized in other aspects of a person's daily life.

The COVID-19 pandemic quickly illustrated that primary care can be delivered outside the traditional office visit. As the pandemic swept the nation and prompted a need to socially distance—for the safety of both clinicians and individuals—telehealth adoption in primary care increased by nearly 50 percent, with clinicians in both rural and urban settings seeing increases (Bosworth et al., 2020; Mann et al., 2020; Mehrotra et al., 2020). Even before, interest in use of telehealth services was increasing for both clinicians and individuals (AMA, 2020; Martinez et al., 2018; Orlando et al., 2019). Pandemic-related policy changes reduced barriers to telehealth access and promoted its use for primary and specialty care (Bashshur et al., 2020; CMS, 2020b). In addition, many professional medical societies endorse telehealth services and provide guidance for medical practice in this evolving landscape (AANP, 2019; CDC, 2020; Committee on Pediatric Workforce, 2015; Joint Task Force for the Development of Telepsychology Guidelines for Psychologists, 2013). See Chapter 7 for more about telehealth services.

A report from the U.S. Department of Health and Human Services (HHS) notes that even after Medicare in-person primary care visits resumed in May 2020, demand was steady for telehealth visits (Bosworth et al., 2020). A 2020 survey by McKinsey found that 48 percent of individuals who used telehealth during the pandemic were satisfied with the care they received, and 37 percent were likely to use telehealth in the future (Cordina et al., 2020). While in-person, patient–clinician interactions will remain necessary, and likely preferred by many people, the pandemic accelerated openness to telehealth in ways previously unseen from policy makers, clinicians, and individuals alike.

Where telehealth has been unable to meet people's needs, including testing for and treating COVID-19 itself, primary care teams have partnered with health departments, academic institutions, local governments, and others to create opportunities for care. This includes developing drive-through testing sites and respiratory diagnostic centers that preserve personal protective equipment, especially important in federally designated shortage areas, and protecting both team members and individuals from potential spread (Barzin et al., 2020; Ton et al., 2020). The disruption and forced innovation brought about by COVID-19 could lead to purposeful changes in primary care delivery and enable better person-centered care if policy makers and payers make it a priority.

Partnerships Among Primary Care, Public Health, and Community-Based Organizations

Having primary care teams embedded within communities and partnering with public health and community-based organizations is not a new idea in the United States. In the late nineteenth century, dispensaries were established to provide medical care to the poor in neighborhood settings (Rosenberg, 1974). Although dispensaries were short-lived due to concerns about direct competition with private physicians (Burrow, 1977), their creation was prompted by a recognition that social conditions were influencing health and that health care services, informed by social medicine ideals, should be moved out of the hospital into the community (Janes, 1876; Rosen, 1947, 1949).

In the early twentieth century, many U.S. cities were proposing to organize and coordinate networks of health centers in each district that would serve defined geographic communities, adhere to the notion that a neighborhood should be identified and assessed, and recognize that unique health services should be targeted toward the special needs of each individual community (Davis, 1927; Hiscock, 1935; Pomeroy, 1929; Schmacke, 1998; Wilinsky, 1933). This period also featured a growing realization that community members should be involved in care delivery.

While district centers were created and called for services *in* the community, *for* the community, and *by* the community, most were limited to only offering public health and preventive services that complemented care already offered by private physicians, thus creating the chasm between modern day primary care and public health (Burrow, 1977; Winslow, 1919, 1929). One exception was the Indian Health Service (IHS), which implemented a more comprehensive model that combined primary care and public health in the late 1950s; it proved effective in promoting healthy behaviors, preventing disease (Nutting et al., 1979), and improving quality of care (Shorr and Nutting, 1977).

In 1966, the U.S. government produced *Health Is a Community Affair* (National Commission on Community Health Services, 1967). This 3-year study of healthy communities reviewed the evidence supporting the effectiveness of partnerships between primary care, public health, and communities and described the notion of "communities of solution" as an approach to health care defined by problems to be solved rather than geographic locales, specific delivery systems, or governmental agencies. A community of solution comprises people who come together to address an important problem or seize an opportunity to improve health, and it envisions primary care teams collaborating with many diverse partners, depending on the nature of the problems and the community. In addition to community members and public health professionals, each unique community of solution would include many other public and private partners and community-based organizations (Gotler et al., 2020; Griswold et al., 2013; The Folsom Group, 2012; Westfall, 2013).

Community participation in primary care was formalized as an important concept in the Alma-Ata Declaration of 1978.[7] Community-oriented care was recognized by the Institute of Medicine in 1983 as an important aspect of high-quality primary care and further emphasized in *Primary Care: America's Health in a New Era* (IOM, 1996). More recently, the ACA created new incentives for primary care to pursue community-based population health care. The October 2018 Global Conference on Primary Health Care in Astana, Kazakhstan, and resulting Astana Declaration reasserted this commitment to people-centered care and the role of community as well as both primary care and primary health care to achieving it (WHO and Ministry of Healthcare Republic of Kazakhstan, 2018; WHO and UNICEF, 2018).

Health Centers

Health centers provide high-quality, locally tailored, comprehensive primary care services and gynecologic, behavioral health, preventive health (including dental, cancer screening, family planning, and immunizations), vision and eye care, and diagnostic laboratory and radiologic services. They also offer case management services,[8] referrals to specialty care and social

---

[7] The Declaration of Alma-Ata was adopted at the International Conference on Primary Health Care in what was then known as Alma-Ata in the Soviet Socialist Republic (today, it is known as Almaty, Kazakhstan). The conference and declaration called for national and international action to strengthen primary health care throughout the world (International Conference on Primary Health Care, 1978). The Declaration is available at https://www.who.int/publications/almaata_declaration_en.pdf (accessed October 5, 2020).

[8] In 42 CFR § 440.169 (2009), the Centers for Medicare & Medicaid Services (CMS) defines case management services as "services furnished to assist individuals … in gaining access to needed medical, social, educational, and other services" (which does not include "the direct delivery of underlying medical, educational, social, or other services").

services, and transportation and translation services. The care delivered by health centers, which include FQHCs, health care for people who are homeless, health centers for residents of public housing, school-based health clinics, and migrant health centers, is based on tenets of community-oriented primary care and represents the largest segment of the primary care system.

Health centers are descendants of the original neighborhood health centers, which started in 1965 as two demonstration projects of the Office of Economic Opportunity Community Action Program to provide health and social services access points in poor and medically underserved communities and promote community empowerment (CHroniCles, 2020; Levitan, 1974). Congress passed an amendment to the original Economic Opportunity Act in 1966 to provide further funding for the planning of operation of more "comprehensive health service programs" (Anderson et al., 1976, p. 13). By 1972, more than 100 neighborhood health centers and other comprehensive health service projects had been initiated with grant assistance from the Office of Economic Opportunity (Zwick, 1972).

FQHCs are health centers that receive Health Resources and Services Administration (HRSA) Health Center Program federal grant funding to improve the health of underserved populations (HRSA, 2020a). Today, more than 1,400 FQHCs operate nearly 13,000 delivery sites. They serve nearly 30 million people, including more than 398,000 veterans, one-third of all people living in poverty, 20 percent of those living in rural locations, and more than 10 percent of all children (HRSA, 2020b). Delivery sites include tribal or urban American Indian and Alaska Native areas, remote sites connected to a community health center, and sites deemed "look-alikes" that meet the requirements of FQHCs but do not receive federal grant funding (Rural Health Information Hub, 2019).

Rural health clinics (RHCs) are Centers for Medicare & Medicaid Services (CMS)-certified clinics in rural Medically Underserved Areas or Health Professional Shortage Areas and provide primary care services. RHCs, like FQHCs, must meet Medicare and Medicaid health and safety standards in 42 CFR Part 491; however, RHCs are not subject to many of the other FQHC requirements and may be privately owned (CMS, 2019).

One key community-oriented feature of health centers is that all are required to have at least 51 percent of their governing boards of directors composed of people in the community who are served by the health center and reflect the demographic characteristic of its population (HRSA, 2020a; Taylor, 2004). This requirement ensures that the people served—who are often from under-represented communities that rarely are included in organization-level decision making—have a voice in how services are delivered. In practice, some evidence indicates that the demographics of patients on health center governing boards are not always representative of the patient population overall and that they seldom hold executive positions on the board (Wright, 2013, 2015). Nevertheless, including patients in the system-wide decision-making process is a practical way to engage the community and ensure that its needs are addressed in the health centers' daily operations.

Health centers are also required to complete a community needs assessment every 3 years, which includes a review of barriers (including transportation) and unmet health needs of the medically underserved (including the ratio of primary care physicians relative to the population, health indexes for the population served, the poverty level, and other demographic factors in demand for services, such as the percent of the population over age 65). In addition, they must make and maintain a reasonable effort to build and sustain relationships with other clinicians and services, such as hospitals and specialists, within their catchment areas to help facilitate seamless coordination with services that are not offered within the health centers themselves. They must also annually assess the geographic boundaries of their patient population (HRSA, 2018). In some communities, the community needs assessment is coordinated with those mandated for nonprofit hospitals and accredited public health departments with the goal of also coordinating their collective response to identified needs—an approach recommended by *Primary Care and Public Health: Exploring Integration to Improve Population Health* (IOM, 2012).

Health centers are financially accessible to the communities they serve. They are required to provide services to everyone, regardless of insurance status or ability to pay out of pocket. Uninsured individuals pay on a board-approved sliding scale based on income and family size. Revenue streams for health centers include Medicaid, Medicare, private insurance, and out-of-pocket payments. Medicare and Medicaid largely use a bundled, prospective payments system (PPS) that pays health centers per visit, not per service rendered. This allows for more flexibility and efficiency because health centers are not ordinarily covered by Medicaid FFS payments. However, the PPS rates have not kept up with inflation or the recent expansion of health center services in recent years and now only cover about 82 percent of the cost to care for Medicaid recipients (NACHC, 2020b). Similarly, while FQHCs provide services for 16 percent of Medicaid recipients, less than 2 percent of Medicaid payments go to them. Still, there is evidence that Medicaid beneficiary costs at FQHCs are lower than in other settings. A study of Medicaid beneficiaries comparing those who primarily receive primary care at FQHCs to those who seek care elsewhere found that costs were 24 percent lower for FQHC users. They also had fewer hospital admissions, fewer visits overall, and spent less on inpatient and specialty care (Nocon et al., 2016).

Evidence indicates that health centers have reduced access and outcome disparities across racial and ethnic groups, income, and insurance status

(NACHC, 2020a; Politzer et al., 2001). Their enabling services, such as transportation, nutrition assistance, health education, and housing, play a particularly important role in improving access. One recent nationally representative study found that among HRSA-funded health center clients, those who used enabling services had nearly twice as many visits and were more likely to get routine check-ups, receive preventive care and flu shots, and report higher patient satisfaction than those who did not (Yue et al., 2019). Health centers also outperform other delivery settings across a wide array of measures spanning quality and outcomes, patient satisfaction, and cost-effectiveness (NACHC, 2020a).

While the number of health centers has increased since the passage of the ACA, the expansion was largely in urban areas and less likely in areas that were rural or had more than 20 percent of the population below the federal poverty level (Chang et al., 2019). This suggests that improving access to health care for financially disadvantaged populations will require increasing the number of health centers to reach them; however, this is proving more difficult to achieve, as workforce shortages in primary care have contributed to a greater percentage of health centers reporting budgeted but unfilled positions for primary care physicians, registered nurses or licensed practical nurses, and licensed mental health clinicians (Lewis et al., 2019). One strategy health centers have employed to counter this is the Teaching Health Center Graduate Medical Education program, which places physician and dental trainees in health centers, mostly in primary care settings and rural or underserved areas (HRSA, 2021).

Health centers partner with the communities in which they operate in a variety of ways—from designing communication materials that community members want to working with local health departments to optimize and widen services offered and populations served (Mader et al., 2019; NACHC and NACCHO, 2010). Initiatives such as the Migrant Clinicians Network also work with health centers to help improve access and reduce disparities among vulnerable migrant populations (MCN, 2021). These models of partnership have improved health outcomes for millions of Americans and been shown to reduce access to care disparities for disadvantaged populations (HRSA, 2020b; Jones et al., 2013).

Indian Health Service

An agency within HHS, the IHS provides health care to approximately 2.6 million American Indian and Alaska Native people from more than 574 federally recognized tribes in 37 states (IHS, 2020a). Its primary care clinics include federal, tribal, and Urban Indian Health organizations that provide comprehensive care across the lifespan in rural areas, on reservations, and, increasingly, in urban population centers (IHS, 2020b). Many

IHS-affiliated clinics serve as safety net clinics to both IHS beneficiaries and non-beneficiaries within their communities, and some are also designated FQHCs (IHS, 2005, 2020c). The vast majority of IHS primary care is administered by tribes through self-determination contracts rather than by the federal government, with more than 60 percent of IHS appropriations administered by tribes (IHS, 2020b). Self-determination is at the heart of person-centered, family-centered, and community-oriented primary care. It enhances the mission of the IHS, which is to raise the physical, mental, social, and spiritual health of American Indian and Alaska Native people to the highest level. As recognized in the 2019 IHS strategic plan, ensuring the availability and accessibility of high-quality, culturally appropriate, primary, and preventive care services to all beneficiaries best supports accomplishing the IHS mission (IHS, 2019).

Despite many Tribal and Urban Indian Health Programs serving as "the glue that holds their communities together," the IHS is chronically underfunded and provides health care services to less than half the eligible population (UCLA American Indian Studies Center, 2016; Urban Indian Health Commission, 2007, p. 7). This underfunding contributes to the persistent health disparities among the American Indian and Alaska Native population (Warne and Frizzell, 2014). A 2018 U.S. Government Accountability Office (GAO) report found that IHS, as an agency, spends approximately $4,000 per beneficiary, which represents less than 50 and 30 percent of the amount spent by the VA ($10,692) and Medicare ($13,185), respectively (GAO, 2018b). A separate GAO report found that in part as a result of its inability to match market-rate salaries, IHS struggles to fill vacancies for clinicians, which negatively affects patient access and quality of care (GAO, 2018a). Evidence also suggests IHS could be more systematic in assessing community needs (GAO, 2020). Despite these significant limitations and challenges, many Tribal and Urban Indian Health Programs have found ways to thrive and deliver comprehensive and holistic community-oriented health care to their communities to achieve the IHS mission. SCF's Nuka System of Care represents the gold standard for tribal health organizations seeking to transform care for their own people and communities, as evidenced by its outcomes achievements and multiple quality awards (Gottlieb, 2013).

School-Based Health Center Partnerships

The nearly 2,600 school-based health centers (SBHCs) represent another example of effective partnerships between community organizations and primary care that have increased access (Love et al., 2019b). Some 6.3 million students nationwide have access to care at an SBHC from an interprofessional team of clinicians, including primary care and mental health clinicians, in collaboration with the school community. SBHCs often function as a partnership between the school and the community's health organization, such as a health center, hospital, or local health department. Specific SBHC services vary based on community needs and resources as determined through collaborations among the community, the school district, and local health care clinicians. Sixty-two percent of SBHCs have provided services to individuals other than the students in their schools, including faculty and school personnel, family members of student users, out-of-school youth, and others in the broader community. This enhanced access to care, including primary care, has reduced health care disparities for disadvantaged populations and improved oral health outcomes (Love et al., 2019b).

In recent years, SBHCs have begun using telehealth to further expand their reach into communities and enhance the effectiveness of their services. More than half the SBHCs offering telehealth serve rural communities, where access to care is often limited by clinician shortages and transportation issues, and approximately three-quarters are staffed by primary care clinicians only, with the remainder staffed by primary care and mental health care clinicians (Love et al., 2019a).

Nurse-Managed Health Centers

Nurse-managed health centers (NMHCs) deliver whole-person primary care and are led and primarily staffed by advanced practice registered nurses (APRNs). The estimated 250 NMHCs in the United States serve more than 1.5 million medically underserved people, typically in low-income urban and rural areas (Esperat et al., 2012; IOM, 2011). Most NMHCs are affiliated with university-based nursing schools or independent nonprofits, but some are affiliated with FQHCs, SBHCs, or other health centers.

Though NMHCs resemble community health centers in the populations and areas they serve, they are generally ineligible for FQHC status and federal funding due to a governance structure that includes the boards of their founding institutions, rather than the center's patients (Hansen-Turton et al., 2010). To enable federal support, section 5208 of the ACA established a federal program to fund NMHCs, earmarking $50 million to be distributed that year via one-time grants and noting that "such sums as may be necessary for each of the fiscal years 2011 through 2014."[9] Through HRSA, nearly $15 million in grants was awarded to 10 NMHCs, which provided care to more than 94,000 patients and trained more than 900 APRNs (Cooper, n.d.; Hansen-Turton, 2012). However, in an effort to

---

[9] Patient Protection and Affordable Care Act, Public Law 111-148, § 5208 (March 23, 2010).

decrease overall spending, federal funding stopped there and the program was not renewed (Carthon et al., 2015).

Settings of Care for Older Adults

Older adults may need to receive primary care in a variety of settings outside of a traditional primary care practice. Residents of nursing homes often have complex care needs and include individuals who need post-acute care (after a hospital stay) and those who are long-term stay residents. Care of the nursing home resident includes assessment and management of both acute and chronic physical and psychosocial health care needs, coordination of needed health care services, the management of transitions between different health care settings, and advance care planning, among other services (Unwin et al., 2010). Increasingly, medical care in nursing homes is provided by nurse practitioners (NPs) and physician assistants (Teno et al., 2017).

Some older adults are home bound and thus rely on home-based care. The Independence at Home model provides comprehensive primary care services to Medicare beneficiaries with severe chronic illness and disability within their own homes (CMS, 2020a). The VA also has a home-based primary care program that serves veterans in their homes (VA, 2020).

Across settings, the Geriatric Resources for Assessment and Care of Elders (GRACE) model focuses on primary care for low-income older adults (Counsell et al., 2006). An NP paired with a social worker—the support team—leads the GRACE model, and the two professionals work together with an interdisciplinary team (including a geriatrician, pharmacist, physical therapist, mental health social worker, and community services liaison) to develop a care plan. The support team then works directly with the primary care physician to implement the plan. The model includes in-home visits by the support team, and plays a particularly important role in continuity of care during care transitions (Bielaszka-DuVernay, 2011). The GRACE model has been associated with satisfaction among primary care physicians (Counsell et al., 2009) and improved quality of care and quality of life (Counsell et al., 2006). For high-risk patients, the model has been associated with reduced hospitalization rates (Counsell et al., 2007).

Payment

Each of the previous levers requires supportive policies and payment arrangements. FFS payment covers the vast majority of primary care payment in the United States today and is a major challenge for primary care practices when partnering with communities, including the use of community members like CHWs and promotores de salud. Currently, CHWs are paid through a patchwork of funding options, such as Medicaid demonstration waivers, health homes, Medicaid managed care plans, and grants (Lloyd et al., 2020). This gap would be addressed by a comprehensive payment model that supports the organization and delivery of primary care services that fits community needs, as outlined in Chapter 9. For example, if certain communities want to expand their CHW workforce and integrate CHWs into their primary care teams, this comprehensive payment would allow for flexible allocation of resources and not depend on billing for each individual service provided by only certain members of the care team (e.g., physician, NP) under certain conditions (e.g., billable in-person visit code). In addition, incremental financing options could more adequately fund CHWs and other primary care–community partnerships. One example is a policy initiative currently under consideration that would support creating an optional Medicaid benefit to fund CHWs and be linked to evidence-informed standards for hiring, training, and deploying them (Biden, 2020).

FINDINGS AND CONCLUSIONS

Moving from patient-centered care to a person-centered, family-centered, and community-oriented approach represents an evolution of primary care to focus on individual people in the context of their lived experiences, their family, their social worlds, and their community. The relationship between the person seeking care (and their family) and the interprofessional team is an essential component of this shift. Building and maintaining this relationship in what is currently a disease-focused system, and achieving personalized, prioritized, and coordinated care for all people and families in communities, will require a system that supports developing and sustaining strong individual and community relationships in primary care to build a foundation for dismantling the pervasive systemic inequities in health care. Supporting and expanding delivery models, particularly those for the underserved (such as health centers), and empaneling populations will help ensure that all Americans have a usual source of primary care. Creating opportunities for individuals, families, and communities to participate in the organizational decision making at health care organizations and that related to the care itself will help the nation to reduce health disparities, particularly in underserved populations, and support achieving health equity for all populations.

Instead of responding to whole-health needs using a community-oriented approach, clinicians and health care organizations are rewarded for preventing, diagnosing, and treating diseases and performing procedures, prescribing medications, and providing care based on traditional biomedical models. Multiple levers can help shift primary care toward community-oriented models, including data systems, interprofessional care teams, care delivery settings, and partnerships between primary care, public health, and community-based organizations. All of these levers can be influenced by policy changes and innovative payment models.

As the United States grapples with the effects of the COVID-19 pandemic, levels of unemployment not seen since the Great Depression, and a reckoning of its long-standing history of racism and injustice, primary care will have to transform to meet current demands. This is an opportunity to radically reimagine it so that it is built around the people it serves, their families, and their communities, paid in ways that support this approach, and grounded in relationship-centered care, equity, and social justice. Until the barriers to innovation and sustainability are removed, it will be challenging to achieve high-quality, high-value primary care for all communities. Without success in expanding and supporting primary care's ability to address the needs of not only individuals but families and communities, the nation will be challenged to meet the health care needs of all communities, particularly underserved populations.

REFERENCES

AAFP (American Academy of Family Physicians). 2018. *Survey takes hard look at physician-patient conversations.* https://www.aafp.org/news/practice-professional-issues/20181107 doc-patientcomms.html (accessed August 24, 2020).

AANP (American Association of Nuse Practitioners). 2019. *Position statement: Telehealth.* Austin, TX: American Association of Nurse Practitioners.

Adamson, M. 2011. The patient-centered medical home: An essential destination on the road to reform. *American Health & Drug Benefits* 4(2):122–124.

Adler, N. E., and D. H. Rehkopf. 2008. U.S. disparities in health: Descriptions, causes, and mechanisms. *Annual Review of Public Health* 29(1):235–252.

Adler, N. E., M. M. Glymour, and J. Fielding. 2016. Addressing social determinants of health and health inequalities. *JAMA* 316(16):1641–1642.

AHRQ (Agency for Healthcare Research and Quality). 2017. *Physician burnout.* Rockville, MD: Agency for Healthcare Research and Quality.

AHRQ. 2018. *Guide to improving patient safety in primary care settings by engaging patients and families.* Rockville, MD: Agency for Healthcare Research and Quality.

AIR (American Institute for Research). 2013. *Empanelment implementation guide.* Washington, DC: American Institute for Research.

Alexander, J. A., G. R. Cohen, C. G. Wise, and L. A. Green. 2013. The policy context of patient centered medical homes: Perspectives of primary care providers. *Journal of General Internal Medicine* 28(1):147–153.

Alsan, M., O. Garrick, and G. Graziani. 2019. Does diversity matter for health? Experimental evidence from Oakland. *American Economic Review* 109(12):4071–4111.

Alsan, M., M. Wanamaker, and R. R. Hardeman. 2020. The Tuskegee study of untreated syphilis: A case study in peripheral trauma with implications for health professionals. *Journal of General Internal Medicine* 35(1):322–325.

AMA (American Medical Association). 2016. *Point-of care registries: Proactively manage chronic care conditions.* https://edhub.ama-assn.org/steps-forward/module/2702745 (accessed May 6, 2020).

AMA. 2020. *AMA digital health research: Physicians' motivations and requirements for adopting digital health and attitudinal shifts from 2016–2019.* Chicago, IL: American Medical Association.

American Geriatrics Society Expert Panel on the Care of Older Adults with Multimorbidity. 2012. Patient-centered care for older adults with multiple chronic conditions: A stepwise approach from the American Geriatrics Society: American Geriatrics Society expert panel on the care of older adults with multimorbidity. *Journal of the American Geriatrics Society* 60(10):1957–1968.

Anderson, E. J., L. R. Judd, J. T. May, and P. K. New. 1976. *The neighborhood health center program: Its growth and problems: An introduction.* Washington, DC: National Association of Community Health Centers.

Andrades, M., S. Kausar, and A. Ambreen. 2013. Role and influence of the patient's companion in family medicine consultations: "The patient's perspective." *Journal of Family Medicine and Primary Care* 2(3):283–287.

Andres, C., S. Spenceley, L. L. Cook, R. Wedel, and T. Gelber. 2016. Improving primary care: Continuity is about relationships. *Canadian Family Physician* 62(2):116–119.

Arizona Prevention Research Center. 2015. *National community health worker advocacy survey.* Tucson, AZ: University of Arizona.

Artiga, S., and E. Hinton. 2018. *Beyond health care: The role of social determinants in promoting health and health equity.* https://www.kff.org/racial-equity-and-health-policy/issue-brief/beyond-health-care-the-role-of-social-determinants-in-promoting-health-and-health-equity (accessed January 21, 2021).

Bailey, M. J., and A. Goodman-Bacon. 2015. The war on poverty's experiment in public medicine: Community health centers and the mortality of older Americans. *American Economic Review* 105(3):1067–1104.

Barzin, A., D. A. Wohl, and T. P. Daaleman. 2020. Development and implementation of a COVID-19 respiratory diagnostic center. *Annals of Family Medicine COVID-19 Collection* 18(5):464.

Bashshur, R., C. R. Doarn, J. M. Frenk, J. C. Kvedar, and J. O. Woolliscroft. 2020. Telemedicine and the COVID-19 pandemic, lessons for the future. *Telemedicine and e-Health* 26(5):571–573.

Batista, R., K. Pottie, L. Bouchard, E. Ng, P. Tanuseputro, and P. Tugwell. 2018. Primary health care models addressing health equity for immigrants: A systematic scoping review. *Journal of Immigrant and Minority Health* 20(1):214–230.

Beasley, J. W., T. H. Hankey, R. Erickson, K. C. Stange, M. Mundt, M. Elliott, P. Wiesen, and J. Bobula. 2004. How many problems do family physicians manage at each encounter? A WREN study. *Annals of Family Medicine* 2(5):405–410.

Bergman, D., C. Bethell, N. Gombojav, S. Hassink, and K. C. Stange. 2020. Physical distancing with social connectedness. *Annals of Family Medicine* 18(3):272–277.

Biden, J. 2020. *The Biden plan for mobilizing American talent and heart to create a 21st century caregiving and education workforce.* https://medium.com/@JoeBiden/the-biden-plan-for-mobilizing-american-talent-and-heart-to-create-a-21st-century-caregiving-and-af5ba2a2dfeb (accessed August 17, 2020).

Bielaszka-DuVernay, C. 2011. The GRACE model: In-home assessments lead to better care for dual eligibles. *Health Affairs* 30(3):431–434.

Bitton, A., J. Fifield, H. Ratcliffe, A. Karlage, H. Wang, J. H. Veillard, D. Schwarz, and L. R. Hirschhorn. 2019. Primary healthcare system performance in low-income and middle-income countries: A scoping review of the evidence from 2010 to 2017. *BMJ Global Health* 4:e001551.

Black, R. E., C. E. Taylor, S. Arole, A. Bang, Z. A. Bhutta, A. M. R. Chowdhury, B. R. Kirkwood, N. Kureshy, C. F. Lanata, J. F. Phillips, M. Taylor, C. G. Victora, Z. Zhu, and H. B. Perry. 2017. Comprehensive review of the evidence regarding the effectiveness of community-based primary health care in improving maternal, neonatal and child health: 8. Summary and recommendations of the expert panel. *Journal of Global Health* 7(1):010908.

Blaum, C. S., J. Rosen, A. D. Naik, C. D. Smith, L. Dindo, L. Vo, K. Hernandez-Bigos, J. Esterson, M. Geda, R. Ferris, D. Costello, D. Acampora, T. Meehan, and M. E. Tinetti. 2018. Feasibility of implementing patient priorities care for older adults with multiple chronic conditions. *Journal of the American Geriatrics Society* 66(10):2009–2016.

Bodenheimer, T., E. H. Wagner, and K. Grumbach. 2002. Improving primary care for patients with chronic illness. *JAMA* 288(14):1775–1779.

Bodenheimer, T., A. Ghorob, R. Willard-Grace, and K. Grumbach. 2014. The 10 building blocks of high-performing primary care. *Annals of Family Medicine* 12(2):166–171.

Bogart, L. M., G. J. Wagner, H. D. Green, Jr., M. G. Mutchler, D. J. Klein, B. McDavitt, S. J. Lawrence, and C. L. Hilliard. 2016. Medical mistrust among social network members may contribute to antiretroviral treatment nonadherence in African Americans living with HIV. *Social Science & Medicine* 164:133–140.

Bor, J., G. H. Cohen, and S. Galea. 2017. Population health in an era of rising income inequality: USA, 1980-2015. *The Lancet* 389(10077):1475–1490.

Borrell-Carrió, F., A. L. Suchman, and R. M. Epstein. 2004. The biopsychosocial model 25 years later: Principles, practice, and scientific inquiry. *Annals of Family Medicine* 2(6):576–582.

Bosworth, A., J. Ruhter, L. W. Samson, S. Sheingold, C. Taplin, W. Tarazi, and R. Zuckerman. 2020. *Medicare beneficiary use of telehealth visits: Early data from the start of the COVID-19 pandemic.* Washington, DC: Office of the Assistant Secretary for Planning and Evaluation, U.S. Department of Health and Human Services.

Botelho, R. J., B. H. Lue, and K. Fiscella. 1996. Family involvement in routine health care: A survey of patients' behaviors and preferences. *Journal of Family Practice* 42(6):572–576.

Boyd, C. M., J. Darer, C. Boult, L. P. Fried, L. Boult, and A. W. Wu. 2005. Clinical practice guidelines and quality of care for older patients with multiple comorbid diseases: Implications for pay for performance. *JAMA* 294(6):716–724.

Braddock, C. H., 3rd, L. Snyder, R. L. Neubauer, G. S. Fischer, American College of Physicians Ethics, Professionalism and Human Rights Committee, and the Society of General Internal Medicine Ethics Committee. 2013. The patient-centered medical home: An ethical analysis of principles and practice. *Journal of General Internal Medicine* 28(1):141–146.

Braveman, P. 2014. What are health disparities and health equity? We need to be clear. *Public Health Reports* 129(Suppl 2):5–8.

Braveman, P., and L. Gottlieb. 2014. The social determinants of health: It's time to consider the causes of the causes. *Public Health Reports* 129(Suppl 2):19–31.

Braveman, P. A., S. Kumanyika, J. Fielding, T. Laveist, L. N. Borrell, R. Manderscheid, and A. Troutman. 2011. Health disparities and health equity: The issue is justice. *American Journal of Public Health* 101(Suppl 1):S149–S155.

Brown, E. J., S. Kangovi, C. Sha, S. Johnson, C. Chanton, T. Carter, and D. T. Grande. 2015. Exploring the patient and staff experience with the process of primary care. *Annals of Family Medicine* 13(4):347–353.

Brown, J. B., P. Brett, M. Stewart, and J. N. Marshall. 1998. Roles and influence of people who accompany patients on visits to the doctor. *Canadian Family Physician* 44:1644–1650.

Brownlee, B., and N. Van Borkulo. 2013. *Empanelment: Establishing patient–provider relationships.* Seattle, WA: Qualis Health, The MacColl Center for Health Care Innovation at the Group Health Research Institute.

Buchmueller, T., and C. S. Carpenter. 2010. Disparities in health insurance coverage, access, and outcomes for individuals in same-sex versus different-sex relationships, 2000–2007. *American Journal of Public Health* 100(3):489–495.

Burnham, A. C. 1920. *The community health problem.* New York: The Macmillan Company.

Burrow, J. G. 1977. *Organized medicine in the progressive era: The move toward monopoly.* Baltimore, MD: The Johns Hopkins University Press.

Campbell, J. D., M. Brooks, P. Hosokawa, J. Robinson, L. Song, and J. Krieger. 2015. Community health worker home visits for Medicaid-enrolled children with asthma: Effects on asthma outcomes and costs. *American Journal of Public Health* 105(11):2366–2372.

Carthon, J. M. B., H. Barnes, and D. A. Sarik. 2015. Federal polices influence access to primary care and nurse practitioner workforce. *The Journal for Nurse Practitioners* 11(5):526–530.

CDC (Centers for Disease Control and Prevention). 2020. *Using telehealth to expand access to essential health services during the COVID-19 pandemic.* https://www.cdc.gov/coronavirus/2019-ncov/hcp/telehealth.html#edn6 (accessed December 21, 2020).

Cené, C. W., L. B. Haymore, F. C. Lin, J. Laux, C. D. Jones, J. R. Wu, D. DeWalt, M. Pignone, and G. Corbie-Smith. 2015. Family member accompaniment to routine medical visits is associated with better self-care in heart failure patients. *Chronic Illness* 11(1):21–32.

Chang, C. H., J. P. W. Bynum, and J. D. Lurie. 2019. Geographic expansion of federally qualified health centers 2007–2014. *Journal of Rural Health* 35(3):385–394.

Chaudhri, S., K. C. Zweig, P. Hebbar, S. Angell, and A. Vasan. 2019. Trauma-informed care: A strategy to improve primary healthcare engagement for persons with criminal justice system involvement. *Journal of General Internal Medicine* 34(6):1048–1052.

Chen, J., C. D. Mullins, P. Novak, and S. B. Thomas. 2016. Personalized strategies to activate and empower patients in health care and reduce health disparities. *Health Education & Behavior* 43(1):25–34.

Chokshi, D. A., and L. Cohen. 2018. Progress in primary care—from Alma-Ata to Astana. *JAMA* 320(19):1965–1966.

CHroniCles. 2020. *Community health centers: Chronicling their history and broader meaning.* https://www.chcchronicles.org/stories/community-health-centers-chronicling-their-history-and-broader-meaning (accessed July 17, 2020).

Clay, A. M., and B. Parsh. 2016. Patient- and family-centered care: It's not just for pediatrics anymore. *AMA Journal of Ethics* 18(1):40–44.

Clayman, M. L., D. Roter, L. S. Wissow, and K. Bandeen-Roche. 2005. Autonomy-related behaviors of patient companions and their effect on decision-making activity in geriatric primary care visits. *Social Science & Medicine* 60(7):1583–1591.

CMS (Centers for Medicare & Medicaid Services). 2019. Chapter 13—rural health clinic (RHC) and federally qualified health center (FQHC) services. In *Medicare benefit policy manual.* Baltimore, MD: Centers for Medicare & Medicaid Services. https://www.cms.gov/Regulations-and-Guidance/Guidance/Manuals/Internet-Only-Manuals-IOMs-Items/CMS012673 (accessed January 12, 2021).

CMS. 2020a. *Independence at home demonstration.* https://innovation.cms.gov/innovation-models/independence-at-home (accessed February 26, 2021).

CMS. 2020b. Interim final rule with comment period: Medicare and Medicaid programs; policy and regulatory revisions in response to the COVID-19 public health emergency as published on April 6, 2020. *Federal Register* 85(66):19230–19292. https://www.federalregister.gov/documents/2020/04/06/2020-06990/medicare-and-medicaid-programs-policy-and-regulatory-revisions-in-response-to-the-covid-19-public (accessed December 18, 2020).

Cohen, J. J., B. A. Gabriel, and C. Terrell. 2002. The case for diversity in the health care workforce. *Health Affairs* 21(5):90–102.

Cole-Kelly, K., and D. Seaburn. 1999. Five areas of questioning to promote a family-oriented approach in primary care. *Families, Systems, & Health* 17(3):341–348.

Cometto, G., N. Ford, J. Pfaffman-Zambruni, E. A. Akl, U. Lehmann, B. McPake, M. Ballard, M. Kok, M. Najafizada, A. Olaniran, O. Ajuebor, H. B. Perry, K. Scott, B. Albers, A. Shlonsky, and D. Taylor. 2018. Health policy and system support to optimise community health worker programmes: An abridged WHO guideline. *The Lancet Global Health* 6(12):e1397–e1404.

Committee on Hospital Care. 2003. Family-centered care and the pediatrician's role. *Pediatrics* 112(3):691–696.

Committee on Hospital Care and IPFCC (Institute for Patient- and Family-Centered Care). 2012. Patient- and family-centered care and the pediatrician's role. *Pediatrics* 129(2): 394–404.

Committee on Pediatric Workforce. 2015. The use of telemedicine to address access and physician workforce shortages. *Pediatrics* 136(1):202.

Cooper, K. n.d. *Affordable Care Act nurse managed health clinics (NMHC): Frequently asked questions.* https://www.hrsa.gov/sites/default/files/grants/healthprofessions/acafaq. pdf (accessed March 9, 2021).

Cooper, L. A., D. L. Roter, R. L. Johnson, D. E. Ford, D. M. Steinwachs, and N. R. Powe. 2003. Patient-centered communication, ratings of care, and concordance of patient and physician race. *Annals of Internal Medicine* 139(11):907–915.

Cordina, J., G. Stein, and E. Levin. 2020. *McKinsey consumer healthcare insights.* https://www. mckinsey.com/industries/healthcare-systems-and-services/our-insights/helping-us-healthcare-stakeholders-understand-the-human-side-of-the-covid-19-crisis (accessed December 18, 2020).

Cornelius, T., N. Moise, J. L. Birk, D. Edmondson, and B. P. Chang. 2018. The presence of companions during emergency department evaluation and its impact on perceptions of clinician-patient communication. *Emergency Medicine Journal* 35(11):701–703.

Coster, J. E., J. K. Turner, D. Bradbury, and A. Cantrell. 2017. Why do people choose emergency and urgent care services? A rapid review utilizing a systematic literature search and narrative synthesis. *Academic Emergency Medicine* 24(9):1137–1149.

Counsell, S. R., C. M. Callahan, A. B. Buttar, D. O. Clark, and K. I. Frank. 2006. Geriatric Resources for Assessment and Care of Elders (GRACE): A new model of primary care for low-income seniors. *Journal of the American Geriatrics Society* 54(7):1136–1141.

Counsell, S. R., C. M. Callahan, D. O. Clark, W. Tu, A. B. Buttar, T. E. Stump, and G. D. Ricketts. 2007. Geriatric care management for low-income seniors: A randomized controlled trial. *JAMA* 298(22):2623–2633.

Counsell, S. R., C. M. Callahan, W. Tu, T. E. Stump, and G. W. Arling. 2009. Cost analysis of the Geriatric Resources for Assessment and Care of Elders care management intervention. *Journal of the American Geriatrics Society* 57(8):1420–1426.

Cyril, S., B. J. Smith, A. Possamai-Inesedy, and A. M. Renzaho. 2015. Exploring the role of community engagement in improving the health of disadvantaged populations: A systematic review. *Global Health Action* 8:29842.

Daniels, E. C., B. D. Powe, T. Metoyer, G. McCray, P. Baltrus, and G. S. Rust. 2012. Increasing knowledge of cardiovascular risk factors among African Americans by use of community health workers: The ABCD community intervention pilot project. *Journal of the National Medical Association* 104(3–4):179–185.

Davis, K., S. C. Schoenbaum, and A. M. Audet. 2005. A 2020 vision of patient-centered primary care. *Journal of General Internal Medicine* 20(10):953–957.

Davis, M. M. 1927. Goal-posts and yardsticks in health center work. *American Journal of Public Health* 17(5):433–440.

Derose, K. P., M. V. Williams, C. A. Branch, K. R. Flórez, J. Hawes-Dawson, M. A. Mata, C. W. Oden, and E. C. Wong. 2019. A community-partnered approach to developing church-based interventions to reduce health disparities among African-Americans and Latinos. *Journal of Racial and Ethnic Health Disparities* 6(2):254–264.

DeVoe, J. E., J. W. Saultz, L. Krois, and C. J. Tillotson. 2009. A medical home versus temporary housing: The importance of a stable usual source of care. *Pediatrics* 124(5):1363–1371.

Driscoll, D. L., V. Hiratsuka, J. M. Johnston, S. Norman, K. M. Reilly, J. Shaw, J. Smith, Q. N. Szafran, and D. Dillard. 2013. Process and outcomes of patient-centered medical care with Alaska Native people at Southcentral Foundation. *Annals of Family Medicine* 11(Suppl 1):S41–S49.

Edgoose, J. Y. C., and J. M. Edgoose. 2017. Finding hope in the face-to-face. *Annals of Family Medicine* 15(3):272–274.

Ekman, I., K. Swedberg, C. Taft, A. Lindseth, A. Norberg, E. Brink, J. Carlsson, S. Dahlin-Ivanoff, I.-L. Johansson, K. Kjellgren, E. Lidén, J. Öhlén, L.-E. Olsson, H. Rosén, M. Rydmark, and K. S. Sunnerhagen. 2011. Person-centered care—ready for prime time. *European Journal of Cardiovascular Nursing* 10(4):248–251.

Ellner, A. L., and R. S. Phillips. 2017. The coming primary care revolution. *Journal of General Internal Medicine* 32(4):380–386.

Enard, K. R., and D. M. Ganelin. 2013. Reducing preventable emergency department utilization and costs by using community health workers as patient navigators. *Journal of Healthcare Management* 58(6):412–427; discussion 428.

Eng, E., M. E. Salmon, and F. Mullan. 1992. Community empowerment: The critical base for primary health care. *Family & Community Health: The Journal of Health Promotion & Maintenance* 15(1):1–12.

Engel, G. L. 2012. The need for a new medical model: A challenge for biomedicine. *Psychodynamic Psychiatry* 40(3):377–396.

Epstein, L., J. Gofin, R. Gofin, and Y. Neumark. 2002. The Jerusalem experience: Three decades of service, research, and training in community-oriented primary care. *American Journal of Public Health* 92(11):1717–1721.

Esperat, M. C. R., T. Hanson-Turton, M. Richardson, A. Tyree Debisette, and C. Rupinta. 2012. Nurse-managed health centers: Safety-net care through advanced nursing practice. *Journal of the American Academy of Nurse Practitioners* 24(1):24–31.

Etz, R. S. 2016. People are primary: A perspective from the Keystone IV conference. *Journal of the American Board of Family Practice* 29(Suppl 1):S40–S44.

Feagin, J., and Z. Bennefield. 2014. Systemic racism and U.S. health care. *Social Science & Medicine* 103:7–14.

Fertig, A. R., P. S. Corso, and D. Balasubramaniam. 2012. Benefits and costs of a free community-based primary care clinic. *Journal of Health and Human Services Administration* 34(4):456–470.

Finkelstein, A., A. Zhou, S. Taubman, and J. Doyle. 2020. Health care hotspotting—a randomized, controlled trial. *New England Journal of Medicine* 382(2):152–162.

Flocke, S. A., M. A. Goodwin, and K. C. Stange. 1998. The effect of a secondary patient on the family practice visit. *Journal of Family Practice* 46(5):429–434.

Fortuna, R. J., W. Johnson, J. S. Clark, S. Messing, S. Flynn, and S. R. Judge. 2020. Impact of patient-centered medical home transformation on providers, staff, and quality. *Population Health Management*. Epub ahead of print.

Friedberg, M. W., E. C. Schneider, M. B. Rosenthal, K. G. Volpp, and R. M. Werner. 2014. Association between participation in a multipayer medical home intervention and changes in quality, utilization, and costs of care. *JAMA* 311(8):815–825.

GAO (U.S. Government Accountability Office). 2018a. *Indian Health Service: Agency faces ongoing challenges filling provider vacancies*. Washington, DC: U.S. Government Accountability Office.

GAO. 2018b. *Indian Health Service: Spending levels and characteristics of IHS and three other federal health care programs.* Washington, DC: U.S. Government Accountability Office.

GAO. 2020. *Indian Health Service: Actions needed to improve oversight of federal facilities' decision-making about the use of funds.* Washington, DC: U.S. Government Accountability Office.

Garcia, M. E., A. B. Bindman, and J. Coffman. 2019. Language-concordant primary care physicians for a diverse population: The view from California. *Health Equity* 3(1):343–349.

Garfield, C., and S. Kangovi. 2019. Integrating community health workers into health care teams without coopting them. *Health Affairs Blog* (May 10). https://www.healthaffairs.org/do/10.1377/hblog20190507.746358/full (accessed January 21, 2021).

Geiger, H. J. 2002. Community-oriented primary care: A path to community development. *American Journal of Public Health* 92(11):1713–1716.

Gofin, J., R. Gofin, and J. P. Stimpson. 2015. Community-oriented primary care (COPC) and the Affordable Care Act: An opportunity to meet the demands of an evolving health care system. *Journal of Primary Care & Community Health* 6(2):128–133.

Gold, R., A. Bunce, S. Cowburn, J. V. Davis, J. C. Nelson, C. A. Nelson, E. Hicks, D. J. Cohen, M. A. Horberg, G. Melgar, J. W. Dearing, J. Seabrook, N. Mossman, and J. Bulkley. 2019. Does increased implementation support improve community clinics' guideline-concordant care? Results of a mixed methods, pragmatic comparative effectiveness trial. *Implementation Science* 14(1):100.

Gotler, R. S., L. A. Green, and R. S. Etz. 2020. What 1966 can teach us about the future of primary care: The case for communities of solution. *Milbank Quarterly Opinion.* https://www.milbank.org/quarterly/opinions/what-1966-can-teach-us-about-the-future-of-primary-care-the-case-for-communities-of-solution (accessed June 10, 2020).

Gottlieb, K. 2013. The Nuka system of care: Improving health through ownership and relationships. *International Journal of Circumpolar Health* 72.

Green, L. A., and J. C. Puffer. 2010. Family medicine at 40 years of age: The journey to transformation continues. *Journal of the American Board of Family Medicine* 23:S1–S4.

Greene, S. M., L. Tuzzio, and D. Cherkin. 2012. A framework for making patient-centered care front and center. *The Permanente Journal* 16(3):49–53.

Griswold, K. S., S. E. Lesko, J. M. Westfall, and G. Folsom. 2013. Communities of solution: Partnerships for population health. *Journal of the American Board of Family Medicine* 26(3):232–238.

Hansen-Turton, T. 2012. *Nurse-managed health clinics provided badly needed primary care—but without funding, they and their patients are at risk.* https://www.rwjf.org/en/blog/2012/01/nurse-managed-health-clinics-provided-badly-needed-primary-carebut-without-funding-they-and-their-patients-are-at-risk.html (accessed March 9, 2021).

Hansen-Turton, T., D. N. Bailey, N. Torres, and A. Ritter. 2010. Nurse-managed health centers. *American Journal of Nursing* 110(9):23–26.

Health centres of tomorrow. 1947. *The Lancet* 249(6436):32–33.

Helfrich, C. D., E. D. Dolan, J. Simonetti, R. J. Reid, S. Joos, B. J. Wakefield, G. Schectman, R. Stark, S. D. Fihn, H. B. Harvey, and K. Nelson. 2014. Elements of team-based care in a patient-centered medical home are associated with lower burnout among VA primary care employees. *Journal of General Internal Medicine* 29(Suppl 2):S659–S666.

Hiscock, I. V. 1935. The development of neighborhood health services in the United States. *Milbank Quarterly* 13(1):30–51.

Holden, K. B., J. Hopkins, A. Belton, K. Butty, D. C. Tabor, and D. Satcher. 2019. Leveraging science to advance health equity: A regional health policy research center's approach. *Ethnicity & Disease* 29(Suppl 2):323–328.

Hollander-Rodriguez, J., and J. E. DeVoe. 2018. Family medicine's task in population health: Defining it and owning it. *Family Medicine* 50(9):659–661.

Hone, T., J. Macinko, and C. Millett. 2018. Revisiting Alma-Ata: What is the role of primary health care in achieving the sustainable development goals? *The Lancet* 392(10156): 1461–1472.

HRSA (Health Resources and Services Administration). 2018. *Health center program compliance manual.* https://bphc.hrsa.gov/programrequirements/compliancemanual/introduction.html (accessed August 27, 2020).

HRSA. 2020a. *Health center program.* https://bphc.hrsa.gov/programrequirements (accessed July 30, 2020).

HRSA. 2020b. *Health center program: Impact and growth.* https://bphc.hrsa.gov/about/healthcenterprogram (accessed February 17, 2021).

HRSA. 2021. *Teaching Health Center Graduate Medical Education (THCGME) program.* https://bhw.hrsa.gov/grants/medicine/thcgme (accessed March 30, 2021).

Hughes, L. S., R. L. Phillips, Jr., J. E. DeVoe, and A. W. Bazemore. 2016. Community vital signs: Taking the pulse of the community while caring for patients. *Journal of the American Board of Family Practice* 29(3):419–422.

Hunt, B. R., and M. S. Hurlbert. 2016. Black:white disparities in breast cancer mortality in the 50 largest cities in the United States, 2005–2014. *Cancer Epidemiology* 45:169–173.

Igel, L. H., and B. H. Lerner. 2016. Moving past individual and "pure" autonomy: The rise of family-centered care. *AMA Journal of Ethics* 18(1):56–62.

IHS (Indian Health Service). 2005. Part 2—services to Indians and others (Chapter 4 Other beneficiaries). In *Indian health manual.* Rockville, MD: Indian Health Service.

IHS. 2019. Notice: Indian Health Service strategic plan fiscal year 2019–2023 as published on February 28, 2019. *Federal Register* 84(40):6796–6807. https://www.federalregister.gov/documents/2019/02/28/2019-03486/indian-health-service-strategic-plan-fiscal-year-2019-2023 (accessed December 18, 2020).

IHS. 2020a. *About IHS.* https://www.ihs.gov/aboutihs (accessed December 14, 2020).

IHS. 2020b. *IHS profile.* https://www.ihs.gov/newsroom/factsheets/ihsprofile (accessed December 14, 2020).

IHS. 2020c. *Office of Urban Indian Health programs.* https://www.ihs.gov/urban (accessed December 14, 2020).

Institute for Clinical Systems Improvement. 2014. *Building community relations: Real-life examples.* Princeton, NJ: Robert Wood Johnson Foundation.

International Conference on Primary Health Care. 1978. *Declaration of Alma-Ata.* Alma-Ata, USSR: World Health Organization.

IOM (Institute of Medicine). 1983. *Community oriented primary care: New directions for health services delivery.* Washington, DC: National Academy Press.

IOM. 1996. *Primary care: America's health in a new era.* Washington, DC: National Academy Press.

IOM. 2001. *Crossing the quality chasm: A new health system for the 21st century.* Washington, DC: National Academy Press.

IOM. 2008. *Retooling for an aging America: Building the health care workforce.* Washington, DC: The National Academies Press.

IOM. 2011. *The future of nursing: Leading change, advancing health.* Washington, DC: The National Academies Press.

IOM. 2012. *Primary care and public health: Exploring integration to improve population health.* Washington, DC: The National Academies Press.

Izquierdo, A., M. Ong, E. Pulido, K. B. Wells, M. Berkman, B. Linski, V. Sauer, and J. Miranda. 2018. Community partners in care: 6- and 12-month outcomes of community engagement versus technical assistance to implement depression collaborative care among depressed older adults. *Ethnicity & Disease* 28(Suppl 2):339–348.

Jackson, C. S., and J. N. Gracia. 2014. Addressing health and health-care disparities: The role of a diverse workforce and the social determinants of health. *Public Health Reports* 129(Suppl 2):57–61.

Janes, E. H. 1876. Health of tenement populations and the sanitary requirements of their dwelling. *Reports and Papers of the American Public Health Association in the Years 1874–1875* 2:115–124.

Joint Learning Network for Universal Health Coverage, Ariadne Labs, and Comagine Health. 2019. *Empanelment: A foundational component of primary health care.* Ariadne Labs, Comagine Health.

Joint Task Force for the Development of Telepsychology Guidelines for Psychologists. 2013. *Guidelines for the practice of telepsychology.* Washington, DC: American Psychological Association.

Jolley, J., and L. Shields. 2009. The evolution of family-centered care. *Journal of Pediatric Nursing* 24(2):164–170.

Jones, E., L. Shi, A. S. Hayashi, R. Sharma, C. Daly, and Q. Ngo-Metzger. 2013. Access to oral health care: The role of federally qualified health centers in addressing disparities and expanding access. *American Journal of Public Health* 103(3):488–493.

Jones, K. A., S. Do, L. Porras-Javier, S. Contreras, P. J. Chung, and T. R. Coker. 2018. Feasibility and acceptability in a community-partnered implementation of "CenteringParenting" for group well-child care. *Academic Pediatrics* 18(6):642–649.

Kangovi, S., F. K. Barg, T. Carter, K. Levy, J. Sellman, J. A. Long, and D. Grande. 2014a. Challenges faced by patients with low socioeconomic status during the post-hospital transition. *Journal of General Internal Medicine* 29(2):283–289.

Kangovi, S., N. Mitra, D. Grande, M. L. White, S. McCollum, J. Sellman, R. P. Shannon, and J. A. Long. 2014b. Patient-centered community health worker intervention to improve posthospital outcomes: A randomized clinical trial. *JAMA Internal Medicine* 174(4):535–543.

Kangovi, S., N. Mitra, D. Grande, H. Huo, R. A. Smith, and J. A. Long. 2017. Community health worker support for disadvantaged patients with multiple chronic diseases: A randomized clinical trial. *American Journal of Public Health* 107(10):1660–1667.

Kark, S. L., and E. Kark. 1999. *Promoting community health: From Pholela to Jerusalem.* Johannesburg, ZA: Witwatersrand University Press.

Kark, S. L., and H. L. Riche. 1944. A health study of South African Bantu school children. *South African Medical Journal* 18:100–103.

Kennedy, I. 2003. Patients are experts in their own field. *BMJ* 326(7402):1276–1277.

Kokorelias, K. M., M. A. M. Gignac, G. Naglie, and J. I. Cameron. 2019. Towards a universal model of family centered care: A scoping review. *BMC Health Services Research* 19(1):564.

Kramer, B. J., B. Creekmur, M. N. Mitchell, and D. Saliba. 2018. Expanding home-based primary care to American Indian reservations and other rural communities: An observational study. *Journal of the American Geriatrics Society* 66(4):818–824.

Kravitz, R. L., and M. D. Feldman. 2017. Reinventing primary care: Embracing change, preserving relationships. *Journal of General Internal Medicine* 32(4):369–370.

Krist, A. H., D. Shenson, S. H. Woolf, C. Bradley, W. R. Liaw, S. F. Rothemich, A. Slonim, W. Benson, and L. A. Anderson. 2013. Clinical and community delivery systems for preventive care: An integration framework. *American Journal of Preventive Medicine* 45(4):508–516.

Kuhlthau, K. A., S. Bloom, J. Van Cleave, A. A. Knapp, D. Romm, K. Klatka, C. J. Homer, P. W. Newacheck, and J. M. Perrin. 2011. Evidence for family-centered care for children with special health care needs: A systematic review. *Academic Pediatrics* 11(2):136–143.

Landon, B. E., K. Grumbach, and P. J. Wallace. 2012. Integrating public health and primary care systems: Potential strategies from an IOM report. *JAMA* 308(5):461–462.

Leppin, A. L., K. Schaepe, J. Egginton, S. Dick, M. Branda, L. Christiansen, N. M. Burow, C. Gaw, and V. M. Montori. 2018. Integrating community-based health promotion programs and primary care: A mixed methods analysis of feasibility. *BMC Health Services Research* 18(1):72.

Levitan, S. 1974. Healing the poor in their backyard. In *Neighborhood health centers*, edited by R. Hollister, B. Kramer, and S. Bellin. Lexington, MA: Lexington Books. P. 54.

Lewis, C., Y. Getachew, M. K. Abrams, and M. M. Doty. 2019. *Changes at community health centers, and how patients are benefiting: Results from the Commonwealth Fund national survey of federally qualified health centers, 2013–2018.* https://www.commonwealth-fund.org/publications/issue-briefs/2019/aug/changes-at-community-health-centers-how-patients-are-benefiting (accessed November 24, 2020).

Liss, D. T., P. A. Fishman, C. M. Rutter, D. Grembowski, T. R. Ross, E. A. Johnson, and R. J. Reid. 2013. Outcomes among chronically ill adults in a medical home prototype. *American Journal of Managed Care* 19(10):e348–e358.

Lloyd, J., K. Moses, and R. Davis. 2020. *Recognizing and sustaining the value of community health workers and promotores.* Hamilton, NJ: Center For Health Care Strategies.

Love, H., N. Panchal, J. Schlitt, C. Behr, and S. Soleimanpour. 2019a. The use of tele-health in school-based health centers. *Global Pediatric Health* 6:2333794X19884194. 2333794X19884194.

Love, H. E., J. Schlitt, S. Soleimanpour, N. Panchal, and C. Behr. 2019b. Twenty years of school-based health care growth and expansion. *Health Affairs* 38(5):755–764.

Mader, K., J. M. Sammen, C. Klene, J. Nguyen, M. Simpson, S. L. Ruland, and J. M. Westfall. 2019. Community-designed messaging interventions to improve cost-of-care conversations in settings serving low-income, Latino populations. *Annals of Internal Medicine* 170(Suppl 9):S79–S86.

Malat, J., M. van Ryn, and D. Purcell. 2009. Blacks' and whites' attitudes toward race and nativity concordance with doctors. *Journal of the National Medical Association* 101(8):800–807.

Mann, D. M., J. Chen, R. Chunara, P. A. Testa, and O. Nov. 2020. COVID-19 transforms health care through telemedicine: Evidence from the field. *Journal of the American Medical Informatics Association* 27(7):1132–1135.

Martin, J. C., R. F. Avant, M. A. Bowman, J. R. Bucholtz, J. R. Dickinson, K. L. Evans, L. A. Green, D. E. Henley, W. A. Jones, S. C. Matheny, J. E. Nevin, S. L. Panther, J. C. Puffer, R. G. Roberts, D. V. Rodgers, R. A. Sherwood, K. C. Stange, and C. W. Weber. 2004. The future of family medicine: A collaborative project of the family medicine community. *Annals of Family Medicine* 2(Suppl 1):S3–S32.

Martinez, K. A., M. Rood, N. Jhangiani, L. Kou, S. Rose, A. Boissy, and M. B. Rothberg. 2018. Patterns of use and correlates of patient satisfaction with a large nationwide direct to consumer telemedicine service. *Journal of General Internal Medicine* 33(10):1768–1773.

Martinez-Bianchi, V., B. Frank, J. Edgoose, L. Michener, M. Rodriguez, L. Gottlieb, B. Reddick, C. Kelly, K. Yu, S. Davis, J. Carr, J. W. Lee, K. L. Smith, R. D. New, and J. Weida. 2019. Addressing family medicine's capacity to improve health equity through collaboration, accountability and coalition-building. *Family Medicine* 51(2):198–203.

MCN (Migrant Clinicians Network). 2021. *Our story.* https://www.migrantclinician.org/about/our-story (accessed March 10, 2021).

McGinnis, J. M., P. Williams-Russo, and J. R. Knickman. 2002. The case for more active policy attention to health promotion. *Health Affairs* 21(2):78–93.

Mehrotra, A., M. Chernew, D. Linetsky, H. Hatch, and D. Cutler. 2020. *What impact has COVID-19 had on outpatient visits?* New York: The Commonwealth Fund.

Mitchell, P., M. Wynia, R. Golden, B. McNellis, S. Okun, C. E. Webb, V. Rohrbach, and I. Von Kohorn. 2012. *Core principles & values of effective team-based health care. NAM Perspectives.* Discussion Paper, National Academy of Medicine, Washington, DC.

Montague, E., and O. Asan. 2014. Dynamic modeling of patient and physician eye gaze to understand the effects of electronic health records on doctor-patient communication and attention. *International Journal of Medical Informatics* 83(3):225–234.

Morse, M., A. Finnegan, B. Wispelwey, and C. Ford. 2020. Will COVID-19 pave the way for progressive social policies? Insights from critical race theory? *Health Affairs Blog* (July 2). https://www.healthaffairs.org/do/10.1377/hblog20200630.184036/full (accessed August 17, 2020).

MSM (Morehouse School of Medicine). 2021. *Southeast regional clinicians network membership.* https://www.msm.edu/Research/research_centersandinstitutes/NCPC/divisions/research/sercn-membership.php (accessed March 2, 2021).

Mullan, F., and L. Epstein. 2002. Community-oriented primary care: New relevance in a changing world. *American Journal of Public Health* 92(11):1748–1755.

NACHC (National Association of Community Health Centers). 2020a. *Community health center chartbook.* Bethesda, MD: National Association of Community Health Centers.

NACHC. 2020b. *The facts about Medicaid's FQHC prospective payment system (PPS).* National Association of Community Health Centers.

NACHC and NACCHO (National Association of County and City Health Officials). 2010. *Partnerships between federally qualified health centers and local health departments for engaging in the development of a community-based system of care.* Bethesda, MA: National Association of Community Health Centers.

Naik, A. D., L. N. Dindo, J. R. Van Liew, N. E. Hundt, L. Vo, K. Hernandez-Bigos, J. Esterson, M. Geda, J. Rosen, C. S. Blaum, and M. E. Tinetti. 2018. Development of a clinically feasible process for identifying individual health priorities. *Journal of the American Geriatrics Society* 66(10):1872–1879.

NASEM (National Academies of Sciences, Engineering, and Medicine). 2017. *Communities in action: Pathways to health equity.* Washington, DC: The National Academies Press.

NASEM. 2019a. *Integrating social care into the delivery of health care: Moving upstream to improve the nation's health.* Washington, DC: The National Academies Press.

NASEM. 2019b. *Investing in interventions that address non-medical, health-related social needs: Proceedings of a workshop.* Washington, DC: The National Academies Press.

National Center for Medical-Legal Partnership. 2017. *Helping families keep their heat and lights on.* https://medical-legalpartnership.org/utility-story (accessed November 2, 2020).

National Commission on Community Health Services. 1967. *Health is a community affair: Report of the National Commission on Community Health Services.* Cambridge, MA: Harvard University Press.

NCQA (National Committee for Quality Assurance). 2020. *Patient-centered medical home (PCMH).* https://www.ncqa.org/programs/health-care-providers-practices/patient-centered-medical-home-pcmh (accessed June 2, 2020).

Nimmon, L., and T. Stenfors-Hayes. 2016. The "handling" of power in the physician-patient encounter: Perceptions from experienced physicians. *BMC Medical Education* 16.

Nocon, R. S., S. M. Lee, R. Sharma, Q. Ngo-Metzger, D. B. Mukamel, Y. Gao, L. M. White, L. Shi, M. H. Chin, N. Laiteerapong, and E. S. Huang. 2016. Health care use and spending for Medicaid enrollees in federally qualified health centers versus other primary care settings. *American Journal of Public Health* 106(11):1981–1989.

Nutting, P. A., J. E. Barrick, and S. C. Logue. 1979. The impact of a maternal and child health care program on the quality of prenatal care: An analysis by risk group. *Journal of Community Health* 4(4):267–279.

O'Brien, M. J., C. H. Halbert, R. Bixby, S. Pimentel, and J. A. Shea. 2010. Community health worker intervention to decrease cervical cancer disparities in Hispanic women. *Journal of General Internal Medicine* 25(11):1186–1192.

Ockene, J. K., E. A. Edgerton, S. M. Teutsch, L. N. Marion, T. Miller, J. L. Genevro, C. J. Loveland-Cherry, J. E. Fielding, and P. A. Briss. 2007. Integrating evidence-based clinical and community strategies to improve health. *American Journal of Preventive Medicine* 32(3):244–252.

ODPHP (Office of Disease Prevention and Health Promotion). 2020. *Access to primary care.* https://www.healthypeople.gov/2020/topics-objectives/topic/social-determinants-health/interventions-resources/access-to-primary (accessed November 2, 2020).

Okun, S., S. Schoenbaum, D. Andrews, P. Chidambaran, V. Chollette, J. Gruman, S. Leal, B. A. Bown, P. H. Mitchel, C. Parry, W. Prins, R. Ricciardi, M. A. Simon, R. Stock, D. C. Strasser, C. E. Webb, M. K. Wynia, and D. Henderson. 2014. *Patients and health care teams forging effective partnerships. NAM Perspectives.* Discussion Paper, National Academy of Medicine.

Ong, M. K., L. Jones, W. Aoki, T. R. Belin, E. Bromley, B. Chung, E. Dixon, M. D. Johnson, F. Jones, P. Koegel, D. Khodyakov, C. M. Landry, E. Lizaola, N. Mtume, V. K. Ngo, J. Perlman, E. Pulido, V. Sauer, C. D. Sherbourne, L. Tang, E. Vidaurri, Y. Whittington, P. Williams, A. Lucas-Wright, L. Zhang, M. Southard, J. Miranda, and K. Wells. 2017. A community-partnered, participatory, cluster-randomized study of depression care quality improvement: Three-year outcomes. *Psychiatric Services* 68(12):1262–1270.

Orlando, J. F., M. Beard, and S. Kumar. 2019. Systematic review of patient and caregivers' satisfaction with telehealth videoconferencing as a mode of service delivery in managing patients' health. *PLOS ONE* 14(8):e0221848.

Osborn, H. A., J. T. Glicksman, M. G. Brandt, P. C. Doyle, and K. Fung. 2017. Primary care specialty career choice among Canadian medical students: Understanding the factors that influence their decisions. *Canadian Family Physician* 63(2):e107–e113.

Park, M., T. T. Giap, M. Lee, H. Jeong, M. Jeong, and Y. Go. 2018. Patient- and family-centered care interventions for improving the quality of health care: A review of systematic reviews. *International Journal of Nursing Studies* 87:69–83.

Peikes, D., A. Zutshi, J. Genevro, K. Smith, M. Parchman, and D. Meyers. 2015. *Early evidence on the patient-centered medical home.* Rockville, MD: Agency for Healthcare Quality and Research.

Pettoello-Mantovani, M., A. Campanozzi, L. Maiuri, and I. Giardino. 2009. Family-oriented and family-centered care in pediatrics. *Italian Journal of Pediatrics* 35(1):12.

PHCPI (Primary Health Care Performance Initiative). 2019. *Population health management: Empanelment.* Primary Health Care Performance Initiative.

Philip, S., D. Govier, and S. Pantely. 2019. *Patient-centered medical home: Developing the business case from a practice perspective.* Seattle, WA: Milliman, National Committee for Quality Assurance.

Phillips, R. L., D. J. Cohen, A. Kaufman, W. P. Dickinson, and S. Cykert. 2019. Facilitating practice transformation in frontline health care. *Annals of Family Medicine* 17(Suppl 1):S2–S5.

Politzer, R. M., J. Yoon, L. Shi, R. G. Hughes, J. Regan, and M. H. Gaston. 2001. Inequality in America: The contribution of health centers in reducing and eliminating disparities in access to care. *Medical Care Research and Review* 58(2):234–248.

Pollack, S. M. 2019. Pay for relationship: A novel solution to the primary care crisis. *NEJM Catalyst.*

Pomeroy, J. L. 1929. Health center development in Los Angeles County. *JAMA* 93(20):1546–1550.

Possemato, K., L. O. Wray, E. Johnson, B. Webster, and G. P. Beehler. 2018. Facilitators and barriers to seeking mental health care among primary care veterans with posttraumatic stress disorder. *Journal of Traumatic Stress* 31(5):742–752.

Puffer, J. C., J. Borkan, J. E. DeVoe, A. Davis, R. L. Phillips, Jr., L. A. Green, and J. W. Saultz. 2015. Envisioning a new health care system for America. *Family Medicine* 47(8):598–603.

Reid, R. J., K. Coleman, E. A. Johnson, P. A. Fishman, C. Hsu, M. P. Soman, C. E. Trescott, M. Erikson, and E. B. Larson. 2010. The group health medical home at year two: Cost savings, higher patient satisfaction, and less burnout for providers. *Health Affairs (Project Hope)* 29(5):835–843.

Rhodes, P., C. Sanders, and S. Campbell. 2014. Relationship continuity: When and why do primary care patients think it is safer? *British Journal of General Practice* 64(629):e758–e764.

Rimmer, A. 2020. Can patients use family members as non-professional interpreters in consultations? *BMJ* 368:m447.

Rock, R. M., W. R. Liaw, A. H. Krist, S. Tong, D. Grolling, J. Rankin, and A. W. Bazemore. 2019. Clinicians' overestimation of their geographic service area. *Annals of Family Medicine* 17(Suppl 1):S63–S66.

Rosen, G. 1947. What is social medicine? A genetic analysis of the concept. *Bulletin of the History of Medicine* 21(5):674–733.

Rosen, G. 1949. The idea of social medicine in America. *Canadian Medical Association Journal* 61(3):316–323.

Rosen, G. 1971. Public health: Then and now. The first neighborhood health center movement—its rise and fall. *American Journal of Public Health* 61(8):1620–1637.

Rosenberg, C. E. 1974. Social class and medical care in nineteenth-century America: The rise and fall of the dispensary. *Journal of the History of Medicine and Allied Science* 29(1):32–54.

Rosland, A.-M., J. D. Piette, H. Choi, and M. Heisler. 2011. Family and friend participation in primary care visits of patients with diabetes or heart failure: Patient and physician determinants and experiences. *Medical Care* 49(1):37–45.

Rural Health Information Hub. 2019. *Federally qualified health centers (FQHCs) and the health center program.* https://www.ruralhealthinfo.org/topics/federally-qualified-health-centers (accessed November 24, 2020).

Rust, G. S., V. Murray, H. Octaviani, E. D. Schmidt, J. P. Howard, V. Anderson-Grant, and K. Willard-Jelks. 1999. Asthma care in community health centers: A study by the Southeast Regional Clinicians' Network. *JAMA* 91(7):398–403.

Rust, G., E. Daniels, D. Satcher, J. Bacon, H. Strothers, and T. Bornemann. 2005. Ability of community health centers to obtain mental health services for uninsured patients. *JAMA* 293(5):554–556. https://jamanetwork.com/journals/jama/fullarticle/200284 (accessed February 2, 2020).

Saha, S., and M. C. Beach. 2020. Impact of physician race on patient decision making and ratings of physicians: A randomized experiment using video vignettes. *Journal of General Internal Medicine* 35(4):1084–1091.

Saha, S., M. Komaromy, T. D. Koepsell, and A. B. Bindman. 1999. Patient-physician racial concordance and the perceived quality and use of health care. *Archives of Internal Medicine* 159(9):997–1004.

Saha, S., S. H. Taggart, M. Komaromy, and A. B. Bindman. 2000. Do patients choose physicians of their own race? *Health Affairs* 19(4):76–83.

Sarinopoulos, I., D. L. Bechel-Marriott, J. M. Malouin, S. Zhai, J. C. Forney, and C. L. Tanner. 2017. Patient experience with the patient-centered medical home in Michigan's statewide multi-payer demonstration: A cross-sectional study. *Journal of General Internal Medicine* 32(11):1202–1209.

Sayers, S. L., T. White, C. Zubritsky, and D. W. Oslin. 2006. Family involvement in the care of healthy medical outpatients. *Family Practice* 23(3):317–324.

Schilling, L. M., L. Scatena, J. F. Steiner, G. A. Albertson, C. T. Lin, L. Cyran, L. Ware, and R. J. Anderson. 2002. The third person in the room: Frequency, role, and influence of companions during primary care medical encounters. *Journal of Family Practice* 51(8):685–690.

Schmacke, N. 1998. Health promotion through neighborhood health centers: A tribute to George Rosen on the 20th anniversary of his death. *Health Promotion International* 13(2):151–154.

Schwenk, T. L. 2014. The patient-centered medical home: One size does not fit all. *JAMA* 311(8):802–803.

Scott, J. G., D. Cohen, B. Dicicco-Bloom, W. L. Miller, K. C. Stange, and B. F. Crabtree. 2008. Understanding healing relationships in primary care. *Annals of Family Medicine* 6(4):315–322.

Seervai, S. 2020. *How community health workers put patients in charge of their health.* https:// www.commonwealthfund.org/publications/podcast/2020/may/how-community-health-workers-put-patients-charge-their-health (accessed June 12, 2020).

Shen, M. J., E. B. Peterson, R. Costas-Muñiz, M. H. Hernandez, S. T. Jewell, K. Matsoukas, and C. L. Bylund. 2018. The effects of race and racial concordance on patient-physician communication: A systematic review of the literature. *Journal of Racial and Ethnic Health Disparities* 5(1):117–140.

Shorr, G. I., and P. A. Nutting. 1977. A population-based assessment of the continuity of ambulatory care. *Medical Care* 15(6):455–464.

Shukor, A. R., S. Edelman, D. Brown, and C. Rivard. 2018. Developing community-based primary health care for complex and vulnerable populations in the Vancouver coastal health region: Healthconnection clinic. *The Permanente Journal* 22:18-010.

Singer, M. 1989. The coming of age of critical medical anthropology. *Social Science & Medicine* 28(11):1193–1203.

SNOCAP-USA (State Networks of Colorado Ambulatory Practices and Partners), E. E. Stewart, N. Taylor-Post, L. Nichols, E. W. Staton, and A. Schleunin. 2014. Community connections: Linking primary care patients to local resources for better management of obesity. Rockville, MD: Agency for Healthcare Research and Quality. https://www.ahrq. gov/ncepcr/tools/obesity-kit/index.html (accessed November 24, 2020).

Starfield, B. 2009. Primary care and equity in health: The importance to effectiveness and equity of responsiveness to peoples' needs. *Humanity & Society* 33(1–2):56–73.

Starfield, B. 2011. Is patient-centered care the same as person-focused care? *The Permanente Journal* 15:63–69.

Starfield, B. 2012. Primary care: An increasingly important contributor to effectiveness, equity, and efficiency of health services. SESPAS report 2012. *Gaceta Sanitaria* 26(Suppl 1):20–26.

Starfield, B., L. Shi, and J. Macinko. 2005. Contribution of primary care to health systems and health. *Milbank Quarterly* 83(3):457–502.

Stephens, G. G. 2010. Remembering 40 years, plus or minus. *Journal of the American Board of Family Practice* 23(Suppl 1):S5–S10.

Sullivan, E. E., and A. Ellner. 2015. Strong patient-provider relationships drive healthier outcomes. *Harvard Business Review.* https://hbr.org/2015/10/strong-patient-provider-relationships-drive-healthier-outcomes (accessed January 12, 2021).

Susser, M., Z. Stein, M. Cormack, and M. Hathorn. 1955. Medical care in a South African township. *The Lancet* 268(6870):912–915.

Taylor, J. 2004. *The fundamentals of communith health centers.* Washington, DC: The George Washington University.

Teno, J. M., P. L. Gozalo, A. N. Trivedi, S. L. Mitchell, J. N. Bunker, and V. Mor. 2017. Temporal trends in the numbers of skilled nursing facility specialists from 2007 through 2014. *JAMA Internal Medicine* 177(9):1376–1378.

The Folsom Group. 2012. Communities of solution: The Folsom Report revisited. *Annals of Family Medicine* 10(3):250–260.

The Larry A. Green Center and PCC (Primary Care Collaborative). 2020. *Quick COVID-19 primary care survey: Patient series 1 fielded May 4–11, 2020.* https://www.green-center. org/covid-survey (accessed January 21, 2021).

Tinetti, M. E., T. R. Fried, and C. M. Boyd. 2012. Designing health care for the most common chronic condition—multimorbidity. *JAMA* 307(23):2493–2494.

Ton, A. N., T. Jethwa, K. Waters, L. L. Speicher, and D. Francis. 2020. COVID-19 drive through testing: An effective strategy for conserving personal protective equipment. *American Journal of Infection Control* 48(6):731–732.

UCLA (University of California, Los Angeles) American Indian Studies Center. 2016. *Access to care among American Indians and Alaska Natives in Los Angeles.* https://www.aisc. ucla.edu/research/pb4.aspx (accessed December 14, 2020).

Unwin, B. K., M. Porvaznik, and G. D. Spoelhof. 2010. Nursing home care: Part I. Principles and pitfalls of practice. *American Family Physician* 81(10):1219–1227.

Urban Indian Health Commission. 2007. *Invisible tribes: Urban Indians and their health in a changing world.* Seattle, WA: Urban Indian Health Commission.

VA (U.S. Department of Veterans Affairs). 2020. *What is home based primary care?* https:// www.va.gov/GERIATRICS/pages/Home_Based_Primary_Care.asp (accessed February 26, 2021).

van den Berk-Clark, C., E. Doucette, F. Rottnek, W. Manard, M. A. Prada, R. Hughes, T. Lawrence, and F. D. Schneider. 2018. Do patient-centered medical homes improve health behaviors, outcomes, and experiences of low-income patients? A systematic review and meta-analysis. *Health Services Research* 53(3):1777–1798.

van Weel, C. 2011. Person-centred medicine in the context of primary care: A view from the world organization of family doctors (WONCA). *Journal of Evaluation in Clinical Practice* 17(2):337–338.

Wagner, E. H., K. Coleman, R. J. Reid, K. Phillips, M. K. Abrams, and J. R. Sugarman. 2012. The changes involved in patient-centered medical home transformation. *Primary Care: Clinics in Office Practice* 39(2):241–259.

Wald, L. D. 1911. *The house on Henry Street.* New York: Henry Holt & Co.

Wang, E. A., C. S. Hong, S. Shavit, R. Sanders, E. Kessell, and M. B. Kushel. 2012. Engaging individuals recently released from prison into primary care: A randomized trial. *American Journal of Public Health* 102(9):e22–e29.

Warne, D., and L. B. Frizzell. 2014. American Indian health policy: Historical trends and contemporary issues. *American Journal of Public Health* 104(Suppl 3):S263–S267.

Wells, K. B., K. E. Watkins, B. Hurley, L. Tang, F. Jones, and J. Gilmore. 2018. Commentary: Applying the community partners in care approach to the opioid crisis. *Ethnicity & Disease* 28(Suppl 2):381–388.

Westfall, J. M. 2013. Cold-spotting: Linking primary care and public health to create communities of solution. *Journal of the American Board of Family Medicine* 26(3):239–240.

Westfall, J. M., R. Roper, A. Gaglioti, and D. E. Nease, Jr. 2019. Practice-based research networks: Strategic opportunities to advance implementation research for health equity. *Ethnicity & Disease* 29(Suppl 1):113–118.

Whitehead, L., E. Jacob, A. Towell, M. Abu-Qamar, and A. Cole-Heath. 2018. The role of the family in supporting the self-management of chronic conditions: A qualitative systematic review. *Journal of Clinical Nursing* 27(1–2):22–30.

WHO (World Health Organization). 2016. *Framework on integrated, people-centered health services.* Geneva, Switzerland: World Health Organization.

WHO. 2020a. *Social determinants of health.* https://www.who.int/health-topics/social-determinants-of-health (accessed November 2, 2020).

WHO. 2020b. *World Health Organization health systems strengthening glossary.* Geneva, Switzerland: World Health Organization.

WHO and Ministry of Healthcare Republic of Kazakhstan. 2018. *Global Conference on Primary Health Care. 25–26 October 2018—Astana, Kazakhstan.* https://www.who. int/news-room/events/detail/2018/10/25/default-calendar/global-conference-on-primary-health-care (accessed March 24, 2019).

WHO and UNICEF (United Nations Children's Fund). 2018. *Declaration of Astana.* Astana, Kazakhstan: World Health Organization and United Nations Children's Fund.

Wiggins, N., S. Kaan, T. Rios-Campos, R. Gaonkar, E. Morgan, and J. Robinson. 2013. Preparing community health workers for their role as agents of social change: Experience of the community capacitation center. *Journal of Community Practice* 21:186–202.

Wilinsky, C. 1933. *Health units of Boston, 1924–1933.* Boston, MA: City of Boston Printing Department.

Williams, D. R., J. A. Lawrence, and B. A. Davis. 2019a. Racism and health: Evidence and needed research. *Annual Review of Public Health* 40:105–125.

Williams, D. R., J. A. Lawrence, B. A. Davis, and C. Vu. 2019b. Understanding how discrimination can affect health. *Health Services Research* 54(Suppl 2):1374–1388.

Winslow, C.-E. A. 1919. The health center movement. *Modern Medicine* 1(4).

Winslow, C.-E. A. 1929. *The life of Hermann M. Biggs: M.D., D. Sc., LL. D., physician and statesman of the public health.* Philadelphia, PA: Lea & Febiger.

Wolff, J. L., and C. M. Boyd. 2015. A look at person- and family-centered care among older adults: Results from a national survey [corrected]. *Journal of General Internal Medicine* 30(10):1497–1504.

Wolff, J. L., and D. L. Roter. 2011. Family presence in routine medical visits: A meta-analytical review. *Social Science & Medicine* 72(6):823–831.

Wright, B. 2013. Who governs federally qualified health centers? *Journal of Health Politics, Policy and Law* 38(1):27–55.

Wright, B. 2015. Do patients have a voice? The social stratification of health center governing boards. *Health Expectations* 18(3):430–437.

Xierali, I. M., and M. A. Nivet. 2018. The racial and ethnic composition and distribution of primary care physicians. *Journal of Health Care for the Poor and Underserved* 29(1):556–570.

Yoon, J., E. Chang, L. V. Rubenstein, A. Park, D. M. Zulman, S. Stockdale, M. K. Ong, D. Atkins, G. Schectman, and S. M. Asch. 2018. Impact of primary care intensive management on high-risk veterans' costs and utilization: A randomized quality improvement trial. *Annals of Internal Medicine* 168(12):846–854.

Youngclaus, J., and L. Roskovensky. 2018. An updated look at the economic diversity of U.S. Medical students. *AAMC in Brief* 18(5).

Yue, D., N. Pourat, X. Chen, C. Lu, W. Zhou, M. Daniel, H. Hoang, A. Sripipatana, and N. A. Ponce. 2019. Enabling services improve access to care, preventive services, and satisfaction among health center patients. *Health Affairs* 38(9):1468–1474.

Zhang, X., B. Hailu, D. C. Tabor, R. Gold, M. H. Sayre, I. Sim, B. Jean-Francois, C. A. Casnoff, T. Cullen, V. A. Thomas, Jr., L. Artiles, K. Williams, P.-T. Le, C. F. Aklin, and R. James. 2019. Role of health information technology in addressing health disparities: Patient, clinician, and system perspectives. *Medical Care* 57.

Zwick, D. I. 1972. Some accomplishments and findings of neighborhood health centers. *The Milbank Memorial Fund Quarterly* 50(4):387–420.

5

Integrated Primary Care Delivery

Integrated primary care delivery is a foundational strategy for health care organizations to support a culture of high-quality, person- and family-centered primary care built on trusted, accessible, and continuous relationships (see Chapter 2 for the committee's definition of high-quality primary care). This chapter outlines the implementation facilitators needed to support the adoption, implementation, and sustainability of integrated delivery structures and processes of health care organizations that enable improved health outcomes and promote population health and health equity.

Integrated care has been defined as care that is coordinated across professionals, facilities, and support systems; continuous over time and between visits; and tailored to personal and family needs, values, and preferences (Singer et al., 2011). It encompasses a diverse set of methods and models that aim to facilitate improved patient experiences through enhanced coordination and continuity of care (Rocks et al., 2020). When applied to primary care, a functional definition of integrated care is care that results when a primary care team and another team or organization or service external to primary care work together with patients and families "using a systematic and cost-effective approach" to provide person- and family-centered care for a defined population (AHRQ, 2013, p. 2). Examples include integrating primary care with behavioral health, pharmacy, and oral health services and with public health and services to address social determinants of health (SDOH) (NASEM, 2019a). The professionals and staff for these joint services are integrated directly into primary care practices through an interprofessional team-based approach to care.

THE GOALS OF INTEGRATED CARE DELIVERY

The main reasons to integrate interprofessional team-based methods into primary care are to expand the impact of primary care, grow its capacity to comprehensively address a broader range of whole-person health needs, and establish effective, shared linkages with families, community organizations, and specialist resources over time (Bitton et al., 2018). The rationale for this integration is that primary care is where most people seek any health care and where they are most likely to develop sustained, healing relationships focused on well-being that can contribute to overall population health (Buckley et al., 2013; Colwill et al., 2016; Ellner and Phillips, 2017; Flieger, 2017; Frey, 2010; Gottlieb, 2013; Green and Puffer, 2016; Kravitz and Feldman, 2017). It is also the venue that delivers most mental health care, and visits to primary care often involve issues related to other family members or social needs (Gard et al., 2020; Pinto and Bloch, 2017; Pinto et al., 2016; Xierali et al., 2013). Implementing integrated, team-based care with high fidelity has been shown to improve health care quality and cost outcomes (IOM, 2011; Reiss-Brennan et al., 2016; Yogman et al., 2018) and may help achieve health equity by including social and health services that meet all communities' needs (Browne et al., 2012; Satcher and Rachel, 2017). Integrated team-based primary care can also help alleviate clinician burnout (NASEM, 2019b).

To guide its work reviewing innovative integration solutions and developing an implementation plan to achieve integration, the committee adopted the Comprehensive Theory of Integration (Singer et al., 2020) as a guiding principle. This theory defines and distinguishes several aspects of integration (see Figure 5-1):

- Structural integration: physical, operational, financial, or legal ties
- Functional integration: formal, written policies and protocols for activities that coordinate and support accountability and decision making
- Normative integration: a common culture and a specific culture of integration
- Interpersonal integration: collaboration or teamwork
- Process (or clinical) integration: organizational actions or activities intended to integrate care services into a single process across people, functions, activities, and operating units over time

The committee focuses its recommendations on implementing the structures and processes that support normative, interpersonal, process, and clinical integration to advance whole-person integrated care. Elements of structural and functional integration are the focus of policy makers and

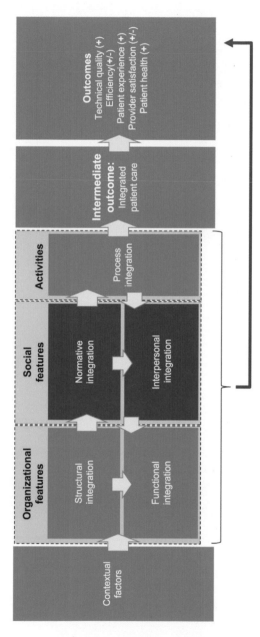

FIGURE 5-1 Comprehensive Theory of Integration.
SOURCE: Singer et al., 2020.

industry leaders (Singer et al., 2020; Valentijn et al., 2015) and covered in subsequent chapters.

Achieving normative, cultural, and process integration for primary care delivery requires health care organizations to design and implement a number of key components and capabilities (see Table 5-1). Several evidence-based structures and processes ("coordinating mechanisms") facilitate integrated primary care delivery (Weaver et al., 2018) (see Table 5-2).

The structures and processes of integrated primary care systems must be nimble enough to allow people to seek care, either in person or virtually, while still providing high-quality, whole-person care for individuals and families. Furthermore, institutional leaders must design and plan for coordinating the needs of integrated primary care with the needs of its communities by thoughtful monitoring. For example, a pediatric-focused integrated primary care system might invest more heavily in community partnerships with Head Start Centers, other preschools, and the local public schools, while a system that serves a largely older, Black adult population may invest more heavily in developing community partnerships with churches and coordinating with long-term care facilities. Effective integrated primary care needs to be tailored not only at the level of the individual and family but also for the population that it serves (see Chapter 4 for more on community partnerships).

Southcentral Foundation

Despite few fully integrated, community-specific primary care systems in the United States, some examples do exist that show their potential for assuring integrated, person-centered primary care. One such example, the Southcentral Foundation (SCF), provides comprehensive, integrated health care for nearly 65,000 Alaska Native and American Indian people in and near Anchorage, Alaska. SCF's Nuka System of Care was designed to align with its vision of "a Native Community that enjoys physical, mental, emotional, and spiritual wellness" (Gottlieb, 2013) (see Chapter 4 for more on SCF's emphasis on relationship-based care). SCF uses a team-based approach to care that is inclusive of team members outside of the traditional clinician, including experts in complementary or integrative medical care and traditional healing practices who provide support throughout the care system and via dedicated clinics in Anchorage (SCF, 2020).

The Nuka integrated primary care team supports structural, normative, and process integration; its core includes a primary care clinician, certified medical assistant, registered nurse case manager, and case management support. An integrated team with clinical behavioral health consultants, pharmacists, registered dietitians, midwives, and advanced practice clinicians supports the core team, with additional expertise, such as integrative

TABLE 5-1 Components of Integrated Primary Care Delivery and Key Capabilities

Key Components of Integrated Care	How the Integrated Care Component Works	Key Capabilities
Interprofessional team-based care (normative integration)	A practice team tailored to the whole-person primary care needs of each person/family (A key element of this practice team is the family navigator, health coach, care coordinator, community health worker, or other team member with the responsibility of providing culturally relevant support, coordination, and service to the person and family.)	1. With a suitable range of expertise both within and outside of primary care (e.g., behavioral health) and role functions (e.g., clinician, coordinator, coach) 2. With shared operations, workflows, and practice culture 3. With formal on-the-job training
Population-based care (process and functional integration)	With a shared population and mission, and a panel of patients in common for total health outcomes	1. A standard set of metrics to guide workflows, data analysis of cost and quality impact of integration
Care management (structural, process, and interpersonal integration)	Using a systematic clinical approach and a system that enables the clinical approach to function	1. Employing methods to identify those members of the population who need or may benefit from care 2. Engaging individuals and families in identifying their needs for care and the particular members of the team to provide it 3. Using an explicit, unified, and shared care plan
Supported by seven facilitators of high-quality primary care • Digital health • Payment • Quality measures and accountability • Interprofessional teams • Leadership • Research • Policy, laws, and regulations	Practice operations, leadership alignment, community partnerships, and business model address all six facilitators	1. Clinic operational systems and process (including technology and data systems) 2. Operations and partnership with non-clinical entities for integration 3. Alignment on purposes, incentives, leadership 4. Sustainable business model

continued

TABLE 5-1 Continued

Key Components of Integrated Care	How the Integrated Care Component Works	Key Capabilities
Supported by implementation framework	Continuous quality improvement and measurement of effectiveness and adoption over time	1. Routine collection of prioritized integrated team measures 2. Periodic examination of and reporting of outcomes and adoption progress with necessary action

SOURCES: Adapted from AHRQ, 2013; Talen and Valeras, 2013; Yonek et al., 2020.

medicine, brought in when needed. All interprofessional team members and support staff, regardless of position, are on board with cultural and organizational training to instill the Nuka philosophy and the basics of quality improvement methods (Gottlieb et al., 2008). The end result is that the primary care team integrates over multiple levels with the wide range of expertise and resources needed to provide whole-person primary care that includes prevention, chronic disease management, acute care, behavioral health, oral care, vision care, and culturally relevant traditional healing.

Intermountain Healthcare

Intermountain Healthcare is a fully integrated delivery system that has consistently produced high-quality outcomes and lower cost through its normative culture of clinical and operational team integration (Reiss-Brennan et al., 2016). Based in Idaho, Nevada, and Utah, Intermountain delivers more than half of all health care in the region through an organized network of 180 primary care clinics, 24 hospitals, and a health insurance plan. Its medical group employs and supports diverse teams of clinicians, but the majority of care is provided by independent, community-based practices. These practices are connected through standard quality metrics and clinical work processes and paid through fee-for-service (FFS) reimbursement. Intermountain has sustained a clinical evidence-based culture designed to help people live the healthiest lives possible and demonstrated improvements in clinical quality and lower costs (James and Savitz, 2011). This integration is built on a common shared culture of high-quality, collaborative teams organized around professional values that focus on individuals' needs, using continuously improved workflows, and robust outcome and process data that drive a single care process model that integrates people, functions, and operations. Intermountain's integration efforts, including the innovative transformation of traditional primary care to an integrated team-based care

TABLE 5-2 Coordinating Mechanisms That Can Support Integrated Primary Care Delivery Through Improved Normative, Interpersonal, and Process Integration

Coordinating Mechanism	Example
Designated role to coordinate care across settings (can be inside or outside of clinic)	• Care coordinators • Patient navigators • Community health workers • Transition teams
Plans and rules	• Treatment plans • Survivorship plans • Protocols • Schedules
Routines	• Team meetings • Huddles/structured team communication • Training/simulation • Multidisciplinary rounding • Callouts (non-hierarchical communication for safety)
Proximity (virtual and real)	• Face-to-face or virtual meeting/interaction • In-person or virtual designated workspaces/colocation • Embedded team support (onsite or virtual navigators)

SOURCE: Adapted from Weaver et al., 2018.

process model for identifying and managing chronic physical and mental health conditions, have produced clinical and cost improvements. Its robust data integration and analytic processes captured the evidence needed for leadership to determine that the $22.19 maximum per-person per-year cost of implementing integrated team-based care in primary care was lower than the overall savings to the whole system ($115.09 per person, per year) and that scaling the innovation held promise for a long-term return on investment for both people seeking care and clinicians (Reiss-Brennan et al., 2016).

Both the SCF Nuka and Intermountain integrated delivery systems have strong structural and functional integration foundations that support their clinical and operational leadership, governance accountability, and investment in promoting cultures of whole-person integrated care while managing overall health care costs continuously over time.

The Blueprint for Health

Launched by the Department of Vermont Health Access in 2003, the Vermont Blueprint for Health (Blueprint) is another example of an integrated primary care system that aims to improve structural, normative, and process integration. The Blueprint is a statewide, whole-population health initiative that supports delivery system reforms in majority rural and "micropolitan" locations (Jones et al., 2016). In addition to supporting primary care practice transformation for patient-centered medical homes (PCMHs), the Blueprint includes important inter-organizational relationships to improve structural integration:

- Community collaboratives that provide leadership by identifying local priorities and allocating resources;
- Community health teams (CHTs) that provide care coordination across health and social services in conjunction with two partner programs: the Vermont Chronic Care Initiative and Support and Services at Home, which integrates subsidized housing for Medicare beneficiaries (RTI International et al., 2017);
- Hub and Spoke, a program for opioid use disorder treatment that partners more than 85 primary care and specialty practices with trainings and resources from the Vermont Department of Health's Division of Alcohol and Drug Abuse Programs, including two CHT team members licensed in mental health or substance abuse; and
- The Women's Health Initiative, designed to improve access to family planning and contraception and support healthy families in both PCMH and obstetrics/gynecology settings, launched in 2017 (AHS, 2019).

The Blueprint also supports process and normative integration by providing education and training programs in the form of a self-management program for community members. It created the Integrated Communities Care Management Learning Collaborative for improving cross-organization care coordination and care management (State of Vermont, 2020).

In 2011, Medicare joined as a payer, and until 2016, Blueprint participated in the Centers for Medicare & Medicaid Services' Multi-Payer Advanced Primary Care Practice Demonstration (RTI International et al., 2017). In the first 2 years, the Blueprint used demonstration funds to hire additional staff for practices and CHTs, including behavioral health specialists, case managers, wellness nurses, social workers, dieticians, pharmacists, and health coaches. During the demonstration, the Blueprint realized $64 million in Medicare net savings relative to comparison PCMH practices, largely attributed to reductions in inpatient and outpatient expenditures; however, it also incurred $40 million in additional Medicaid spending (RTI International et al., 2017), likely the result of the initial increased access and thus increased health care use for a population that previously had high levels of unmet need. Nonetheless, overall medical expenditures decreased by around $5.8 million for every $1 million spent on the Blueprint (Jones et al., 2016). CHTs and Support and Services at Home teams contributed to improved integration by facilitating care continuity and specialist visits and offering services related to population health and chronic disease management that practices were unable to provide on their own (RTI International et al., 2017). These teams improved normative and process integration and helped reduce hospital readmission rates.

Project ECHO (Extension for Community Healthcare Outcomes)

An important example of remote integration, Project ECHO connects governments, academic medical centers, nongovernmental organizations, and centers of excellence around the world to "telementor" clinicians for the purpose of training, enabling collaborative problem solving and co-management of cases, and ultimately improving quality of care in underserved communities (UNM, 2021b). Originally designed by the University of New Mexico for the treatment of hepatitis C, today it operates in 45 countries (UNM, 2021a) and has been used to disseminate clinical training on cancer screening, addiction management, perinatal care, COVID-19 treatment, and many other primary care domains (Archbald-Pannone et al., 2020; Coulson and Galvin, 2020; Francis et al., 2020; Komaromy et al., 2016; Nethan et al., 2020).

With its hub-and-spoke model, Project ECHO enables regular, bidirectional knowledge sharing and collaboration between geographically isolated care team members, fostering new local partnerships, or facilitating the development of new services where they were previously unavailable or insufficient. Project ECHO has been successful, with outcomes including increased knowledge and self-efficacy among clinicians, decreased feelings of professional isolation, increased safety and improved treatment outcomes for patients, and greater ability to enact practice transformation projects (Arora et al., 2008; McDonnell et al., 2020).

The Program of All-Inclusive Care for the Elderly

The Program of All-Inclusive Care for the Elderly (PACE) is a voluntary, community-based medical and social services program available to individuals eligible for nursing home care and living within PACE service areas (CMS, 2021a). PACE is designed to provide whole-person and continuous care to older adults with chronic care needs with the goal of maintaining independent living in their homes for as long as possible. Seen as an effective model of integrated delivery, the program provides all Medicare and Medicaid covered services, including primary care services and health plan management, dentistry, prescription drugs and medication management, nursing care, rehabilitation services, personal and in-home care, specialty services, nutritional counseling, social work counseling, transportation services, and recreation services (CMS, 2021b). Aside from the specialty services, which are provided by referral, the rest of these services operate under the same umbrella. All members of the team—from drivers to those providing recreational services—are trained to observe participants and report their observations to clinical staff. Most participants are dually eligible for Medicare and Medicaid, and PACE financing comes from both programs in prospective capitated payments.

PACE has demonstrated success for participants in reduced hospital use, an increased number of days in the community, fewer unmet needs, and better health overall (Boult and Wieland, 2010; Gonzalez, 2017; Hirth et al., 2009; Meret-Hanke, 2011). However, a 2014 review noted that it is challenging to conduct a rigorous, comparative evaluation of the program and that much of the published research of PACE is weak (Ghosh et al., 2014). The review found PACE offered no cost savings for Medicare and was more costly for Medicaid than other forms of care. Cost studies overall, however, have been somewhat mixed (e.g., a 2014 study found that PACE Medicaid capitation payments demonstrated savings compared to projected FFS estimates for equivalent long-term care) (Wieland et al., 2013). There are currently 138 PACE programs across 31 states (NPA, 2021).

Although the demonstrated outcomes of the aforementioned whole-person, community-specific integrated care delivery models are limited to those systems, considerable evidence exists for more targeted innovations of integration that specifically address the broader national primary care burden of those with mental health and social needs. The sections that follow provide evidence-based practices for integrating behavioral health and social needs in primary care and promising trends for best practice integration for oral and public health. This integration of services allows primary care to shift to a focus on whole-person care, equitable across settings, and supports sustained team relationships that take into account a more complete view of health and well-being in the context of community experiences.

Behavioral Health Integration

The evidence for primary care integration is strongest for a behavioral health–primary care model (Asarnow et al., 2015b; Coventry et al., 2015; McGinty and Daumit, 2020; Miller et al., 2014). Mental health is a growing, costly global priority that has been exacerbated by the COVID-19 pandemic (Holingue et al., 2020). Primary care has historically been the de facto mental health system for many individuals in the United States (Mitchell et al., 2009). Behavioral health concerns are often identified and managed within primary care, and integrating mental and physical health through innovative screening, diagnosis, and team management in primary care increases the likelihood that whole-person care—including behavioral health needs—can be addressed equitably, efficiently, and effectively (Anderson et al., 2015; Foy et al., 2019; Hodgkinson et al., 2017; Miller and Druss, 2013; Miller et al., 2014; Reiss-Brennan, 2014; Reiss-Brennan et al., 2016; Wissow et al., 2016; Xierali et al., 2013). Individuals and families prefer to address their emotional and physical concerns through trusted primary care relationships (NAMI, 2011; Parker et al., 2020) and to be treated as a whole person, not just a disease (Croghan and Brown, 2010; NAMI, 2011). The continuum of the degree of behavioral health–primary care integration between clinicians affects processes of care (Ramanuj et al., 2019). Structural integration ranges from simple coordination and co-location, where the clinicians may be physically nearby without integration within the care process, to collaborative care (Asarnow et al., 2015a). In collaborative care, primary care and behavioral health professionals work together, often with a care manager or coordinator, to care for a shared population such that patients experience a single organized system that treats the whole person (Gerrity, 2016).

Integrated models of primary care and behavioral health can improve normative and process integration; studies have shown that mental and behavioral health team integration produces better health outcomes and lower costs for adults (Archer et al., 2012; Gilbody et al., 2006; Huffman et al., 2014; Katon and Guico-Pabia, 2011; Katon et al., 2010; Reiss-Brennan et al., 2016; Unützer et al., 2013) and improved outcomes for children and adolescents (Asarnow et al., 2015b; Platt et al., 2018).

When served at primary care clinics at which mental health is a routine part of the medical visit, compared to traditional primary care, patients had improved quality of care, lower rates of emergency department (ED) visits, fewer hospital admissions, and lower overall costs for chronic medical conditions (Reiss-Brennan et al., 2016). A meta-analysis of randomized controlled trials of integrated primary care–behavioral health models for children and adolescents demonstrated better outcomes for the integrated care model compared with usual care. The strongest effects were seen for collaborative care models in which primary care clinicians, care managers, and mental health specialists work in a team-based approach to care (Asarnow et al., 2015b). Research has also demonstrated that integrated team-based care is highly effective for patients from ethnic minority groups and reduces health disparities for those populations (Areán et al., 2005; Ell et al., 2009, 2010; Holden et al., 2014; Miranda et al., 2003).

Pediatric populations have fewer complex, high-cost cases with complex medical and behavioral health needs compared to adult populations, making the short-term return on investment (ROI) of integration more elusive. However, the ability to affect adult trajectories of health by transforming primary care to address the social, developmental, and behavioral levers of health more comprehensively during childhood and adolescence can have a much larger effects on ROI over the long term, which would be true for not only health care but also other sectors, such as education, justice, and the workforce.

When compared with FFS Medicaid, a pediatric accountable care organization (ACO) with primary care and behavioral health integration, a population health focus, and an emphasis on care coordination demonstrated a lower rate of cost growth without reducing quality measures or outcomes of care (Kelleher et al., 2015). Integrated care for children and adolescents likely requires a set of supports unique from that for adult care, particularly during expansion. For example, child mental health concerns are inextricably linked to parental mental health and family psychosocial needs, making it imperative to include mechanisms to address and treat parents' and family mental health needs, social needs, and parent–child interaction (Wissow et al., 2020). Furthermore, child mental health is more likely to require more-intensive behavioral treatments and greater investment in team members who can provide these more time-intensive, family-inclusive interventions (Shonkoff and Fisher, 2013), rather than isolated medication management, as may be more typical of adult behavioral health integrated care.

Integrating behavioral health and primary care has been shown to have value for the care of older adults as well. For example, the Improving Mood: Promoting Access to Collaborative Treatment model of depression care for older adults in primary care settings has been associated with better health outcomes, better quality of life, and equal or lower health care costs (Fann et al., 2009; Grympa et al., 2006; Katon et al., 2006; Unützer et al., 2002, 2008). Older adults may be more willing to accept screenings or treatment within a primary care practice rather than being referred to a specialty clinic (Bartels et al., 2004; Samuels et al., 2015). Furthermore, a study of the Primary Care Research in Substance Abuse and Mental Health for the Elderly model showed that primary care clinicians thought that "older adults were more likely to experience greater convenience with less stigma if the mental health services were integrated within the primary care setting" (Gallo et al., 2004, p. 307).

Oral Health Integration

Opportunities to integrate oral health services within primary care settings can benefit high-quality whole-person care for people of all ages. Oral health is an essential component of whole health, given that oral disease negatively affects overall health (HHS, 2000). Young children typically do not make a first visit to a dental office until they are 4 or 5 years old, although recommendations are to do so by the first birthday and cost of care is lower for children with an earlier dental visit (Kolstad et al., 2015).

The American Academy of Pediatrics (AAP) recommends at least 12 preventive care visits in the first 5 years (AAP, 2017, 2020), offering multiple opportunities to provide oral health promotion messages, screen for early childhood caries, and apply preventive fluoride varnish in accordance with recommendations of the United States Preventive Services Task Force and AAP (Clark et al., 2020; Moyer, 2014; Segura et al., 2014). That adults are more likely to visit a physician than a dentist in a given year is another opportunity for preventive interventions and oral health condition management (Lutfiyya et al., 2019). Oral health services offered in the primary care setting improve access, decrease the likelihood of needing general anesthesia for pediatric dental concerns (Meyer et al., 2020) and for seeking dental care services at EDs.

In 2020, 59 million Americans lived in 6,296 federally designated dental shortage areas (HRSA, 2020), with many of these areas in rural regions where primary care medical services are available. These primary care sites may offer the best opportunity for screening and primary oral health prevention services for many people. Integration is feasible in rural practices using public health nurses and dental hygienists as part of a primary care team (Dahlberg et al., 2019; Gnaedinger, 2018). Offering preventive oral health services in the medical home has been shown to increase availability for rural individuals and those of underserved racial/ethnic groups with historically less access (Elani et al., 2020; Kranz et al., 2014).

Primary care–oral health integration is in an early stage of development. Advancing structural integration of dentistry into primary care requires implementation strategies that address systemic barriers in both fields. The most prominent such barrier is that dentistry remains the most siloed of the health professions, with services overwhelmingly delivered by small private offices that are dentist centered and operating independently, meaning less of a professional drive to integrate. In the primary care setting, to accomplish even a basic expansion of oral health services requires additional physician and allied staff education and competencies related to oral health. Other barriers to integration include a low priority because of a lack of understanding of the impact of oral health on health in general, Medicare coverage for dental services, and adult Medicaid coverage in many states (Atchison et al., 2018a).

The best integration of primary care and oral health appears to occur when health systems clearly define and view dental care as central to a broad definition of health care and oral health as an essential part of overall health. A series of case studies of medical and dental integration (Maxey et al., 2017) found it was successful when physicians embraced the importance of oral health and championed integration within their clinics. One model gaining acceptance embeds dental hygienists into pediatric practice (Braun and Cusick, 2016), obstetric practices, and diabetes clinics

(Atchison et al., 2018b). Increasingly, federally qualified health centers (FQHCs) are making room for dental health integration, but it remains fairly uncommon elsewhere (Highmark Foundation, 2009; Langelier et al., 2015; Maxey, 2014).

Social Needs Integration

In 2014, the Robert Wood Johnson Foundation highlighted that medical care has only a fraction of impact on health as compared to other determinants, such as environment and social circumstances (McGovern, 2014). The evidence is clear that social and economic supports, as well as the larger societal structures that support differential access to them, have strong and lasting impact on the health and well-being of individuals, families, and communities (Fichtenberg et al., 2020). However, the evidence of how these SDOH can be most effectively integrated into health care, and into primary care specifically, is still nascent (Gottlieb et al., 2017). Despite the need for more evidence to understand the intricacies of designing, implementing, and sustaining the integration of social needs into primary care, several evidence-based models can guide this integration. Many models of integrated care systems have focused on addressing SDOH, care coordination, and behavioral health needs with a goal of reducing high-cost care for adults with chronic disease (Herrera et al., 2019; NASEM, 2019a). Others, particularly among pediatric populations, have focused on addressing SDOH as a part of more comprehensive preventive care and primary care services (Fierman et al., 2016).

Identifying families with social needs is a first step in primary care–social needs integration. Studies have demonstrated the ability of screening to identify these individuals and families and provide needed referrals (Andermann, 2018; Garg et al., 2016; Herrera et al., 2019). However, both successful connection to these referral sources and a positive impact on health outcomes have been more difficult to achieve (Fiori et al., 2020; Kangovi et al., 2020). Trials of stand-alone screening and referral programs have often failed to demonstrate robust effects on health outcomes, with some studies showing improved health outcomes only for high-risk populations and others demonstrating no or modest effects (Gottlieb et al., 2017; Lindau et al., 2019; Wu et al., 2019). Overall, screening rates for SDOH are low—only 16 percent of physician practices (including primary care practices) surveyed in 2019 screened patients for food insecurity, housing instability, utility needs, transportation needs, and interpersonal violence. Practices providing care for more economically disadvantaged populations reported screening at higher rates (Fraze et al., 2019).

Results have been more promising when addressing social needs is integrated into primary care settings and part of more comprehensive programs that are relationship based (e.g., use a navigator, community health worker [CHW], or home visitor) and considers additional health and health care needs (Dworkin and Garg, 2019; Gottlieb et al., 2016; Kangovi et al., 2020). For example, an intervention in which CHWs provide tailored social support, navigation, and advocacy to help low-income adults with chronic disease achieve health goals demonstrated positive effects on chronic disease control, such as blood sugar levels and body mass index, and health behaviors, such as tobacco use, patient-perceived quality of care, and hospitalization rates (Kangovi et al., 2018; Lohr et al., 2018). To test another model, researchers conducted a trial of a 2-year, longitudinal, home-based, care management intervention for low-income older adults in community-based health centers using a nurse practitioner and social worker as part of an interprofessional team with the primary care clinician. This approach improved quality of care and reduced acute care use (Counsell et al., 2007). These trials illustrate the importance of integrating social needs as a critical element of care, yet in the context of a longitudinal, relationship-based approach.

There are also several examples of integrating social needs by using CHWs in international settings (Palazuelos et al., 2018). In Brazil, as part of the Family Health Strategy initiative, CHWs are fully integrated into primary care teams and regularly consult physician and nurse team members. The initiative serves approximately two-thirds of the Brazilian population, with a focus on lower-income residents. CHWs make at least one monthly visit to each family, regardless of need, to monitor living conditions and health status, support chronic disease management, triage, and provide basic primary care services. The model enables CHWs to collect high-quality data on each individual and is credited with improving inequity in use and outcomes, improving breastfeeding and immunization rates, and decreasing chronic disease–related hospitalizations (Wadge et al., 2016). In Ghana, the Community-based Health Planning and Services program is built on the notion that community engagement is an essential component of a strong primary care system, deploying nurses (deemed "community health officers") who provide door-to-door primary care services (Awoonor-Williams et al., 2020). The Equipo Básico de Atención Integral de Salud (basic integrated health care teams) are the foundation of Costa Rica's primary care system, provide the majority of primary care in the country, and are fully integrated with public health. The teams include a physician, nurse, technical assistant (similar to a CHW), medical clerk, and pharmacist. The technical assistants are responsible for disease prevention and health promotion, sanitation, data collection, and referrals to physicians and hospitals. They engage in community outreach in churches and schools but also make home visits to a geographically empaneled population where they can assist in addressing SDOH overcoming barriers to care (Pesec et al., 2017).

Within child health, team-based approaches to care have been developed and studied to integrate social needs with developmental and behavioral health needs, care coordination, and preventive care needs, with the ultimate goal of positively impacting the child's—and family's—life course (Coker et al., 2013a; Fierman et al., 2016; Mooney et al., 2014). Multiple delivery models for child preventive health have used a team-based approach, incorporating non-clinicians to provide preventive developmental services, address SDOH, and generally improve parents' confidence and efficacy in supporting their child to reach their full potential for health and well-being (Coker et al., 2013b; Freeman and Coker, 2018). These models have demonstrated improved parenting behaviors, parental mental health, and use of preventive care and decreased ED use (Coker et al., 2016; Mendelsohn et al., 2005; Mimila et al., 2017; Minkovitz et al., 2003, 2007). Integrated models for primary care pediatrics that incorporate social needs, particularly for preventive care visits, use strategies such as group care, and employ CHWs, navigators, and health coaches to ensure that the behavioral health and psychosocial needs of families are met (Freeman and Coker, 2018).

The focus on primary care integration is occurring in multiple settings and across a variety of populations. For example, AAP's Addressing Social Health and Early Childhood Wellness Collaborative is a national initiative to help pediatric primary care practices more effectively implement, measure, and continuously improve integration of key social needs services for families with young children, focusing on screening, counseling, referral, and follow-up related to maternal depression, SDOH, and socioemotional development using quality improvement methodology. It includes a technical assistance and resources center to help practices implement effective screening, referral, and follow-up for these three factors. The collaborative has also established a national learning collaborative of pediatric practices (Flower et al., 2020; Georgia AAP, 2020).

The PACE model of care for older adults described earlier in this chapter also exemplifies the importance of integrating social care needs into the primary care of older adults. In another example, the Ambulatory Integration of the Medical and Social (AIMS) model uses social workers to assess social care needs among patients in primary and specialty care and then integrate needed medical and social care services (Newman et al., 2018). Early evidence suggests that use of the AIMS model may be associated with decreased utilization of health care services (Rowe et al., 2016).

Public Health Integration

Our country's fragmented response to the COVID-19 pandemic is a clear manifestation of our failure to implement the 1996 report's recommendations to improve public health–primary care integration so as to better respond to and manage emergencies and natural disasters. It is apparent from the nation's response to the pandemic that both primary care and public health had insufficient resources to meet the demand for testing, contact tracing, and treatment and that collaboration was generally insufficient to support combining forces. One systemic barrier to integrating public health and primary care is that for decades, national plans for a public health crisis have not included the role of primary care (HHS, 2017; Holloway et al., 2014). As the virus spread, communication and preparedness protocols between public health entities and those providing frontline primary care was insufficient. Primary care as a sector lacked the funding and policy support needed to provide maximum assistance during the pandemic (Ali et al., 2020); in fact, because of financial pressures arising from the pandemic (and the lack of support to offset them), many independent physician practices across the country have closed or are the verge of closing.

Primary care capabilities to respond to the immediate and long-term health consequences of the pandemic, including economic, mental and social health complications, requires a high level of integration between public health agencies and primary care practices. Now that several vaccines have been approved and are being distributed across the United States, public health and primary care integration will be critical for reaching vulnerable subpopulations lacking access to care, navigating potential vaccine shortages, and tracking vaccine receipt, while monitoring the epidemiology of the ongoing spread and mutation of the virus.

COVID-19 has impacted racial and ethnic minority populations disproportionately, both directly and indirectly, with staggering increases in morbidity and mortality in Black, Hispanic, and Indigenous populations (Azar et al., 2020; Price-Haywood et al., 2020; Vahidy et al., 2020). As a result of pre-existing and systemic inequities in family wealth, housing access, employment, education, and other key factors that affect families' well-being, Black, Hispanic, Indigenous, and other people of color will disproportionately experience negative, long-term effects on their health and well-being. These communities, more acutely than others, will face an urgent and critical need for integrated, supportive public health and primary care services and interventions to buffer the disproportionate negative health impact of job loss, morbidity and mortality, gaps in education, and increased overall toxic stress during the pandemic and a recovery period.

Despite calls for greater integration of public health and primary care (AAFP Integration of Primary Care and Public Health Work Group, 2015; IOM, 1996, 2012; Welton et al., 1997), primary care practices, public health agencies, and community-based organizations continue to operate separately for the most part, other than large-scale health screening and immunization efforts and literacy promotion and lifestyle modification initiatives (Levesque et al., 2013; Scutchfield et al., 2012). While some progress has been made, including the Centers for Disease Control and Prevention's attempts to integrate population health into graduate medical education competencies and numerous demonstration programs that work toward integration (CDC, 2016), true integration remains limited.

Benefits of Public Health Integration

Public health–primary care integration has many benefits beyond crisis situations. A close partnership can improve the treatment of chronic conditions and increase the effectiveness and enhance dissemination of prevention and health promotion. Integration also increases the capacity of primary care to influence public health, by bringing a larger focus to the health of a community through connected healing and trusted relationships, thereby reaching individuals and their families who otherwise may not access primary care services. Public health nursing programs, such as Nurse–Family Partnerships, show cost-effectiveness for reaching high-risk families (Wu et al., 2017). Schools and day care centers are integration avenues, with opportunities to reach children, adolescents, and their families. Other "third places,"[1] such as senior centers, places of worship, adult day care facilities, barber shops and beauty salons, and libraries, can increase access to services for older adults (Keeton et al., 2012; Northridge et al., 2016; Riley et al., 2016).

Comprehensive Data Integration

Achieving the most effective integration of primary care and public health requires integrating the data that these two sectors produce, which supports process integration protocols within and across settings to monitor and improve outcomes. Cross-sector data integration for enhanced community and population health interventions within primary care is a key area of opportunity, particularly to expand the reach of a traditional primary care setting. Primary care practice data can help public health professionals conduct surveillance and community assessments, while access to public health data for primary care team members can allow them to observe information on community needs beyond the "micro" practice level and conduct proactive risk identification (IOM, 2012). A prime example of this is Hennepin Health in Minnesota, an ACO with four partners: the Hennepin County Human Services and Public Health Department; the Hennepin County Medical Center; NorthPoint Health, an FQHC; and the

---

[1] "Third places" are public places on neutral ground where people may gather, enjoy the company of others, and interact (Oldenburg, 1989).

Metropolitan Health Plan, a nonprofit, county-run Medicaid managed care plan. The technological centerpiece of the ACO includes three elements:

- a unified electronic health record system shared by all partners;
- electronic data dashboards that provide information tailored to team member needs; and
- an integrated data warehouse that incorporates data from health plan claims and enrollment, the electronic health record (EHR), and social service records (Sandberg et al., 2014).

During a 2016 analysis, Hennepin Health—the default option for newly eligible Medicaid beneficiaries in Hennepin County who do not select a plan—was working to incorporate nonmedical information from housing providers, the foster care system, the corrections department, and other local agencies (Hostetter et al., 2016). By sharing data, the ACO could stratify members into risk tiers and send CHWs and social workers to connect those at the highest risk to primary care and the other medical, behavioral, or social services. Often, these individuals likely would not have a relationship with primary care otherwise (Sandberg et al., 2014).

Comparing Hennepin's second and third years of operation, it saw a 9.1 percent overall decrease of ED visits and a 3.3 percent increase of outpatient primary care visits. For members receiving housing assistance through Hennepin, who account for up to 50 percent of members, ED visits fell by 35 percent and outpatient clinic visits, including to primary care, increased by 21 percent (Hostetter et al., 2016). In redesigning the way public health entities interacted with primary care settings in Hennepin County, as opposed to creating new programs or relying on additional funding, Hennepin Health has been able to sustain its integrated partnerships.

Specialist and Hospitalist Integration

Key to high-functioning primary care teams is a readily available system for referral of patients from primary care to specialist care when needed. From 1999 to 2009, referrals in the United States from primary care to specialty care more than doubled from 41 million to 105 million (Barnett et al., 2012). Unfortunately, there is little evidence that effective coordination is the norm between the specialist, primary care team, and the patient. Currently, patients with multiple chronic conditions often receive care from multiple specialty groups, adding to duplication in services, inconvenience with making follow-up appointments across multiple providers, and potential medical error with one specialist being unaware of the treatment protocol being prescribed by another specialist (Vimalananda et al., 2018). Studies have shown that well-coordinated primary and specialty services lead to reductions in acute care and more efficient use of specialty care

(Newman et al., 2019). Three factors could improve this process including clear communication and buy-in between services, EHR interoperability, and engagement of the patient and family in care coordination.

While patients should be referred for specialist care in complex situations, the referral process should not mean that the primary care service is abdicating their role in the management of the patient's condition. Shared responsibility is necessary to have a fully integrated care model. Furthermore, when a primary care team's patient is hospitalized, the team should manage the care or coordinate care with hospitalists to ensure that knowledge of the patient and family is available, coordinate as the patient nears discharge, and manage care post-discharge. Studies have shown that poor care coordination affects patient clinical outcomes and satisfaction with their care. Coordination across settings affects patients' clinical outcomes and satisfaction with their care (Weinberg et al., 2007). Systems should support shared responsibility between the primary care team and the hospital team for inpatient care and for informed transitions back to primary care.

IMPLEMENTATION FACILITATORS: HOW TO INTEGRATE PRIMARY CARE DELIVERY

Even when organizations are successful delivering consistently high quality or value through integrated processes, the approaches they use and lessons they learn are not easily scaled beyond their walls because of the unique structures and resources of the local environment. However, though individual characteristics of these high-performing organizations may differ, they do share four similar delivery habits—repeated behaviors and activities and the ways of thinking that they reflect and engender (Bohmer, 2011)—that are integrated systematically into the organizational culture, workflows, and clinical management focused on outcomes and building value. The leaders of these organizations routinely invest in the following:

1. planning and developing specifications well in advance of implementation, enabling them to integrate operational and clinical decision making with explicit criteria and parse heterogeneous patient populations into clinically meaningful subtypes;
2. infrastructure design of microsystems—staff, information technologies, clinical technologies, physical space, business processes, and policies and procedures supporting patient care—to match their subpopulation with workflows, training, and how they allocate resources to the different members of the clinical team;
3. measurement and oversight designed for internal process controls and performance rather than being driven by the need to report to external regulators, payers, and rating agencies; and

4. self-study to examine positive and negative deviances in care and outcomes, ensure their clinical practices are consistent with latest science, and create new knowledge and innovations (Bohmer, 2011).

When considering how integrated delivery provides the context to achieve high-quality primary care, these habits highlight the normative culture that organizations can promote to support implementing and adopting the following facilitators.

Digital Health Integration

Digital technology with data system integration is a key facilitator of integrated care delivery and foundational to achieving accessible high-quality primary care. As noted in Chapter 1, no other aspect of patient care delivery has changed as much since the 1996 Institute of Medicine (IOM) report as the ubiquitous use of digital technology, which is playing an important role in disrupting the paternalistic status quo of care and transforming primary care into more equitable partnerships between individuals and their primary care team (Meskó et al., 2017). At the same time, digital health technologies support collecting and organizing person-generated health care data that can generate new findings and new analytical tools to improve person-centered care (Sharma et al., 2018). These technologies allow individuals to access their own data, interact remotely with their care team, and even provide real-time monitoring and diagnostic information that can better inform treatment (Buis, 2019).

Digital health tools and innovations can be a critical element of true integrated care delivery. For example, text messaging, telehealth, and app-based tools can extend the services, and thus impact, of a single primary care visit (Coker et al., 2019; Levin et al., 2011; Stockwell et al., 2012; van Grieken et al., 2017). See Chapter 7 for more on digital health in primary care.

Accountability Integration

Accountability for developing, implementing, governing, and monitoring integrated team-based care is a critical facilitator for measuring high-quality primary care outcomes. Accountability requires that the normative integration culture values measured self-study and empirical evidence that facilitates improvements over time and demonstrates and quantifies that primary care adds value to the overall health care system. The successful integrated delivery systems noted earlier had explicit processes for accountability and evaluation.

Payment Model Integration

Investing in integrated care to deliver high-quality primary care while reducing cost and the strain on resources remains a promising global solution to disparities in access and reducing overall health care cost. However, the cost-effectiveness of integrated care remains unclear except when integrated delivery systems conducted follow-up assessments for a sufficient time to compensate for implementation costs and reflect long-term benefits (Rocks et al., 2020).

There are limited examples of whole-person, integrated care delivery models with a supportive payment system that researchers have studied rigorously and produced findings to demonstrate improved care and decreased overall costs of care. Partners for Kids, an Ohio ACO, receives a per-member, per-month payment—the average of the age- and gender-adjusted capitated fee for each child enrollee per month—through the five state Medicaid managed care plans. While Partners for Kids takes full financial and clinical risk for its Medicaid enrollees, it also retains any savings from the cost of care. The delivery model incorporated team-based care with non-clinicians, behavioral health integration, care coordination, and a focus on population health. When compared with FFS Medicaid, this program demonstrated a lower rate of cost growth without reducing quality measures or outcomes of care (Kelleher et al., 2015).

Hennepin Health offers a broad array of integrated services, including care coordination, behavioral health, and dental care. Its evaluation of newly onboarded, very low-income adults during Medicaid expansion found that 6 months of continuous enrollment was associated with less use of the ED and hospital and more use of primary and dental care (Vickery et al., 2020).

Integrated Care for Kids (InCK) is a child- and family-centered integrated delivery care model with a matched state payment model for children insured by Medicaid or the Children's Health Insurance Program. The model aims to reduce expenditures and improve the quality of care for children and adolescents from birth to age 21 through prevention, early identification, and treatment of behavioral and physical health needs. Seven states received federal funding at the start of 2020 to launch this system, with a sustainable alternative payment model to support it.[2] Initiatives such as InCK explicitly require a state-specific alternative payment model that aligns payment with care quality and health outcomes and has the goal of long-term sustainability.

While an aligned payment system is integral to short- and long-term sustainability of integrated primary care delivery, it is also critical to have

---

[2] Additional information is available at https://innovation.cms.gov/innovation-models/integrated-care-for-kids-model (accessed February 14, 2021).

the financial resources to support design and implementation activities and the initial start-up of an integrated primary care practice. In fact, barriers to implementing integrated primary care delivery include the high start-up costs for cultural and quality transformation; hiring and training the primary care team, including team members focused on chronic and preventive care (Peikes et al., 2014); and hiring team members who deliver behavioral health services (Beil et al., 2019).

Implementing Team-Based Integrated Primary Care at the Practice and Clinic Levels

Meeting the committee's definition of high-quality primary care (see Chapter 2) requires coordinated integrated care delivery structures and processes. Integrated care delivery galvanizes the shift of primary care from a procedural service to the relational provision of whole-person care that produces person, family, and community health and well-being.

Integration on a structural level that includes interprofessional teams that provide whole-person care to individuals and families is required for success. Creating the structural elements of integration is generally the first step for primary care practices and clinics. Implementing these structural elements can begin with asking the basic question of what range of services to include in an integrated model of care (e.g., behavioral health, social services, oral health care, pharmacy services, complex care coordination) to meet the needs of the population and then developing an understanding of the interprofessional team needed to provide, coordinate, and engage individuals and families in this care (e.g., care coordinators, CHWs, therapists) (Starfield, 1998). The team members will likely need to develop external partnerships with community resources outside of the traditional health care team (e.g., schools, day care centers, pharmacies). Finally, once the range of services, team, composition, and community partnerships have been established for high-quality primary care, a practice must determine what supportive structural elements. These can include a governance structure to hold leadership accountable to ensuring that primary care addresses community needs, information systems and workflow to support team communication and coordination while keeping the individual and family central to care, and financing that can support the independent contributions of each team member to meet the specific needs of individuals and families (see Figure 5-2).

Many practices and clinics will face challenges paying for many of the structures needed for team-based integrated care. Without these structures, however, practices will not fully develop the processes needed for high-quality primary care. Prior to the widespread use of hybrid payment models that better support team-based integrated care, some practices will be able to capitalize on the efficiencies gained in team-based care that shift preventive care, chronic care management, and social needs support to other team members, which can allow primary care clinicians to use their time more efficiently to address more complex medical needs.

Small practices, especially those in rural settings, may have additional challenges of finding personnel, independent of payment mechanisms, for integrated team-based care. These practices will likely rely more on external community partnerships for a more virtual integration of behavioral health, social needs, oral health, and public health. Small practices without the space, personnel, or resources to support the team necessary for integrated care can also band together to benefit from economies of scale (Mostashari, 2016) by sharing centralized personnel and other necessary resources that are otherwise not available at the practice level for team-based integrated care. The exponential expansion of telehealth and virtual visits also provides a feasible option for care delivery using shared resources across practices. For example, small- and medium-sized practices that participate in independent practice associations and physician–hospital organizations are more likely to have care management processes for adults with chronic conditions (Casalino et al., 2013). Practices may also consider incorporating CHWs (Kangovi et al., 2020) or pharmacists into their primary care to meet the needs of individuals and families.

Research Integration

As alluded to above, several areas for care delivery integration would benefit from more research, such as to establish the training requirements for effectively translating behavioral health interventions for primary care settings and community-based delivery that is more culturally relevant and logistically feasible for individuals and families (e.g., matching the number of therapeutic contacts and non-face-to-face formats for specified behavioral health interventions). Research should also be conducted to help primary care settings have a more adaptable framework for implementing integrated care that can meet their internal business and community-specific needs and determine how to best take advantage of the expanding role of digital and eHealth tools in integrated care. It is also critical that all research focused on continuous relationships and care integration be targeted to the populations that face the widest health inequities as a means of reducing these inequities (Lion and Raphael, 2015).

Leadership Integration

Strong, committed, and collective leadership is one of the most important facilitators of building and leading teams of practices through the

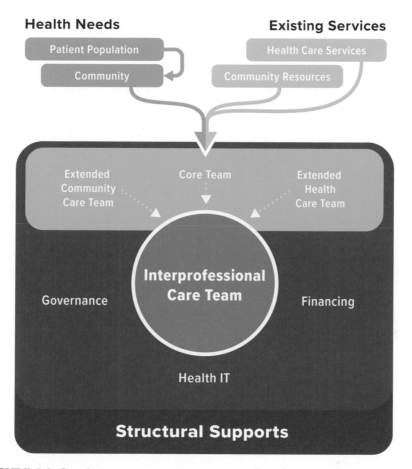

FIGURE 5-2 Creating a structure to support team-based integrated care.
NOTE: IT = information technology.

inherently challenging processes of culture change and integrating whole-person care across settings. While Chapter 1 discussed how the lack of leadership at local, state, and national levels played a central role in the failure of the 1996 IOM recommendations to take hold in primary care, leadership at the practice level is also important for successful transformation to person- and family-centered and community-oriented practice. One study found, for example, that practices with higher leadership scores had higher odds of making changes (Donahue et al., 2013). A systematic review, however, found little research on the effectiveness of clinical leadership on integrated primary care practice and outcomes for individuals (Nieuwboer et al., 2019). What research has identified are two important leadership styles that appear to contribute to fostering integrated care: collective leadership that influences team members based on social interactions (Forsyth and Mason, 2017) and transformational leadership that achieves change through charisma and motivational approaches that get staff to achieve more than what is expected of them and challenges staff to look beyond self-interest (Dionne et al., 2014).

Several research groups and organizations have created programs for developing leaders to support team-based primary care. One effort funded by the Robert Wood Johnson Foundation developed the 12-month Emerging Leaders program to "demonstrate the relevance of an interdisciplinary cohort approach to leadership development; model a new way of working across silos in teams"; and enhance multiple aspects of leadership development, including confidence and skill development (Coleman et al., 2019, p. 2). One element was the policy of reimbursing practices for the expense of covering staff who participated. At the organizational level, the American Academy of Family Physicians has established the Primary Care Leadership Collaborative,[3] which supports medical student teams committed to advancing primary care and improving the health of their communities.

Policy, Laws, and Regulations

Health centers are leaders in adoption of specific PCMH elements that can facilitate implementing integrated care. These elements include onsite behavioral health or social workers, an onsite care coordinator/patient navigator, routine comprehensive health assessments, including SDOH, referrals based on SDOH, and clinical tools and resources to address SDOH (Rittenhouse et al., 2020). To enable this level of integration, the Health Resources and Services Administration's policies stipulate providing critical resources: technical assistance, a related national cooperative agreement with the National Committee for Quality Assurance (NCQA) to facilitate certification, funds to pay for certification, and financial incentives, including increased payments for quality for health centers that were NCQA recognized. The onsite availability of these services (behavioral health, social work) represents a structural facilitator for implementing integrated primary care delivery, but it is not sufficient to achieve sustained implementation of integrated care. From the Theory of Integration discussed earlier, these health centers would possess the organizational features of structural integration and then need ongoing measurement and monitoring to further implement the functional, normative, interpersonal, and process elements of integration to achieve integrated primary care.

---

[3] Additional information is available at https://www.aafp.org/students-residents/medical-students/fmig/pclc.html (accessed February 14, 2021).

FINDINGS AND CONCLUSIONS

Evidence supports structures and processes that incorporate the elements necessary for optimal, whole-person health, including integrating behavioral health services, oral health care, social needs, and population and public health. While many structures of primary care integration are still underdeveloped, the evidence is convincing that behavioral health integration for both child and adult populations is effective at improving clinical outcomes and lowering costs and should be advanced, scaled, and accessible immediately. This evidence is evolving for social, public health, and oral health integration as well. Several examples of integrated high-quality primary care include functional integration across various areas and demonstrate evidence of improved clinical outcomes and higher quality of care without large spending increases and sometimes even reduced costs in the short run (Kelleher et al., 2015). The most successful models, and thus sustainable ones, are likely to have payment systems and a leadership structure that promote a strong culture of functional integration and the production of high-quality outcomes. Integration, however, is not one size fits all—practices and systems should strive to integrate services based on the needs of the community they serve. Practices in locations where resources are scant can partner with each other to pool resources, connect virtually to needed services, and consider including additional team members such as CHWs or pharmacists into their practices.

For primary care integration to advance, payment systems will need to move away from FFS and toward mandatory hybrid models or other alternative models, including ACO models, in which organizations can reap the financial benefits of improving health and well-being, and provide incentives to invest in start-up costs associated with planning, specifying, and designing the infrastructure of an effective integrated delivery system that thrives on interprofessional teams for high-quality care. These payment models must also consider the long-term savings in investments in prevention, health promotion, coordinated and whole-person and family-centered chronic care management, and early diagnostic and treatment services, which may impact sectors outside of health care, including education, social services, and the justice system. Thus, new payment models, including value-based payment, must account for and incentivize these additional outcomes.

In addition to policies and payment structures not explicitly supporting integrated primary care delivery, care transformation and value-based payment initiatives can have downsides. Clinicians may game performance to avoid penalties (Sjoding et al., 2015) and incur high administrative costs to report measures for external incentive programs (Casalino et al., 2016).

Hybrid payment with multi-payer alignment would reduce administrative burden (including data collection) and limit the need for condition-specific, value-based payments, while encouraging expanded use of CHWs, health coaches, and other staff who can support integrated care delivery.

Aligned structures, policies, and leadership are not sufficient for sustainable integrated care; each delivery system must create clear systematic implementation processes, including clinical and operational workflows that allow teams to work together to meet the individual and complex medical, social, and behavioral health needs of individuals and families. These processes will often include digital or eHealth innovations and a clear system for data collection, measurement, and "self-study" continuous improvement, which will produce innovations equitably matched to improve health at the community or population level.

Innovative integrated care delivery models will likely continue to expand in the private sector, particularly as the for-profit, direct-to-consumer industry of personalized and concierge health care grows. However, to stop the continued growth of health inequities for low-income, Black, brown, and Indigenous communities, it will be important to develop and implement policies, payment structures, and other facilitators that will advance health equity and allow everyone to receive high-quality, integrated primary care. If primary care remains the largest platform for continuous, relationship-based care in the United States, one that considers the needs and preferences of individuals, families, and communities, then this essential function of providing health care value requires significant investment in implementing already proven integrated delivery methods and structures for all.

REFERENCES

AAFP (American Academy of Family Physicians) Integration of Primary Care and Public Health Work Group. 2015. *Integration of primary care and public health (position paper).* https://www.aafp.org/about/policies/all/integration-primary-care.html (accessed November 20, 2020).

AAP (American Academy of Pediatrics). 2017. *Bright futures: Guidelines for health supervision of infants, children and adolescents*, 4th ed. Itasca, IL: American Academy of Pediatrics.

AAP. 2020. *Recommendations for preventive pediatric health care.* Itasca, IL: American Academy of Pediatrics.

AHRQ (Agency for Healthcare Research and Quality). 2013. *Lexicon for behavioral health and primary care integration.* Rockville, MD: Agency for Healthcare Research and Quality.

AHS (Vermont Agency of Human Services). 2019. *Blueprint for health 101.* Montpelier, VT: Vermont Agency of Human Services.

Ali, M. K., D. J. Shah, and C. Del Rio. 2020. Preparing primary care for COVID-20. *Journal of General Internal Medicine.* Epub ahead of print.

Andermann, A. 2018. Screening for social determinants of health in clinical care: Moving from the margins to the mainstream. *Public Health Reviews* 39:19.

Anderson, L. E., M. L. Chen, J. M. Perrin, and J. Van Cleave. 2015. Outpatient visits and medication prescribing for U.S. children with mental health conditions. *Pediatrics* 136(5):e1178–e1185.

Archbald-Pannone, L. R., D. A. Harris, K. Albero, R. L. Steele, A. F. Pannone, and J. B. Mutter. 2020. COVID-19 collaborative model for an academic hospital and long-term care facilities. *Journal of the American Medical Directors Association* 21(7):939–942.

Archer, J., P. Bower, S. Gilbody, K. Lovell, D. Richards, L. Gask, C. Dickens, and P. Coventry. 2012. Collaborative care for depression and anxiety problems. *Cochrane Database of Systematic Reviews* 10:CD006525.

Areán, P. A., L. Ayalon, E. Hunkeler, E. H. Lin, L. Tang, L. Harpole, H. Hendrie, J. W. Williams, Jr., and J. Unützer. 2005. Improving depression care for older, minority patients in primary care. *Medical Care* 43(4):381–390.

Arora, S., C. Fassler, L. Marsh, T. Holmes, G. Murata, S. Kalishman, D. Dion, J. Scaletti, W. Pak, and T. Peterson. 2008. *Project ECHO: Extension for Community Healthcare Outcomes.* Rockville, MD: Agency for Healthcare Research and Quality.

Asarnow, J. R., K. E. Hoagwood, T. Stancin, J. E. Lochman, J. L. Hughes, J. M. Miranda, T. Wysocki, S. G. Portwood, J. Piacentini, D. Tynan, M. Atkins, and A. E. Kazak. 2015a. Psychological science and innovative strategies for informing health care redesign: A policy brief. *Journal of Clinical Child and Adolescent Psychology* 44(6):923–932.

Asarnow, J. R., M. Rozenman, J. Wiblin, and L. Zeltzer. 2015b. Integrated medical-behavioral care compared with usual primary care for child and adolescent behavioral health: A meta-analysis. *JAMA Pediatrics* 169(10):929–937.

Atchison, K. A., R. G. Rozier, and J. A. Weintraub. 2018a. *Integration of oral health and primary care: Communication, coordination, and referral. NAM Perspectives.* Discussion Paper, National Academy of Medicine, Washington, DC.

Atchison, K. A., J. A. Weintraub, and R. G. Rozier. 2018b. Bridging the dental-medical divide: Case studies integrating oral health care and primary health care. *Journal of the American Dental Association* 149(10):850–858.

Awoonor-Williams, J. K., E. Tadiri, and H. Ratcliffe. 2020. Translating research into practice to ensure community engagement for successful primary health care service delivery: The case of CHPS in Ghana. *PHCPI.* https://improvingphc.org/translating-research-practice-ensure-community-engagement-successful-primary-health-care-service-delivery-case-chps-ghana (accessed November 18, 2020).

Azar, K. M. J., Z. Shen, R. J. Romanelli, S. H. Lockhart, K. Smits, S. Robinson, S. Brown, and A. R. Pressman. 2020. Disparities in outcomes among COVID-19 patients in a large health care system in California. *Health Affairs* 39(7):1253–1262.

Barnett, M. L., Z. Song, and B. E. Landon. 2012. Trends in physician referrals in the United States, 1999–2009. *Archives of Internal Medicine* 172(2):163–170.

Bartels, S. J., E. H. Coakley, C. Zubritsky, J. H. Ware, K. M. Miles, P. A. Areán, H. Chen, D. W. Oslin, M. D. Llorente, G. Costantino, L. Quijano, J. S. McIntyre, K. W. Linkins, T. E. Oxman, J. Maxwell, and S. E. Levkoff. 2004. Improving access to geriatric mental health services: A randomized trial comparing treatment engagement with integrated versus enhanced referral care for depression, anxiety, and at-risk alcohol use. *American Journal of Psychiatry* 161(8):1455–1462.

Beil, H., R. K. Feinberg, S. V. Patel, and M. A. Romaire. 2019. Behavioral health integration with primary care: Implementation experience and impacts from the State Innovation Model Round 1 states. *Milbank Quarterly* 97(2):543–582.

Bitton, A., J. H. Veillard, L. Basu, H. L. Ratcliffe, D. Schwarz, and L. R. Hirschhorn. 2018. The 5S-5M-5C schematic: Transforming primary care inputs to outcomes in low-income and middle-income countries. *BMJ Global Health* 3(Suppl 3):e001020.

Bohmer, R. M. 2011. The four habits of high-value health care organizations. *New England Journal of Medicine* 365(22):2045–2047.

Boult, C., and G. D. Wieland. 2010. Comprehensive primary care for older patients with multiple chronic conditions: "Nobody rushes you through." *JAMA* 304(17):1936–1943.

Braun, P. A., and A. Cusick. 2016. Collaboration between medical providers and dental hygienists in pediatric health care. *Journal of Evidence Based Dental Practice* 16:59–67.

Browne, A. J., C. M. Varcoe, S. T. Wong, V. L. Smye, J. Lavoie, D. Littlejohn, D. Tu, O. Godwin, M. Krause, K. B. Khan, A. Fridkin, P. Rodney, J. O'Neil, and S. Lennox. 2012. Closing the health equity gap: Evidence-based strategies for primary health care organizations. *International Journal for Equity in Health* 11(1).

Buckley, D. I., P. McGinnis, L. J. Fagnan, R. Mardon, J. Johnson, Maurice, and C. Dymek. 2013. *Clinical-community relationships evaluation roadmap.* Rockville, MD: Agency for Healthcare Research and Quality.

Buis, L. 2019. Implementation: The next giant hurdle to clinical transformation with digital health. *Journal of Medical Internet Research* 21(11):e16259.

Casalino, L. P., F. M. Wu, A. M. Ryan, K. Copeland, D. R. Rittenhouse, P. P. Ramsay, and S. M. Shortell. 2013. Independent practice associations and physician-hospital organizations can improve care management for smaller practices. *Health Affairs* 32(8):1376–1382.

Casalino, L. P., D. Gans, R. Weber, M. Cea, A. Tuchovsky, T. F. Bishop, Y. Miranda, B. A. Frankel, K. B. Ziehler, M. M. Wong, and T. B. Evenson. 2016. U.S. physician practices spend more than $15.4 billion annually to report quality measures. *Health Affairs* 35(3):401–406.

CDC (Centers for Disease Control and Prevention). 2016. *Advancing integration of population health into graduate medical education.* https://www.cdc.gov/csels/dsepd/academic-partnerships/wip/milestone.html (accessed August 5, 2020).

Clark, M. B., M. A. Keels, and R. L. Slayton. 2020. Fluoride use in caries prevention in the primary care setting. *Pediatrics* 146(6):e2020034637.

CMS (Centers for Medicare & Medicaid Services). 2021a. *Program of all-inclusive care for the elderly.* https://www.medicaid.gov/medicaid/long-term-services-supports/program-all-inclusive-care-elderly/index.html (accessed February 11, 2021).

CMS. 2021b. *Programs of all-inclusive care for the elderly benefits.* https://www.medicaid.gov/medicaid/long-term-services-supports/pace/programs-all-inclusive-care-elderly-benefits/index.html (accessed February 11, 2021).

Coker, T. R., T. Thomas, and P. J. Chung. 2013a. Does well-child care have a future in pediatrics? *Pediatrics* 131(Suppl 2):S149–S159.

Coker, T. R., A. Windon, C. Moreno, M. A. Schuster, and P. J. Chung. 2013b. Well-child care clinical practice redesign for young children: A systematic review of strategies and tools. *Pediatrics* 131(Suppl 1):S5–S25.

Coker, T. R., S. Chacon, M. N. Elliott, Y. Bruno, T. Chavis, C. Biely, C. D. Bethell, S. Contreras, N. A. Mimila, J. Mercado, and P. J. Chung. 2016. A parent coach model for well-child care among low-income children: A randomized controlled trial. *Pediatrics* 137(3):e20153013.

Coker, T. R., L. Porras-Javier, L. Zhang, N. Soares, C. Park, A. Patel, L. Tang, P. J. Chung, and B. T. Zima. 2019. A telehealth-enhanced referral process in pediatric primary care: A cluster randomized trial. *Pediatrics* 143(3).

Coleman, K., E. H. Wagner, M. D. Ladden, M. Flinter, D. Cromp, C. Hsu, B. F. Crabtree, and S. McDonald. 2019. Developing emerging leaders to support team-based primary care. *The Journal of Ambulatory Care Management* 42(4).

Colwill, J. M., J. J. Frey, M. A. Baird, J. W. Kirk, and W. W. Rosser. 2016. Patient relationships and the personal physician in tomorrow's health system: A perspective from the Keystone IV conference. *Journal of the American Board of Family Medicine* 29(Suppl 1):S54–S59.

Coulson, C. C., and S. Galvin. 2020. Navigating perinatal care in western North Carolina: Access for patients and providers. *North Carolina Medical Journal* 81(1):41–44.

Counsell, S. R., C. M. Callahan, D. O. Clark, W. Tu, A. B. Buttar, T. E. Stump, and G. D. Ricketts. 2007. Geriatric care management for low-income seniors: A randomized controlled trial. *JAMA* 298(22):2623–2633.

Coventry, P., K. Lovell, C. Dickens, P. Bower, C. Chew-Graham, D. McElvenny, M. Hann, A. Cherrington, C. Garrett, C. J. Gibbons, C. Baguley, K. Roughley, I. Adeyemi, D. Reeves, W. Waheed, and L. Gask. 2015. Integrated primary care for patients with mental and physical multimorbidity: Cluster randomised controlled trial of collaborative care for patients with depression comorbid with diabetes or cardiovascular disease. *BMJ* 350:h638.

Croghan, T. W., and J. D. Brown. 2010. *Integrating mental health treatment into the patient centered medical home*. Rockville, MD: Agency for Healthcare Research and Quality.

Dahlberg, D., D. B. Hiott, and C. C. Wilson. 2019. Implementing pediatric fluoride varnish application in a rural primary care medical office: A feasibility study. *Journal of Pediatric Health Care* 33(6):702–710.

Dionne, S. D., A. Gupta, K. L. Sotak, K. A. Shirreffs, A. Serban, C. Hao, D. H. Kim, and F. J. Yammarino. 2014. A 25-year perspective on levels of analysis in leadership research. *Leadership Quarterly* 25(1):6–35.

Donahue, K. E., J. R. Halladay, A. Wise, K. Reiter, S.-Y. D. Lee, K. Ward, M. Mitchell, and B. Qaqish. 2013. Facilitators of transforming primary care: A look under the hood at practice leadership. *Annals of Family Medicine* 11(Suppl 1):S27–S33.

Dworkin, P. H., and A. Garg. 2019. Considering approaches to screening for social determinants of health. *Pediatrics* 144(4):e20192395.

Elani, H. W., I. Kawachi, and B. D. Sommers. 2020. Changes in emergency department dental visits after Medicaid expansion. *Health Services Research* 55(3):367–374.

Ell, K., W. Katon, L. J. Cabassa, B. Xie, P. J. Lee, S. Kapetanovic, and J. Guterman. 2009. Depression and diabetes among low-income Hispanics: Design elements of a socioculturally adapted collaborative care model randomized controlled trial. *International Journal of Psychiatry in Medicine* 39(2):113–132.

Ell, K., M. P. Aranda, B. Xie, P. J. Lee, and C. P. Chou. 2010. Collaborative depression treatment in older and younger adults with physical illness: Pooled comparative analysis of three randomized clinical trials. *American Journal of Geriatric Psychiatry* 18(6):520–530.

Ellner, A. L., and R. S. Phillips. 2017. The coming primary care revolution. *Journal of General Internal Medicine* 32(4):380–386.

Fann, J. R., M. Y. Fan, and J. Unützer. 2009. Improving primary care for older adults with cancer and depression. *Journal of General Internal Medicine* 24(Suppl 2):S417–S424.

Fichtenberg, C., J. Delva, K. Minyard, and L. M. Gottlieb. 2020. Health and human services integration: Generating sustained health and equity improvements. *Health Affairs* 39(4):567–573.

Fierman, A. H., A. F. Beck, E. K. Chung, M. M. Tschudy, T. R. Coker, K. B. Mistry, B. Siegel, L. J. Chamberlain, K. Conroy, S. G. Federico, P. J. Flanagan, A. Garg, B. A. Gitterman, A. M. Grace, R. S. Gross, M. K. Hole, P. Klass, C. Kraft, A. Kuo, G. Lewis, K. S. Lobach, D. Long, C. T. Ma, D. Messito, D. Navsaria, K. R. Northrip, C. Osman, M. D. Sadof, A. B. Schickedanz, and J. Cox. 2016. Redesigning health care practices to address childhood poverty. *Academic Pediatrics* 16(Suppl 3):S136–S146.

Fiori, K. P., C. D. Rehm, D. Sanderson, S. Braganza, A. Parsons, T. Chodon, R. Whiskey, P. Bernard, and M. L. Rinke. 2020. Integrating social needs screening and community health workers in primary care: The community linkage to care program. *Clinical Pediatrics* 59(6):547–556.

Flieger, S. P. 2017. Implementing the patient-centered medical home in complex adaptive systems: Becoming a relationship-centered patient-centered medical home. *Health Care Management Review* 42(2):112–121.

Flower, K. B., S. Massie, K. Janies, J. B. Bassewitz, T. R. Coker, R. J. Gillespie, M. M. Macias, T. M. Whitaker, J. Zubler, D. Steinberg, L. DeStigter, and M. F. Earls. 2020. Increasing early childhood screening in primary care through a quality improvement collaborative. *Pediatrics* 146(3):e20192328.

Forsyth, C., and B. Mason. 2017. Shared leadership and group identification in healthcare: The leadership beliefs of clinicians working in interprofessional teams. *Journal of Interprofessional Education & Practice* 31(3):291–299.

Foy, J. M., C. M. Green, and M. F. Earls. 2019. Mental health competencies for pediatric practice. *Pediatrics* 144(5).

Francis, E., K. Shifler Bowers, G. Buchberger, S. Ryan, W. Milchak, and J. Kraschnewski. 2020. Reducing alcohol and opioid use among youth in rural counties: An innovative training protocol for primary health care providers and school personnel. *JMIR Research Protocols* 9(11):e21015.

Fraze, T. K., A. L. Brewster, V. A. Lewis, L. B. Beidler, G. F. Murray, and C. H. Colla. 2019. Prevalence of screening for food insecurity, housing instability, utility needs, transportation needs, and interpersonal violence by us physician practices and hospitals. *JAMA Network Open* 2(9):e1911514.

Freeman, B. K., and T. R. Coker. 2018. Six questions for well-child care redesign. *Academic Pediatrics* 18(6):609–619.

Frey, J. J., 3rd. 2010. In this issue: Relationships count for patients and doctors alike. *Annals of Family Medicine* 8(2):98–99.

Gallo, J. J., C. Zubritsky, J. Maxwell, M. Nazar, H. R. Bogner, L. M. Quijano, H. J. Syropoulos, K. L. Cheal, H. Chen, H. Sanchez, J. Dodson, and S. E. Levkoff. 2004. Primary care clinicians evaluate integrated and referral models of behavioral health care for older adults: Results from a multisite effectiveness trial (PRISM-E). *Annals of Family Medicine* 2(4):305–309.

Gard, L. A., A. J. Cooper, Q. Youmans, A. Didwania, S. D. Persell, M. Jean-Jacques, P. Ravenna, M. S. Goel, and M. J. O'Brien. 2020. Identifying and addressing social determinants of health in outpatient practice: Results of a program-wide survey of internal and family medicine residents. *BMC Medical Education* 20(1):18.

Garg, A., R. Boynton-Jarrett, and P. H. Dworkin. 2016. Avoiding the unintended consequences of screening for social determinants of health. *JAMA* 316(8):813–814.

Georgia AAP (Georgia Chapter of the American Academy of Pediatrics). 2020. *Addressing Social Health and Early Childhood Wellness (ASHEW) quality improvement learning collaborative.* https://www.gaaap.org/ashew (accessed August 31, 2020).

Gerrity, M. 2016. *Evolving models of behavioral health integration: Evidence update 2010–2015.* New York: Millbank Memorial Fund.

Ghosh, A., C. Orfield, and R. Schmitz. 2014. *Evaluating PACE: A review of the literature.* Washington, DC: U.S. Department of Health and Human Services, Office of Disability, Aging, and Long-Term Care Policy, and Mathematica Policy Research.

Gilbody, S., P. Bower, J. Fletcher, D. Richards, and A. J. Sutton. 2006. Collaborative care for depression: A cumulative meta-analysis and review of longer-term outcomes. *Archives of Internal Medicine* 166(21):2314–2321.

Gnaedinger, E. A. 2018. Fluoride varnish application, a quality improvement project implemented in a rural pediatric practice. *Public Health Nursing* 35(6):534–540.

Gonzalez, L. 2017. A focus on the Program of All-Inclusive Care for the Elderly (PACE). *Journal of Aging & Social Policy* 29(5):475–490.

Gottlieb, K. 2013. The Nuka system of care: Improving health through ownership and relationships. *International Journal of Circumpolar Health* 72.

Gottlieb, K., I. Sylvester, and D. Eby. 2008. Transforming your practice: What matters most. *Family Practice Management* 15(1):32–38.

Gottlieb, L. M., D. Hessler, D. Long, E. Laves, A. R. Burns, A. Amaya, P. Sweeney, C. Schudel, and N. E. Adler. 2016. Effects of social needs screening and in-person service navigation on child health: A randomized clinical trial. *JAMA Pediatrics* 170(11):e162521.

Gottlieb, L. M., H. Wing, and N. E. Adler. 2017. A systematic review of interventions on patients' social and economic needs. *American Journal of Preventive Medicine* 53(5): 719–729.

Green, L. A., and J. C. Puffer. 2016. Reimagining our relationships with patients: A perspective from the Keystone IV conference. *Journal of the American Board of Family Medicine* 29(Suppl 1):S1–S11.

Grypma, L., R. Haverkamp, S. Little, and J. Unützer. 2006. Taking an evidence-based model of depression care from research to practice: Making lemonade out of depression. *General Hospital Psychiatry* 28(2):101–107.

Herrera, C. N., A. Brochier, M. Pellicer, A. Garg, and M. L. Drainoni. 2019. Implementing social determinants of health screening at community health centers: Clinician and staff perspectives. *Journal of Primary Care & Community Health* 10:2150132719887260.

HHS (U.S. Department of Health and Human Services). 2000. *Oral health in America: A report of the surgeon general.* Rockville, MD: U.S. Department of Health and Human Services, National Institute of Dental and Craniofacial Research, National Institutes of Health.

HHS. 2017. *Pandemic influenza plan: 2017 update.* Washington, DC: U.S. Department of Health and Human Services.

Highmark Foundation. 2009. *Safety net providers: Filling the gap, increasing access and improving health outcomes.* Pittsburgh, PA: Highmark Foundation.

Hirth, V., J. Baskins, and M. Dever-Bumba. 2009. Program of All-inclusive Care (PACE): Past, present, and future. *Journal of the American Medical Directors Association* 10(3): 155–160.

Hodgkinson, S., L. Godoy, L. S. Beers, and A. Lewin. 2017. Improving mental health access for low-income children and families in the primary care setting. *Pediatrics* 139(1).

Holden, K., B. McGregor, P. Thandi, E. Fresh, K. Sheats, A. Belton, G. Mattox, and D. Satcher. 2014. Toward culturally centered integrative care for addressing mental health disparities among ethnic minorities. *Psychological Services* 11(4):357–368.

Holingue, C., L. G. Kalb, K. E. Riehm, D. Bennett, A. Kapteyn, C. B. Veldhuis, R. M. Johnson, M. D. Fallin, F. Kreuter, E. A. Stuart, and J. Thrul. 2020. Mental distress in the United States at the beginning of the COVID-19 pandemic. *American Journal of Public Health* 110(11):1628–1634.

Holloway, R., S. A. Rasmussen, S. Zaza, N. J. Cox, and D. B. Jernigan. 2014. *Updated preparedness and response framework for influenza pandemics.* Washington, DC: Centers for Disease Control and Prevention.

Hostetter, M., S. Klein, and D. McCarthy. 2016. *Hennepin Health: A care delivery paradigm for new Medicaid beneficiaries.* New York: The Commonwealth Fund.

HRSA (Health Resources and Services Administration). 2020. *Shortage areas.* https://data. hrsa.gov/topics/health-workforce/shortage-areas (accessed August 20, 2020).

Huffman, J. C., C. A. Mastromauro, S. R. Beach, C. M. Celano, C. M. DuBois, B. C. Healy, L. Suarez, B. L. Rollman, and J. L. Januzzi. 2014. Collaborative care for depression and anxiety disorders in patients with recent cardiac events: The Management of Sadness and Anxiety in Cardiology (MOSAIC) randomized clinical trial. *JAMA Internal Medicine* 174(6):927–935.

IOM (Institute of Medicine). 1996. *Primary care: America's health in a new era.* Washington, DC: National Academy Press.

IOM. 2011. *Advancing oral health in America.* Washington, DC: The National Academies Press.

IOM. 2012. *Primary care and public health: Exploring integration to improve population health.* Washington, DC: The National Academies Press.

James, B. C., and L. A. Savitz. 2011. How Intermountain trimmed health care costs through robust quality improvement efforts. *Health Affairs* 30(6):1185–1191.

Jones, C., K. Finison, K. McGraves-Lloyd, T. Tremblay, M. K. Mohlman, B. Tanzman, M. Hazard, S. Maier, and J. Samuelson. 2016. Vermont's community-oriented all-payer medical home model reduces expenditures and utilization while delivering high-quality care. *Population Health Management* 19(3):196–205.

Kangovi, S., N. Mitra, L. Norton, R. Harte, X. Zhao, T. Carter, D. Grande, and J. A. Long. 2018. Effect of community health worker support on clinical outcomes of low-income patients across primary care facilities: A randomized clinical trial. *JAMA Internal Medicine* 178(12):1635–1643.

Kangovi, S., N. Mitra, D. Grande, J. A. Long, and D. A. Asch. 2020. Evidence-based community health worker program addresses unmet social needs and generates positive return on investment. *Health Affairs* 39(2):207–213.

Katon, W., and C. J. Guico-Pabia. 2011. Improving quality of depression care using organized systems of care: A review of the literature. *The Primary Care Companion for CNS Disorders* 13(1):PCC.10r01019blu.

Katon, W., J. Unützer, M. Y. Fan, J. W. Williams, Jr., M. Schoenbaum, E. H. Lin, and E. M. Hunkeler. 2006. Cost-effectiveness and net benefit of enhanced treatment of depression for older adults with diabetes and depression. *Diabetes Care* 29(2):265–270.

Katon, W. J., E. H. B. Lin, M. Von Korff, P. Ciechanowski, E. J. Ludman, B. Young, D. Peterson, C. M. Rutter, M. McGregor, and D. McCulloch. 2010. Collaborative care for patients with depression and chronic illnesses. *New England Journal of Medicine* 363(27):2611–2620.

Keeton, V., S. Soleimanpour, and C. D. Brindis. 2012. School-based health centers in an era of health care reform: Building on history. *Current Problems in Pediatric and Adolescent Health Care* 42(6):132–156; discussion 157–158.

Kelleher, K. J., J. Cooper, K. Deans, P. Carr, R. J. Brilli, S. Allen, and W. Gardner. 2015. Cost saving and quality of care in a pediatric accountable care organization. *Pediatrics* 135(3):e582–e589.

Kolstad, C., A. Zavras, and R. K. Yoon. 2015. Cost-benefit analysis of the age one dental visit for the privately insured. *Pediatric Dentistry* 37(4):376–380.

Komaromy, M., D. Duhigg, A. Metcalf, C. Carlson, S. Kalishman, L. Hayes, T. Burke, K. Thornton, and S. Arora. 2016. Project ECHO (Extension for Community Healthcare Outcomes): A new model for educating primary care providers about treatment of substance use disorders. *Substance Abuse* 37(1):20–24.

Kranz, A. M., J. Lee, K. Divaris, A. D. Baker, and W. Vann. 2014. North Carolina physician-based preventive oral health services improve access and use among young Medicaid enrollees. *Health Affairs (Project Hope)* 33(12):2144–2152.

Kravitz, R. L., and M. D. Feldman. 2017. Reinventing primary care: Embracing change, preserving relationships. *Journal of General Internal Medicine* 32(4):369–370.

Langelier, M., J. Moore, B. K. Baker, and E. Mertz. 2015. *Case studies of 8 federally qualified health centers: Strategies to integrate oral health with primary care.* Albany, NY: Center for Health Workforce Studies, School of Public Health, SUNY Albany.

Levesque, J.-F., M. Breton, N. Senn, P. Levesque, P. Bergeron, and D. A. Roy. 2013. The interaction of public health and primary care: Functional roles and organizational models that bridge individual and population perspectives. *Public Health Reviews* 35(1):14.

Levin, W., D. R. Campbell, K. B. McGovern, J. M. Gau, D. B. Kosty, J. R. Seeley, and P. M. Lewinsohn. 2011. A computer-assisted depression intervention in primary care. *Psychological Medicine* 41(7):1373–1383.

Lindau, S. T., J. A. Makelarski, E. M. Abramsohn, D. G. Beiser, K. Boyd, C. Chou, M. Giurcanu, E. S. Huang, C. Liao, L. P. Schumm, and E. L. Tung. 2019. CommunityRx: A real-world controlled clinical trial of a scalable, low-intensity community resource referral intervention. *American Journal of Public Health* 109(4):600–606.

Lion, K. C., and J. L. Raphael. 2015. Partnering health disparities research with quality improvement science in pediatrics. *Pediatrics* 135(2):354–361.

Lohr, A. M., M. Ingram, A. V. Nuñez, K. M. Reinschmidt, and S. C. Carvajal. 2018. Community-clinical linkages with community health workers in the United States: A scoping review. *Health Promotion Practice* 19(3):349–360.

Lutfiyya, M. N., A. J. Gross, B. Soffe, and M. S. Lipsky. 2019. Dental care utilization: Examining the associations between health services deficits and not having a dental visit in past 12 months. *BMC Public Health* 19(1):265.

Maxey, H. L. 2014. *Integration of oral health with primary care in health centers.* Bethesda, MD: National Association of Community Health Centers.

Maxey, H. L., C. W. Norwood, and D. L. Weaver. 2017. Primary care physician roles in health centers with oral health care units. *Journal of the American Board of Family Medicine* 30(4):491–504.

McDonnell, M. M., N. C. Elder, R. Stock, M. Wolf, A. Steeves-Reece, and T. Graham. 2020. Project ECHO integrated within the Oregon Rural Practice-Based Research Network (ORPRN). *Journal of the American Board of Family Medicine* 33(5):789–795.

McGinty, E. E., and G. L. Daumit. 2020. Integrating mental health and addiction treatment into general medical care: The role of policy. *Psychiatric Services* 71(11):1163–1169.

McGovern, L. 2014. *The relative contribution of multiple determinants to health.* Bethesda, MD: Project HOPE: The People-to-People Health Foundation.

Mendelsohn, A. L., B. P. Dreyer, V. Flynn, S. Tomopoulos, I. Rovira, W. Tineo, C. Pebenito, C. Torres, H. Torres, and A. F. Nixon. 2005. Use of videotaped interactions during pediatric well-child care to promote child development: A randomized, controlled trial. *Journal of Developmental and Behavioral Pediatrics* 26(1):34–41.

Meret-Hanke, L. A. 2011. Effects of the Program of All-inclusive Care for the Elderly on hospital use. *The Gerontologist* 51(6):774–785.

Meskó, B., Z. Drobni, É. Bényei, B. Gergely, and Z. Győrffy. 2017. Digital health is a cultural transformation of traditional healthcare. *mHealth* 3:38.

Meyer, B. D., R. Wang, M. J. Steiner, and J. S. Preisser. 2020. The effect of physician oral health services on dental use and expenditures under general anesthesia. *JDR Clinical & Translational Research* 5(2):146–155.

Miller, B. F., and B. Druss. 2013. The role of family physicians in mental health care delivery in the United States: Implications for health reform. *Journal of the American Board of Family Medicine* 26(2):111.

Miller, B. F., S. Petterson, B. T. Burke, R. L. Phillips, Jr., and L. A. Green. 2014. Proximity of providers: Colocating behavioral health and primary care and the prospects for an integrated workforce. *American Psychologist* 69(4):443–451.

Mimila, N. A., P. J. Chung, M. N. Elliott, C. D. Bethell, S. Chacon, C. Biely, S. Contreras, T. Chavis, Y. Bruno, T. Moss, and T. R. Coker. 2017. Well-child care redesign: A mixed methods analysis of parent experiences in the parent trial. *Academic Pediatrics* 17(7):747–754.

Minkovitz, C. S., N. Hughart, D. Strobino, D. Scharfstein, H. Grason, W. Hou, T. Miller, D. Bishai, M. Augustyn, K. T. McLearn, and B. Guyer. 2003. A practice-based intervention to enhance quality of care in the first 3 years of life: The Healthy Steps for Young Children program. *JAMA* 290(23):3081–3091.

Minkovitz, C. S., D. Strobino, K. B. Mistry, D. O. Scharfstein, H. Grason, W. Hou, N. Ialongo, and B. Guyer. 2007. Healthy Steps for Young Children: Sustained results at 5.5 years. *Pediatrics* 120(3):e658–e668.

Miranda, J., N. Duan, C. Sherbourne, M. Schoenbaum, I. Lagomasino, M. Jackson-Triche, and K. B. Wells. 2003. Improving care for minorities: Can quality improvement interventions improve care and outcomes for depressed minorities? Results of a randomized, controlled trial. *Health Services Research* 38(2):613–630.

Mitchell, A. J., A. Vaze, and S. Rao. 2009. Clinical diagnosis of depression in primary care: A meta-analysis. *The Lancet* 374(9690):609–619.

Mooney, K., C. Moreno, P. J. Chung, J. Elijah, and T. R. Coker. 2014. Well-child care clinical practice redesign at a community health center: Provider and staff perspectives. *Journal of Primary Care & Community Health* 5(1):19–23.

Mostashari, F. 2016. The paradox of size: How small, independent practices can thrive in value-based care. *Annals of Family Medicine* 14(1):5–7.

Moyer, V. A. 2014. Prevention of dental caries in children from birth through age 5 years: U.S. Preventive Services Task Force recommendation statement. *Pediatrics* 133(6):1102–1111.

NAMI (National Alliance on Mental Illness). 2011. *The family experience with primary care physicians and staff.* Arlington, VA: National Alliance on Mental Illness.

NASEM (National Academies of Sciences, Engineering, and Medicine). 2019a. *Integrating social care into the delivery of health care: Moving upstream to improve the nation's health.* Washington, DC: The National Academies Press.

NASEM. 2019b. *Taking action against clinician burnout: A systems approach to professional well-being.* Washington, DC: The National Academies Press.

Nethan, S. T., R. Hariprasad, R. Babu, V. Kumar, S. Sharma, and R. Mehrotra. 2020. Project ECHO: A potential best-practice tool for training healthcare providers in oral cancer screening and tobacco cessation. *Journal of Cancer Education* 35(5):965–971.

Newman, E. D., P. F. Simonelli, S. M. Vezendy, C. M. Cedeno, and D. D. Maeng. 2019. Impact of primary and specialty care integration via asynchronous communication. *American Journal of Managed Care* 25(1):26–31.

Newman, M., B. Ewald, and R. Golden. 2018. Are social workers missing from your complex care teams? https://www.bettercareplaybook.org/_blog/2018/13/are-social-workers-missing-your-complex-care-teams (accessed February 24, 2021).

Nieuwboer, M. S., R. van der Sande, M. A. van der Marck, M. G. M. Olde Rikkert, and M. Perry. 2019. Clinical leadership and integrated primary care: A systematic literature review. *European Journal of General Practice* 25(1):7–18.

Northridge, M. E., S. S. Kum, B. Chakraborty, A. P. Greenblatt, S. E. Marshall, H. Wang, C. Kunzel, and S. S. Metcalf. 2016. Third places for health promotion with older adults: Using the consolidated framework for implementation research to enhance program implementation and evaluation. *Journal of Urban Health* 93(5):851–870.

NPA (National PACE Association). 2021. *PACEfinder: Find a PACE program in your neighborhood.* https://www.npaonline.org/pace-you/pacefinder-find-pace-program-your-neighborhood (accessed February 11, 2021).

Oldenburg, R. 1989. *The great good place: Cafes, coffee shops, bookstores, bars, hair salons, and other hangouts at the heart of a community.* St. Paul, MN: Paragon House.

Palazuelos, D., P. E. Farmer, and J. Mukherjee. 2018. Community health and equity of outcomes: The partners in health experience. *The Lancet Global Health* 6(5):e491–e493.

Parker, D., R. Byng, C. Dickens, and R. McCabe. 2020. Patients' experiences of seeking help for emotional concerns in primary care: Doctor as drug, detective and collaborator. *BMC Family Practice* 21(1):35.

Peikes, D. N., R. J. Reid, T. J. Day, D. D. F. Cornwell, S. B. Dale, R. J. Baron, R. S. Brown, and R. J. Shapiro. 2014. Staffing patterns of primary care practices in the comprehensive primary care initiative. *Annals of Family Medicine* 12(2):142–149.

Pesec, M., H. L. Ratcliffe, A. Karlage, L. R. Hirschhorn, A. Gawande, and A. Bitton. 2017. Primary health care that works: The Costa Rican experience. *Health Affairs* 36(3):531–538.

Pinto, A. D., and G. Bloch. 2017. Framework for building primary care capacity to address the social determinants of health. *Canadian Family Physician* 63(11):e476–e482.

Pinto, A. D., G. Glattstein-Young, A. Mohamed, G. Bloch, F. H. Leung, and R. H. Glazier. 2016. Building a foundation to reduce health inequities: Routine collection of sociode-mographic data in primary care. *Journal of the American Board of Family Medicine* 29(3):348–355.

Platt, R. E., A. E. Spencer, M. D. Burkey, C. Vidal, S. Polk, A. F. Bettencourt, S. Jain, J. Stratton, and L. S. Wissow. 2018. What's known about implementing co-located paediatric integrated care: A scoping review. *International Review of Psychiatry* 30(6):242–271.

Price-Haywood, E. G., J. Burton, D. Fort, and L. Seoane. 2020. Hospitalization and mortality among black patients and white patients with COVID-19. *New England Journal of Medicine* 382(26):2534–2543.

Ramanuj, P., E. Ferenchik, M. Docherty, B. Spaeth-Rublee, and H. A. Pincus. 2019. Evolving models of integrated behavioral health and primary care. *Current Psychiatry Reports* 21(1):4.

Reiss-Brennan, B. 2014. Mental health integration: Normalizing team care. *Journal of Primary Care & Community Health* 5(1):55–60.

Reiss-Brennan, B., K. D. Brunisholz, C. Dredge, P. Briot, K. Grazier, A. Wilcox, L. Savitz, and B. James. 2016. Association of integrated team-based care with health care quality, utilization, and cost. *JAMA* 316(8):826–834.

Riley, M., A. R. Laurie, M. A. Plegue, and C. R. Richarson. 2016. The adolescent "expanded medical home": School-based health centers partner with a primary care clinic to improve population health and mitigate social determinants of health. *Journal of the American Board of Family Medicine* 29(3):339–347.

Rittenhouse, D. R., J. A. Wiley, L. E. Peterson, L. P. Casalino, and R. L. Phillips. 2020. Meaningful use and medical home functionality in primary care practice. *Health Affairs* 39(11):1977–1983.

Rocks, S., D. Berntson, A. Gil-Salmerón, M. Kadu, N. Ehrenberg, V. Stein, and A. Tsiachristas. 2020. Cost and effects of integrated care: A systematic literature review and meta-analysis. *European Journal of Health Economics* 21:1211–1221.

Rowe, J. M., V. M. Rizzo, G. Shier Kricke, K. Krajci, G. Rodriguez-Morales, M. Newman, and R. Golden. 2016. The Ambulatory Integration of the Medical and Social (AIMS) model: A retrospective evaluation. *Social Work in Health Care* 55(5):347–361.

RTI International, The Urban Institute, and National Academy for State Health Policy. 2017. *Evaluation of the Multi-payer Advanced Primary Care Practice (MAPCP) demonstration: Final report.* Research Triangle Park, NC: RTI International.

Samuels, S., R. Abrams, R. Shengelia, M. C. Reid, R. Goralewicz, R. Breckman, M. A. Anderson, C. E. Snow, E. C. Woods, A. Stern, J. P. Eimicke, and R. D. Adelman. 2015. Integration of geriatric mental health screening into a primary care practice: A patient satisfaction survey. *International Journal of Geriatric Psychiatry* 30(5):539–546.

Sandberg, S. F., C. Erikson, R. Owen, K. D. Vickery, S. T. Shimotsu, M. Linzer, N. A. Garrett, K. A. Johnsrud, D. M. Soderlund, and J. DeCubellis. 2014. Hennepin Health: A safety-net accountable care organization for the expanded Medicaid population. *Health Affairs* 33(11):1975–1984.

Satcher, D., and S. A. Rachel. 2017. Promoting mental health equity: The role of integrated care. *Journal of Clinical Psychology in Medical Settings* 24(3):182–186.

SCF (Southcentral Foundation). 2020. *Services.* https://www.southcentralfoundation.com/services (accessed December 1, 2020).

Scutchfield, F. D., J. L. Michener, and S. B. Thacker. 2012. Are we there yet? Seizing the moment to integrate medicine and public health. *American Journal of Public Health* 102(Suppl 3):S312–S316.

Segura, A., S. Boulter, M. Clark, R. Gereige, D. M. Krol, W. Mouradian, R. Quinonez, F. Ramos-Gomes, R. Slayton, and M. A. Keels. 2014. Maintaining and improving the oral health of young children. *Pediatrics* 134(6):1224–1229.

Sharma, A., R. A. Harrington, M. B. McClellan, M. P. Turakhia, Z. J. Eapen, S. Steinhubl, J. R. Mault, M. D. Majmudar, L. Roessig, K. J. Chandross, E. M. Green, B. Patel, A. Hamer, J. Olgin, J. S. Rumsfeld, M. T. Roe, and E. D. Peterson. 2018. Using digital health technology to better generate evidence and deliver evidence-based care. *Journal of the American College of Cardiology* 71(23):2680–2690.

Shonkoff, J. P., and P. A. Fisher. 2013. Rethinking evidence-based practice and two-generation programs to create the future of early childhood policy. *Development and Psychopathology* 25(4 Pt 2):1635–1653.

Singer, S. J., J. Burgers, M. Friedberg, M. B. Rosenthal, L. Leape, and E. Schneider. 2011. Defining and measuring integrated patient care: Promoting the next frontier in health care delivery. *Medical Care Research and Review* 68(1):112–127.

Singer, S. J., M. Kerrissey, M. Friedberg, and R. Phillips. 2020. A comprehensive theory of integration. *Medical Care Research and Review* 77(2):196–207.

Sjoding, M. W., T. J. Iwashyna, J. B. Dimick, and C. R. Cooke. 2015. Gaming hospital-level pneumonia 30-day mortality and readmission measures by legitimate changes to diagnostic coding. *Critical Care Medicine* 43(5):989–995.

Starfield, B. 1998. *Primary care: Balancing health needs, services, and technology.* Revised edition. New York: Oxford University Press.

State of Vermont. 2020. *Blueprint for health.* https://blueprintforhealth.vermont.gov (accessed August 5, 2020).

Stockwell, M. S., E. O. Kharbanda, R. A. Martinez, M. Lara, D. Vawdrey, K. Natarajan, and V. I. Rickert. 2012. Text4health: Impact of text message reminder-recalls for pediatric and adolescent immunizations. *American Journal of Public Health* 102(2):e15–e21.

Talen, M. R., and A. B. Valeras, eds. 2013. *Integrated behavioral health in primary care: Evaluating the evidence, identifying the essentials.* New York: Springer.

UNM (University of New Mexico). 2021a. *ECHO hubs.* https://hsc.unm.edu/echo/data-marketplace/interactive-dashboards (accessed March 9, 2021).

UNM. 2021b. *Project ECHO: About us.* https://hsc.unm.edu/echo/about-us (accessed March 9, 2021).

Unützer, J., W. Katon, C. Callahan, and J. Williams. 2002. Collaborative care management of late-life depression in the primary care setting. *JAMA* 288(2):2836–2845.

Unützer, J., W. J. Katon, M. Y. Fan, M. C. Schoenbaum, E. H. Lin, R. D. Della Penna, and D. Powers. 2008. Long-term cost effects of collaborative care for late-life depression. *American Journal of Managed Care* 14(2):95–100.

Unützer, J., H. Harbin, M. Schoenbaum, and B. Druss. 2013. *The collaborative care model: An approach for integrating physical and mental health care in Medicaid health homes.* Washington, DC: Centers for Medicare & Medicaid Services.

Vahidy, F. S., J. C. Nicolas, J. R. Meeks, O. Khan, A. Pan, S. L. Jones, F. Masud, H. D. Sostman, R. Phillips, J. D. Andrieni, B. A. Kash, and K. Nasir. 2020. Racial and ethnic disparities in SARS-COV-2 pandemic: Analysis of a COVID-19 observational registry for a diverse U.S. metropolitan population. *BMJ Open* 10(8):e039849.

Valentijn, P. P., D. Ruwaard, H. J. Vrijhoef, A. de Bont, R. Y. Arends, and M. A. Bruijnzeels. 2015. Collaboration processes and perceived effectiveness of integrated care projects in primary care: A longitudinal mixed-methods study. *BMC Health Services Research* 15:463.

van Grieken, A., E. Vlasblom, L. Wang, M. Beltman, M. M. Boere-Boonekamp, M. P. L'Hoir, and H. Raat. 2017. Personalized web-based advice in combination with well-child visits to prevent overweight in young children: Cluster randomized controlled trial. *Journal of Medical Internet Research* 19(7):e268.

Vickery, K. D., N. D. Shippee, J. Menk, R. Owen, D. M. Vock, P. Bodurtha, D. Soderlund, R. A. Hayward, M. M. Davis, J. Connett, and M. Linzer. 2020. Integrated, accountable care for Medicaid expansion enrollees: A comparative evaluation of Hennepin Health. *Medical Care Research and Review* 77(1):46–59.

Vimalananda, V. G., K. Dvorin, B. G. Fincke, N. Tardiff, and B. G. Bokhour. 2018. Patient, primary care provider, and specialist perspectives on specialty care coordination in an integrated health care system. *Journal of Ambulatory Care Management* 41(1):15–24.

Wadge, H., Y. Bhatti, A. Carter, M. Harris, G. Parston, and A. Darzi. 2016. *Brazil's family health strategy: Using communitiy health workers to provide primary care.* Washington, DC: The Commonwealth Fund.

Weaver, S. J., X. X. Che, L. A. Petersen, and S. J. Hysong. 2018. Unpacking care coordination through a multiteam system lens: A conceptual framework and systematic review. *Medical Care* 56(3):247–259.

Weinberg, D. B., J. H. Gittell, R. W. Lusenhop, C. M. Kautz, and J. Wright. 2007. Beyond our walls: Impact of patient and provider coordination across the continuum on outcomes for surgical patients. *Health Services Research* 42(1 Pt 1):7–24.

Welton, W. E., T. A. Kantner, and S. M. Katz. 1997. Developing tomorrow's integrated community health systems: A leadership challenge for public health and primary care. *Milbank Quarterly* 75(2):261–288.

Wieland, D., B. Kinosian, E. Stallard, and R. Boland. 2013. Does Medicaid pay more to a program of all-inclusive care for the elderly (PACE) than for fee-for-service long-term care? *The Journals of Gerontology: Series A, Biological Sciences and Medical Sciences* 68(1):47–55.

Wissow, L. S., N. van Ginneken, J. Chandna, and A. Rahman. 2016. Integrating children's mental health into primary care. *Pediatric Clinics of North America* 63(1):97–113.

Wissow, L. S., R. Platt, and B. Sarvet. 2020. Policy recommendations to promote integrated mental health care for children and youth. *Academic Pediatrics* S1876-2859(20):30489-7.

Wu, J., K. S. Dean, Z. Rosen, and P. A. Muennig. 2017. The cost-effectiveness analysis of nurse-family partnership in the United States. *Journal of Health Care for the Poor and Underserved* 28(4):1578–1597.

Wu, A. W., C. M. Weston, C. A. Ibe, C. F. Ruberman, L. Bone, R. T. Boonyasai, S. Hwang, J. Gentry, L. Purnell, Y. Lu, S. Liang, and M. Rosenblum. 2019. The Baltimore Community-Based Organizations Neighborhood Network: Enhancing Capacity Together (CONNECT) cluster RCT. *American Journal of Preventive Medicine* 57(2):e31–e41.

Xierali, I. M., S. T. Tong, S. M. Petterson, J. C. Puffer, R. L. Phillips, Jr., and A. W. Bazemore. 2013. Family physicians are essential for mental health care delivery. *Journal of the American Board of Family Practice* 26(2):114–115.

Yogman, M. W., S. Betjemann, A. Sagaser, and L. Brecher. 2018. Integrated behavioral health care in pediatric primary care: A quality improvement project. *Clinical Pediatrics* 57(4):461–470.

Yonek, J., C.-M. Lee, A. Harrison, C. Mangurian, and M. Tolou-Shams. 2020. Key components of effective pediatric integrated mental health care models: A systematic review. *JAMA Pediatrics* 174(5):487–498.

6

Designing Interprofessional Teams and Preparing the Future Primary Care Workforce

The ability to deliver high-quality primary care depends on the availability, accessibility, and competence of a primary care workforce assembled in interprofessional teams to effectively meet the health care needs of diverse care-seekers, families, and communities. People with access to high-quality primary care have better health outcomes, including improvements in chronic disease control, receipt of more preventive services, fewer preventable emergency room visits and hospitalizations, improved health equity, improved quality of life, and longer lives (Basu et al., 2019; Shi, 2012; Starfield et al., 2005). These better outcomes are pronounced among the poor and underserved (Beck et al., 2016; Phillips and Bazemore, 2010; Regalado and Halfon, 2001; Seid and Stevens, 2005).

This chapter focuses on the evidence supporting challenges and innovative solutions to creating interprofessional primary care teams that can offset the eroding capacity of primary care clinicians to deliver a broad scope of person- and family-centered care. The chapter will also discuss key design elements of interprofessional teams and highlight the roles that extended care team members and care team members from the community can play in delivering high-quality primary care. The chapter will then address the diversity of the primary care workforce and the education and training needed to prepare a workforce equipped to meet the growing primary care needs of care-seekers, families, and communities.

DESIGNING THE INTERPROFESSIONAL PRIMARY CARE TEAM

A commonly used definition of team-based care is

the provision of health services to individuals, families, and/or their communities by at least two health providers who work collaboratively with patients and their caregivers—to the extent preferred by each patient—to accomplish shared goals within and across settings to achieve coordinated, high-quality care. (IOM, 2011a; Mitchell et al., 2012, p. 5; Okun et al., 2014, p. 46; Schottenfeld et al., 2016)

High-quality primary care is best provided by a team of clinicians and others who are organized, supported, and accountable to meet the needs of the people and the communities they serve. Team-based care improves health care quality, use, and costs among chronically ill patients (Pany et al., 2021; Reiss-Brennan et al., 2016), and it also leads to lower burnout in primary care (Willard-Grace et al., 2014). Well-designed teams can support nurturing, longitudinal, person-centered care (Mitchell et al., 2012; Sullivan and Ellner, 2015).

Integrated, interprofessional team-based care requires leadership at all levels of the organization, decision-making tools, effective communication, and real-time information that supports whole-person care. In combination, these requirements ensure that a competent, trusted group of health care professionals working together adequately addresses physical health, behavioral health, social needs, and oral health (Ellner and Phillips, 2017). See Chapter 5 for more insight into the delivery of integrated care and how to approach integration.

Meeting the Needs of Patients and the Community

Team-based care will look different depending on the health needs and demographics of the population; the setting in which it receives care; the distinct regional, economic, and sociocultural contexts of the community in which that population lives; and the assets of that community. Ideally, the team should reflect the diversity of the patients and community it serves (Katkin et al., 2017), and because the needs of patients and their families will change over time, primary care teams should be able to evolve in response to those changing needs (Bodenheimer, 2019b; Bodenheimer and Smith, 2013; Brownstein et al., 2011; Coker et al., 2013; Fierman et al., 2016; Grumbach et al., 2012; Katkin et al., 2017; Margolius et al., 2012).

Community-oriented primary care, as discussed in Chapter 4, is an approach to care delivery by which services—both health care and community-based resources—are designed and organized to meet the specific needs of a given population and community. This approach involves health facilities or systems completing an epidemiologic assessment of the population to identify its specific health needs, which may include social services in addition to traditional health services (IOM, 1983). Health centers, for example, must complete these assessments every 3 years and often do so in collaboration with hospitals and public health departments (HRSA, 2018). Every 3 years, as a condition of their tax-exempt status, nonprofit hospitals are also required to complete a community health assessment and, based on the results, develop an implementation plan to meet the needs of their populations.[1] Assessments can include a review of the geographic boundaries of the population served; any barriers to care, including transportation and child care; unmet health needs of the medically underserved in that population, including the ratio of primary care physicians (PCPs) relative to the population; health indexes for the population; the population's poverty level; and other demographic factors that affect the demand for services, such as the percentage of the population over age 65. Needs assessments similar to those produced by health centers can guide the efforts of primary care teams in conducting community health assessments of their own and inform the composition of the primary care team to match the specific needs of the community it serves.

The COVID-19 pandemic illustrated the need for primary care practices to adapt quickly to changing needs in their communities. In particular, the pandemic highlighted that expanded access to care is necessary, and many states relaxed or waived scope of practice requirements for advanced practice nurses and pharmacists (Cadogan and Hughes, 2020; Hess et al., 2020; Zolot, 2020). This change has led to reports of improved patient access and opened the door to discussions to permanently rethink team members' scope of practice to better meet community needs and reduce barriers to care (AANP, 2020a; Aruru et al., 2021; Feyereisen and Puro, 2020).

Designing Teams for Success: Structure and Culture

Interprofessional primary care teams should have a structure and a culture (Bodenheimer, 2019a), which are concepts critical to effective team design (Schottenfeld et al., 2016). The typical structure of an interprofessional primary care team includes a core team, an extended health care team, and what the committee refers to as the "extended community care team" (see Figure 6-1 for an overview of the interprofessional team). Each

---

[1] 26 Internal Revenue Code § 501(r). For more information, see https://www.irs.gov/charities-non-profits/charitable-organizations/requirements-for-501c3-hospitals-under-the-affordable-care-act-section-501r (accessed February 27, 2021).

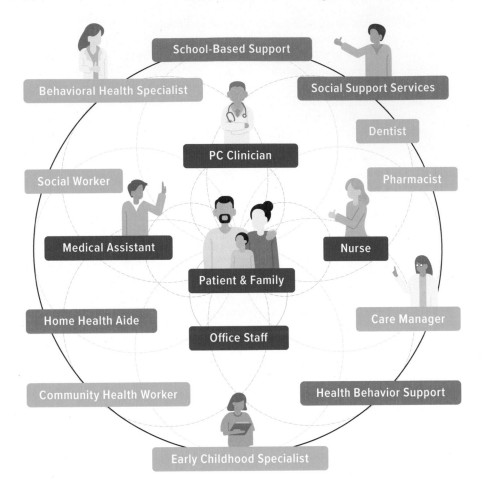

● **Core Team**

● Extended Health Care Team

● **Extended Community Care Team**

FIGURE 6-1 The composition of interprofessional primary care teams.
NOTE: PC = primary care.

segment of the interprofessional primary care team is discussed in more detail later in this chapter.

A defining feature of a care team is its stability. Stability ensures that members of the team *work together consistently* to support one another and that the team includes consistent individuals who care for patients and their families and can form stable relationships with them. The core, extended health care, and the extended community care teams require seamless, coordinated, and integrated care delivery processes to ensure that whole-person care is provided to each person. That only comes when the team composition remains stable over time, which allows team members to learn how to best work with one another in a seamless, coordinated, and integrated manner (see Chapter 4) and the care-seeker to know and trust the multiple members of the team.

Planning strategically and distributing the functions of care across various team members, including health professionals working at the top of their scope of practice and non-clinical personnel assuming responsibility for other functions, helps distribute work tasks and functions to those best prepared to implement them. Primary care clinicians are too busy to assume responsibility for all the functions required to meet every need, and no single clinician can be expected to have the expertise and skills needed to do so and do it well (Bodenheimer, 2019a). Aligning each respective team member's competencies and capabilities with the actual work that must be done not only shifts excess work away from the primary care clinician but places it in the hands of those who are educated and trained to execute those tasks. Doing so creates opportunities for each team member to contribute meaningfully to the work that needs to be done, further strengthening team culture (Bohmer, 2011; Sinsky et al., 2013). While team-based delivery distributes many functions across the team, doing so does not diffuse individual accountability, including that of the primary care clinician who is ultimately accountable for a patient's care.

One successful interprofessional primary care model is the U.S. Department of Veterans Affairs' (VA's) Patient-Aligned Care Team (PACT). This care team model incorporates clinical and support staff who deliver all primary care functions and coordinate the remaining needs, including specialty care. To optimize workflow and enhance continuity of care, staff are organized into "teamlets" that provide care to an assigned panel of about 1,200 patients. A teamlet consists of a PCP, physician assistant (PA) or nurse practitioner (NP), registered nurse (RN) care manager, licensed practical nurse or medical assistant, and administrative clerk (Gardner et al., 2018). PACTs have been associated with a decrease in hospitalizations, specialty care visits, emergency department (ED) use, and increased overall mental health visits but decreased visits with mental health specialists outside of a primary care setting (thanks to the VA's separate Primary

Care-Mental Health Integration program), along with lower levels of staff burnout, higher patient satisfaction and access to care, increases in use of preventive services, and improvements in clinical outcomes for patients with diabetes, heart disease, and hypertension (Bidassie, 2017; Hebert et al., 2014; Leung et al., 2019; Nelson et al., 2014; Randall et al., 2017; Rodriguez et al., 2014).

A study of 23 high-performing primary care practices examined how they distribute functions among the team members, use technology to their advantage, use data to improve outcomes, and bring joy to their work (Sinsky et al., 2013). The study elucidated several important characteristics of high-performing teams:

- They are proactive and provide well-thought-out care, including pre-visit planning and laboratory testing.
- They distribute and share the delivery of care among the team members.
- They share clerical tasks, such as documentation, non-physician order entry, and prescription management, among a variety of team members.
- They enhance communication through a variety of strategies.
- They optimize the function of the team through colocation, team meetings, huddles, and mapping workflow.

The study also found that shifting work from a physician-centric model of care to a shared, team-based model of care results in improved professional satisfaction and a greater joy in practice. Consistent with these findings, evidence is mounting that interprofessional primary care teams can improve care quality, reduce health care costs, decrease clinician burnout, and improve the patient experience, but this requires that teams are truly distributing the work and sharing the care responsibilities (Meyers et al., 2019). Producing and sustaining this effective level of high-functioning teamwork requires leadership that recognizes and rewards team-based care.

In addition to its structure, the team's culture is foundational, relational, and reflective of the mission and vision of the organization or practice. Team culture is reflected in how members function together and value each other's role and how they distribute the tasks among each other to reach quality outcomes. It is well known that the roles and functions of individual team members are often poorly defined, and teams are often under-resourced for the work they need to do, leading to chronic misdistribution of effort, exhaustion of human capital, and often less than optimal care (Hysong et al., 2019; Sinsky and Bodenheimer, 2019). Research also suggests that PCPs, who are most often trained individually in hospital settings, are often unskilled at or uncomfortable in a true team-based environment, reflecting a need to train clinicians in the environment in which they will eventually work (O'Malley et al., 2015).

At the core of primary care team culture is care delivery in the context of personal relationships organized with a purpose to meet the needs of individuals and their families and provide comprehensive, coordinated, and continuous connection toward improving health. Good relationships provide the foundation for high-functioning teams and are critical to providing high-quality care (Gittell, 2008). Establishing effective primary care teams requires explicit emphasis on team design that has a structure, a relational and functional culture, and a design optimized with the care-seeker and community to deliver high-quality primary care.

MEMBERS OF THE PRIMARY CARE TEAM

The care-seeker and family are active and engaged members of the primary care team with a central and invaluable role to play in the assessment, treatment, and implementation stages of the process. Likewise, clinicians are expected to provide care that is person centered and includes listening to, informing, and involving people (IOM, 2001). Person-centered care is the practice of caring for people and their families in ways that are meaningful and valuable to the individual.

The following sections provide an overview of the core, extended health care, and extended community care teams. Each section highlights select team members and describes their roles and contributions on the interprofessional team. The list is by no means exhaustive; it highlights the value that others can bring to an interprofessional primary care team. The level designations the committee makes are not the same in all situations. For example, a community health worker (CHW) or pharmacist may be considered part of the core in many settings.

The Core Team

The core team comprises the patient, their family, and various informal caregivers; primary care clinicians, who may be physicians, PAs, NPs, or RNs; and clinical support staff, such as medical assistants and office staff.

Patients, Family Members, and Caregivers

As noted above, person-centered care requires that patients, their family members, and informal caregivers be considered core members of the primary care team. Honoring the care-seeker's voice is essential to ensure that the care meets the needs and goals for that person and their family. Listening to and incorporating that voice in the delivery and governance of primary care has become a national priority (Bombard et al., 2018; IOM, 2013a). Yet, in practice, decisions about the design, delivery, and governance of primary care are still often made without the input of those who are intended to benefit. This gap is even greater for disadvantaged patients, whose opinions, needs, and preferences may not be valued because of institutional discrimination, limited health literacy, or mistrust.

If fortunate, the patient is surrounded by friends and family members who may, depending on the circumstances, function as informal caregivers and should be included on the primary care team. For children and adolescents, the family is a central element of the care team. Likewise, adults may involve their children or other family members in their care.

The United States has no standard definition for informal caregivers, though typically these are friends and family members who provide support with activities of daily living, medication management, and care coordination. These individuals, while not formally trained or certified, have an intimate knowledge of the patient's background, history, usual state of function, and life circumstances. They are invaluable members of the team because they are crucial to shared decision making with the patient and interprofessional primary care team and can work together to identify and reach shared goals (Park and Cho, 2018; Wyatt et al., 2015). This is particularly important for fulfilling shared goals and care plans for children, adolescents, and adults with complex medical needs (Kuo and Houtrow, 2016). In general, family and other informal caregivers have far more daily contact with the patient than any other member of the health care team and are often an underused authority for supporting self-management and recovery (Andrades et al., 2013; Cené et al., 2015; IOM, 2008; Rosland et al., 2011; Whitehead et al., 2018). Experts recommend that formal health care teams help them to understand the tasks of informal care, assess their capacity, and train and monitor caregivers' performance (Friedman and Tong, 2020; Reinhard et al., 2008).

Estimates suggest that some 53 million Americans care for an ailing or aging loved one, typically without pay (AARP and NAC, 2020). Historically, most informal caregiving was unpaid, but in recent years, several states have created payment programs (Polivka, 2001). The VA also has an assistance program in which eligible caregivers are provided a monthly stipend (VA, 2020).

Primary Care Clinicians

The core team of primary care clinicians generally includes physicians, NPs, and PAs. Today, four major trends are strongly influencing the practice and expansion of interprofessional primary care teams: (1) a widening income gap between primary care and medical subspecialties, (2) pressure to increase efficiencies rather than effectiveness of primary care, (3) general under-resourcing of primary care teams, and (4) scope of practice. Physician practice in primary care in the United States is not the province of one group or specialty but rather includes family medicine, general internal medicine, general pediatrics, geriatrics, and others depending on the definition, each having its own certifying board and professional organization (AAMC, 2019; Jabbarpour et al., 2019). This complexity requires high levels of coordination for each to advocate effectively for primary care—something missing from primary care today. The income gap between primary care and specialties is associated with a declining choice of primary care by physicians in training (COGME, 2010; Phillips et al., 2009; Weida et al., 2010) (see Chapter 9 for more details) and with a growing number of these professionals who do enter primary care leaving it or choosing more lucrative opportunities, such as becoming hospitalists or creating niche practices, such as pain clinics or sleep medicine (Cassel and Reuben, 2011; Miller et al., 2017). The dominant fee-for-service model makes patient throughput volume and minimizing overhead the main drivers of primary care efficiency, typically at the expense of its effectiveness (Phillips et al., 2014), leading to reduction in primary care comprehensiveness, one of its highest value functions. It is also associated with one of the highest rates of burnout among physician specialties (Berg, 2020). The result is an eroding and maldistributed primary care workforce (Basu et al., 2019; Chen et al., 2013a; Petterson et al., 2012).

As noted in Chapter 3, NPs and PAs play an important and growing role in the overall primary care workforce, and graduates from NP primary care programs have shown steady growth in the past decade (AANP, 2020b). Within the primary care team, the role of NPs and PAs may vary state to state as a result of differences in state licensure laws. In 23 states and the District of Columbia NPs can practice without physician supervision; other states require such supervision and have other restrictions limiting NPs' scope of practice (AANP, 2021). In 2016 the VA amended its medical regulations to permit full practice authority for NPs[2] when they are acting within the scope of their VA employment regardless of the location of the VA facility (VA, 2016). There has been less of a push for independent practice among PAs, and 37 states allow the supervising physician and PA at the practice level to determine the scope of practice and establish it through a written agreement between the two (AAFP, 2019). State-to-state variation in scope of practice prevents a unified approach to team-based primary care and creates confusion for patients and families. During the

---

[2] This ruling also applied to nurse specialists and nurse-midwives.

COVID-19 crisis multiple states quickly passed legislation to broaden the scope of NP and PA practice, including broadening their authority or changing supervisory requirements to build clinician capacity to address the surge of care-seekers (AAPA, 2020; Lai et al., 2020).

The resistance to increasing the scope of practice of any members of the core primary care team seems antithetical to the need to increase the number of primary care clinicians to expand access to care, particularly in underserved regions (Bruner, 2016; Buerhaus, 2018; Cawley and Hooker, 2013; Neff et al., 2018; Ortiz et al., 2018; Xue et al., 2018b). *Assessing Progress on the Institute of Medicine Report* The Future of Nursing captured this well, saying, "in new collaborative models of practice, it is imperative that *all* health professionals practice to the full extent of their education and training to optimize the efficiency and quality of services for patients" (NASEM, 2016, p. 48).

While all types of clinicians in the core team often have overlapping roles in care delivery, they each offer unique skills that address different needs. Interprofessional team–based care delivery, supported by compatible payment models, would allow practices to fully use the unique contributions these professionals can make to high-quality patient care. Similarly, allowing NPs and PAs to practice at the top of their licensure would also help facilitate team-based care, alleviate some of the burden on physicians, and improve access to services (IOM, 2011b; NASEM, 2016, 2019b). The solutions recommended by this report would help all three see it as a viable, meaningful career and should be a source of common cause.

Registered Nurses

Nurses have a range of competencies that, if used appropriately, could distribute responsibilities more efficiently in primary care. Nurses in primary care, which has emerged as a distinct professional nursing specialty (Borgès Da Silva et al., 2018; Mastal, 2010; Swan and Haas, 2011), are engaged in clinical responsibilities, such as assessing someone's problems or concerns, planning their care with their families, coordinating care, and evaluating outcomes of the care. Nurses can advocate for patients and their families and offer referrals to optimal health services. Studies have shown that involving nurses in coordinating primary care results in improved patient satisfaction (Borgès Da Silva et al., 2018). Many nurses in primary care deliver health education services to patients and their families, perform procedures that require a professional license (such as administering vaccines), and consult with professional colleagues. Nurses often have key insights into workflow and integration of the care team, often acting in roles focused on staffing workload regulatory issues and quality improvement.

Medical Assistants and Office Managers

Medical assistants are essential staff in primary care and one of the fastest-growing sectors in that workforce (BLS, 2020). Typically, medical assistants are assigned to a partnering clinician and can develop long-term relationships with care-seekers and families. They are often an early point of contact and have familiarized themselves with the patients' personal and medical histories. Their role focuses on preparing patients for visits, helping them flow through the clinic, and ensuring that their primary care clinician has the information and resources needed for a whole-person visit. Experience and evidence have shown that medical assistants are often capable of doing much more. Most medical assistants are adept at using the electronic health record (EHR), and research has shown that with training, they can effectively engage in preventive care tasks, coach care-seekers, and manage population health strategies (Naughton et al., 2013). One caveat to the expanded use of medical assistants is that they have high rates of turnover; it can exceed 50 percent per year as a result of burnout and low satisfaction with compensation and opportunities for growth (Friedman and Neutze, 2020; Skillman et al., 2020).

The office manager is also a valuable member of the primary care team, often serving as the first point of contact for care-seekers and their families. Office managers are responsible for a diverse range of functions, including handling routine financial transactions and reimbursements, ordering supplies, scheduling, coordinating office functions, providing general administrative support, and maintaining records and supporting documents (Sachs Hills, 2004).

The Extended Health Care Team

The extended health care team has emerged in primary care delivery to augment the core team's ability to meet the growing needs and complexity of individuals and the local community (Bodenheimer, 2019a). Depending on need, members of this team can include CHWs, pharmacists, dentists, social workers, behavioral health specialists, lactation consultants, nutritionists, and physical and occupational therapists, who may support several core teams (Bodenheimer and Laing, 2007; Mitchell et al., 2019).

Depending on many factors, including the needs of the individual and family and the availability and accessibility of team members, extended care team members may be integrated fully into the core team. The extended care team will look quite different depending on whether the person seeking care is a child, adolescent, adult, older adult, or someone with complex medical needs. In fact, the composition of that team will likely change over the developmental and aging trajectory. For example, the American Academy of Pediatrics (AAP) has published standards for pediatric team-based care that calls for pediatric-specific models (Katkin et al., 2017).

Following are examples of members of the extended health care team and their value-added role on the interprofessional team. These examples highlight the need for greater engagement of interprofessional team members, but the list is not comprehensive.

Community Health Workers

CHWs, also called "promotores de salud" and "peer mentors," are an important and emerging workforce within primary care. They are unique within the health care workforce because they are defined not by their training or functions but rather by their *identity*. CHWs are individuals who share a common sociocultural background and life experiences with the people they serve, and as their name implies, they come from the community in which they serve (Chernoff and Cueva, 2017; Farrar et al., 2011; IOM, 1983; Palazuelos et al., 2018). As a result, they understand the environment and the community and family contexts that affect the person seeking care.

CHWs often come from and serve disadvantaged populations, and they earn their expertise by virtue of challenging life experiences, such as facing discrimination, living with financial hardship, surviving trauma, having a child with complex medical conditions, or even simply being a parent. The combination of lived expertise and altruism, coupled with appropriate training and work practices, enables CHWs to establish trust, provide nonjudgmental support, and offer practical guidance for a range of social, behavioral, economic, and preventive health needs. Their role can include finding social supports; providing health system navigation, health coaching, and advocacy; and connecting individuals to essential resources, such as food, housing, or medications. A growing body of evidence (CDC, 2014) supports their effectiveness to address underlying socioeconomic determinants of health (Wang et al., 2012); improve chronic disease control (Carrasquillo et al., 2017); promote healthy behavior (Minkovitz et al., 2007); improve access to care (O'Brien et al., 2010); increase use of preventive care services; foster healthy development (Mendelsohn et al., 2005); reduce costly hospitalizations (Campbell et al., 2015), readmission (Kangovi et al., 2014), and ED use (Coker et al., 2016); and save Medicaid as much as $4,200 per beneficiary (Kangovi et al., 2020).

The COVID-19 pandemic has illustrated the role that CHWs play in responding to the needs of the community in which they reside, particularly in addressing the social determinants of health (SDOH) that have been shown to increase the risk of COVID-19 infection (Peretz et al., 2020). In

New York City, for example, health care organizations incorporated CHWs into their interprofessional response to COVID-19. In collaboration with community-based organizations, CHW teams proactively contacted socially isolated patients, connecting them with sources of critically important care and support during the pandemic.

The core challenges for integrating CHWs into primary care relate to quality and financing (Kangovi et al., 2015; WHO, 2018). CHW programs vary in their structure and effectiveness. However, effective programs often share specific program elements that include hiring guidelines, compensation, structured supervision, manageable caseloads, community and clinical integration, and a holistic approach to support (Kangovi et al., 2015). CHWs are paid through a complex patchwork of funding options, such as Medicaid demonstration waivers, health homes, Medicaid managed care plans, and grants (Lloyd et al., 2020).

Behavioral Health Specialists

The U.S. primary care system faces a growing challenge in delivering mental health services to populations it serves (NASEM, 2020). Rates of mental health conditions are rising, fueled in part by increasing rates in children and adolescents, the opioid epidemic, and the COVID-19 pandemic (Beck et al., 2018; Holingue et al., 2020; The Larry A. Green Center and PCC, 2020). The behavioral health workforce includes all providers of prevention and treatment services for mental health or substance abuse disorders, including licensed and certified professionals, case coordinators, and peer advisors.

Behavioral health and mental health specialists working in primary care provide a range of education, consultation, and evidence-based interventions when the team determines that this is needed to improve patient function and achieve identified health goals (Skillman et al., 2016). More specifically, both psychotherapy and pharmacotherapy can be added to the care plan with clear evidence-based protocols for both mental health conditions and chronic medical conditions. An integral part of the role of these team members is ongoing education, training, and consultation with medical team members to increase their comfort and confidence in identifying, treating, and managing comorbid mental and physical conditions and addressing a complexity approach to follow-up and team management to ensure continuity and engagement.

A significant barrier for incorporating behavioral health into primary care is the growing shortage of behavioral health workers; the Health Resources and Services Administration (HRSA) projects 250,000 fewer than will be needed by 2025 (HRSA, 2015). Funding is also an ongoing barrier to using and optimizing behavioral and mental health services in primary care, as lack of insurance coverage and out-of-pocket costs for mental health services are often barriers to care-seekers and their families (Cheney et al., 2018; Cook et al., 2017; Rowan et al., 2013).

A further barrier to integrating behavioral health into primary care is a lack of strategies to develop effective and sustainable models for integration (McDaniel et al., 2014). The VA has evaluated the extent of its success in integrating behavioral health into its primary care model and reported that primary care practices serving smaller populations experienced challenges in providing these services (Cornwell et al., 2018). The challenges of creating effective care models in which behavioral health services are part of the extended primary care team have been described, emphasizing the need to integrate them into interprofessional training and educational curricula (NASEM, 2020; Ramanuj et al., 2019).

Pharmacists

Pharmacists working in primary care assume responsibility as members of the interprofessional care team to optimize medication therapy to ensure that it is safe, effective, affordable, and convenient (PCPCC, 2012; Ramalho de Oliveira et al., 2010). With the increasing prevalence of chronic disease and the resultant use of more medications, helping individuals and the health care team manage medication complexities is essential (Buttorff and Bauman, 2017; Qato et al., 2008). Fragmented care may increase the risk of medication mismanagement, as prescribing happens across many care settings and the lack of interoperability of EHRs further limits the accuracy of medication lists. Illness and death resulting from non-optimized medication therapy led to an estimated 275,000 avoidable deaths in 2016, with a cost of nearly $528.4 billion (Watanabe et al., 2018).

Pharmacist expertise is critical in guiding the team, person, and family in effectively assessing, planning, and managing medication use. The pharmacist works with them to develop an individualized plan that achieves the intended goals of therapy with appropriate follow-up to ensure optimal medication use and outcomes (CMM in Primary Care Research Team, 2018). Pharmacists can also collaborate as members of interprofessional primary care teams to deliver preventive care and chronic disease management in a variety of models, including as embedded practitioners in a primary care practice, through collaborative relationships between medical and community pharmacy practices, or via telehealth.

Research has shown that pharmacists contribute positively to the health of people and communities by delivering services aimed at improving medication use, with impact noticed across all areas of the quadruple aim (McFarland and Buck, 2020; PCPCC, 2012). Pharmacists have also been shown to aid in meeting the public health needs of individuals and communities by providing access to needed point-of-care testing, vaccinations, and essential medications (Berenbrok et al., 2020; Newman et al., 2020).

The greatest challenge to integrating the role of the pharmacist in primary care relates to financing barriers, with payment for clinical pharmacy services not systematically covered by Medicare and Medicaid and payment strategies varying widely state to state. Increasingly, health plans and clinical organizations engaged in risk-based contracting are recognizing pharmacists' important contributions to chronic care management through direct payment strategies or inclusion in value-based payment arrangements (Cothran et al., 2019; Cowart and Olson, 2019; Patwardhan et al., 2012). Expanding awareness of the beneficial effects of integrating pharmacists into primary care teams on clinical, economic, and humanistic outcomes is needed to support the scale and sustainability of the positive collaborations emerging nationwide.

Dental Professionals

Oral health is an essential component of overall health and well-being. Unfortunately, preventable oral diseases, including caries and periodontal disease, remain widespread, affecting overall physical and mental health as well as quality of life for many Americans and disproportionately impacting disadvantaged populations including homeless or incarcerated individuals, persons with disabilities, and Indigenous communities (Peres et al., 2019). When chronic dental conditions are effectively managed with early intervention, health outcomes improve and overall health care costs fall (Cigna, 2016; Jeffcoat et al., 2014; Nasseh et al., 2017; Watt et al., 2019), yet access to affordable dental services continues to be a major concern for many.

Opportunities to improve access to oral health services within primary care settings can benefit people of all ages. Primary care services see children multiple times through the first 5 years of life and thus have an opportunity to provide health promotion messages, screen for early childhood caries, and apply preventive fluoride varnish for high-risk children, in accordance with the United States Preventive Services Task Force recommendations (Moyer, 2014) and AAP best practices (Clark et al., 2020). Likewise, primary care teams can conduct oral cancer screening and refer patients with chronic oral conditions to dental offices.

Integrated models of primary care and dentistry can increase access and improve care coordination (Atchison et al., 2018; NASEM, 2019a). In recent years, HRSA has helped health centers tackle limitations in providing dental services, such as outdated equipment and insufficient space, to improve access to integrated, oral health services in primary care settings (HHS, 2019). In 2018, HRSA-funded health centers served more than 6.4

million patients seeking dental care—an increase of 13 percent since 2016—and provided more than 16.5 million with dental visits. In other settings, however, dental care remains almost entirely siloed from the rest of medical care, in both training and practice (see Chapter 5 for more detail). Payment for dental care is also treated separately, and Medicaid and Medicare spend very little on dental services for adults. Children are entitled to dental coverage through Medicaid, though only a small portion of eligible children are enrolled (Hummel et al., 2015; Simon, 2016). Most dental care in the United States is paid for out of pocket, compared to total health spending, with low-income adults facing the most barriers to obtaining it (Vujicic et al., 2016). As with other extended team members, the lack of coverage for dental service limits full integration of dental services in primary care teams. Payment models that support interprofessional, team-based, preventive care could eliminate this as a barrier (Atchison and Weintraub, 2017; Atchison et al., 2018; Hummel et al., 2015; Nasseh et al., 2014; Watt et al., 2019).

Social Workers

In the primary care setting, social workers may be responsible for assessing and screening patients, engaging and understanding them in their social context, providing behavioral health interventions, helping them and their families navigate the health care system, coordinating care across settings, and connecting clients with resources to address food insecurity, transportation, and other factors that affect SDOH (Cornell et al., 2020). They enable individuals with complex needs to live safely in their communities with effective yet realistic care plans, communication, and support. Although social workers' role in primary care is increasing, many primary care practices do not take advantage of their special training, particularly when working with populations of Black, Indigenous, and people of color and those from lower socioeconomic backgrounds. Given that including social workers in primary care settings improves health outcomes (Cornell et al., 2020; Rehner et al., 2017), the percentage of primary care practices who report working with social workers may increase as public and private payers shift toward value-based payment models that emphasize addressing SDOH.

Other Extended Health Care Team Members

In addition to those described above, many other health care professionals may be part of the extended team and contribute value-added care and services to meet the needs of the person seeking care. Others include care coordinators, care managers, home health care nurses, lactation consultants, nutritionists, and therapists (e.g., physical, occupational).

In addition, the primary care team often collaborates with other critically important medical colleagues and specialists, including psychiatrists, cardiologists, endocrinologists, hospitalists, and integrative medicine specialists. For patients with complex needs, coordinating within this wider team is a significant task for the core team.

The Extended Community Care Team

An essential component of the interprofessional primary care team is the extended community care team, which includes organizations and groups, such as early childhood educators, social support services, healthy aging services, caregiving services, home health aides, places of worship and other ministries, and disability support services. This brings together the community organizations, services, and personnel who are dedicated to ensuring that health care teams, care-seekers, and communities have access to the support services and resources needed to ensure the health and wellness of people and communities. Like the extended care team, the extended community care team will vary with the size and the type of the primary care practice and the needs of the population and the local community, and it should be constantly monitored for clinical fit (Katkin et al., 2017).

Team Size

The size and composition of a primary care team depends on the alignment of several key factors: the complexity and severity of the health and social concerns of the population and community to be served; the availability and accessibility of health professionals and community support networks; and the robust institutional data structures used to efficiently and effectively match, allocate, and monitor resource supply with individual, family, and community needs. Randomly allocated small teams and unwieldy large teams that lack clear, matched, and organized workflows monitored by operational leaders risk failure to optimize and deliver the whole-person benefit of primary care despite the level of population complexity. When primary care teams are poorly defined and resourced, they risk depersonalization, lack of relationship continuity, ongoing communication gaps, and failure to engage meaningfully with people and their families, with their unique individual goals, values, and desired outcomes.

A 2018 study modeled team configurations (and the cost per person) required to deliver high-quality primary care to different adult populations (Meyers et al., 2018). Using a combination of practice-level data from 73 practices and 8 site visits, the authors determined that to deliver high-quality primary care to 10,000 adults, a primary care practice needed about 37 full-time team members, including 6 physicians and 2 NPs or PAs, supported by a mix of nurses, medical assistants, and RNs and licensed clinical social workers to help manage those with more complex chronic needs. Other team members, such as a pharmacist, care coordinator, and office staff, were also included. For a 10,000-person panel with a larger proportion of geriatric individuals, the authors modeled a larger team with about 52 members, more devoted to complex care management. For a 10,000-person panel with high social needs, the team included about 50 members but relatively fewer physicians compared to the other models and with additional members, such as CHWs, behavioral health, and other social supports. The authors' model for a smaller, rural panel of 5,000 included about 22 full-time team members, including a CHW (Meyers et al., 2018).

One method of determining team size is empanelment. As described in Chapter 4, this involves identifying the people in the target population, assigning all individuals in a given population to a primary care team or team member, and reviewing and updating the panel continuously (Bearden et al., 2019; McGough et al., 2018). This allows the clinicians and staff of that team to determine the optimal team size given the panel size and its needs.

Systems of care empanel populations in a variety of ways. In Alaska, for example, the Southcentral Foundation (SCF) Nuka System of Care's panels include around 1,500 patients per care team who empanel voluntarily. SCF approaches the task of empanelment with an entire department devoted to checking empanelment status, guiding the transition and information flow for those who switch, and providing other support to the process (Gottlieb, 2013; PHCPI, 2019). Costa Rica takes a different approach, geographically empaneling all citizens to integrated health care teams that each care for around 4,500 patients (Pesec et al., 2017). In a more hybrid approach, Turkish primary care clinicians empanel geographically to ensure universal access but allow empaneled people to switch clinicians after enrollment (PHCPI, 2019).

The literature describes several methods to determine optimal panel size, including a formulaic approach to balancing appointment supply and demand, a time-based method that accounts for the work required to deliver comprehensive care, and using existing panel sizes to construct normative benchmarks (Kivlahan et al., 2017). Panel sizes vary considerably, with many practices unable to provide accurate estimates, but the consensus is that the old, arbitrary standard of 2,500 patients per physician is too large for a single physician to manage effectively in most situations (Raffoul et al., 2016). Even for an interprofessional team, optimal panel size is often below 2,000 and depends on the degree of task-sharing, organized workflow, and matched skill sets of the team members (Altschuler et al., 2012; Brownlee and Van Borkulo, 2013). For example, the VA established panel sizes in 2009 of 1,200 veterans to a full-time physician's panel[3] and adjusts based on location (VHA, 2017). In general, panel sizes for pediatricians are smaller than for primary care practices serving mostly adults because children under 4 years old visit primary care more frequently in a typical year than adults do (Murray et al., 2007).

Multiple methods exist to determine panel populations if they are not based on strict geography. These usually include variations in classifying active care-seekers, as the priority is to keep people with their normal clinician or team, if they have one. That variation includes how far back a health system looks in appointment history to find active accounts and how many and which types of appointments to qualify as active (AIR, 2013). An additional layer, risk adjustment (see Chapter 9), is another important element of empaneling. Practices may account for characteristics including sex, age, comorbidities, acuity, or other traits based on EHRs, claims, or population health data to attempt to evenly distribute a population's health needs across different panels (Brownlee and Van Borkulo, 2013; Kivlahan and Sinsky, 2018).

In addition to strategies to evenly distribute people, health systems or practices will often stratify populations into subgroups, based on specific criteria, to better align and match needs with team resources (Bohmer, 2011). For example, this process may stratify those who would benefit most from interaction with an integrated, behavioral specialist who may only be onsite twice per week or people with multiple medical and medication complexities who require longer visits with key team members (Bohmer, 2011).

EDUCATING AND TRAINING THE
INTERPROFESSIONAL PRIMARY CARE TEAM

Chapter 3 touched briefly on the pipeline problems for primary care workforce production. This section expands on the major factors influencing the education of that workforce and how it needs to change to prepare the workforce for integrated, interprofessional care. Core to the delivery of primary care are competencies underlying team-based care; how to function in an integrated, interprofessional manner; and how to integrate and coordinate care with community-based care team members. To ensure equitable access to primary care, it is necessary to determine the size of the workforce needed along with the types of team members needed in different communities.

---

[3] Literature typically measures panel size per physician, even in interprofessional team-based care settings. For example, the VA staffs one physician and three supporting team members to a panel. It assigns discipline-specific team members, such as dietitians and social workers, across multiple panels.

Over the past decade, the Institute of Medicine (IOM), the World Health Organization, the Josiah Macy Jr. Foundation, and others have issued repeated recommendations for interprofessional education (Cox and Naylor, 2013; Frenk et al., 2010; IOM, 2013b; NASEM, 2016; WHO, 2010). In 2009, major nursing, medicine, pharmacy, dental, and public health organizations founded the Interprofessional Education Collaborative, and over the next 5 years, the Association of American Medical Colleges (AAMC) partnered with the American Association of Colleges of Nursing, the American Board of Medical Specialties, and the American Psychiatric Association to create resources for early interprofessional training and lifelong learning (IPEC, 2020; Swanberg, 2016). Progress has been made, in that most health care disciplines now have interprofessional competencies as an expectation for all their graduates (HPAC, 2019), and some leading institutions integrate these competencies into their initiatives. For example, the VA Centers of Excellence in Primary Care Education focus on developing and implementing models for interprofessional team-based learning and practice in training settings (Harada et al., 2018), while the American College of Physicians created a standing committee to advise on "plans and strategies to promote high-quality education incorporating interprofessional, interdisciplinary, and patient perspectives and promoting partnership with all members of the health care team" (ACP, 2020).

Interprofessional practice has four major established core competencies— values and ethics for interprofessional practice, roles and responsibilities, interprofessional communication, and teams and teamwork (Schmitt et al., 2011)—and the challenge of achieving those competencies lies in incorporating interprofessional didactic and experiential learning into the already crowded medical and health professional education. Challenges also exist in educating and training students alongside the current workforce, especially in settings where the workforce itself is not functioning as an interprofessional team. Interprofessional education competencies are location agnostic, so there is no guarantee that aspiring primary care–bound health professionals, as well as the existing primary care workforce, have any interprofessional education or training specific to the delivery of primary care.

Integrating interprofessional education and training in primary care is also a challenge because crowded clinics often find that accommodating single students from one discipline is disruptive to the normal workflow. This situation makes it almost impossible to accommodate students from different disciplines rotating together for an interprofessional education practicum. It is much easier to train across professions in the contained environment of academic health centers and on large inpatient units, where teams frequently work side by side, than in multiple primary care clinics that are unlikely to be set up for robust team-based care models. For interprofessional education to take root in primary care, the training and care models need to evolve together, and this will take considerably more investment than is currently available (Sanchez and Hermis, 2019; Shrader et al., 2018). Indeed, changes in the funding model for training clinicians in primary care are necessary before primary care practices can engage in interprofessional educational experiences without believing that educating trainees in team-based care will reduce the productivity of the individual clinician.

Too often, students engage in didactic work that introduces them to interprofessional teams, roles, and mutual respect, followed by clinical training in settings that are not interprofessional and lack teamwork, collaboration, and community engagement. Research over the past 40 years on how people learn shows that what learners do is critical to learning and more important than what they are told (NRC, 2005; Sawyer, 2005). The implication is that while primary care–bound students, and perhaps all health profession students, are acquiring their disciplinary knowledge and skills, their curriculum should simultaneously be embedded in environments in which they can experience and progressively engage in high-quality team care (Billett, 2004; Lave and Wenger, 1991; Peterson, 2019; Swanwick, 2005).

DIVERSITY AND EQUITY IN THE PRIMARY CARE WORKFORCE

Research shows that increasing the diversity of the workforce to more closely match the increasing diversity of the United States is essential for "(1) advancing cultural competency, (2) increasing access to high-quality health care services, (3) strengthening the medical research agenda, and (4) ensuring optimal management of the health care system" (Cohen et al., 2002, p. 91). Having a diverse health care workforce that reflects the population has been shown to improve health equity and reduce health care disparities, increase access to care, improve health care outcomes, strengthen patient communication, and heighten patient satisfaction in underserved and minority populations (COGME, 2016; Cohen et al., 2002; Cooper and Powe, 2004; HRSA, 2006; Poma, 2017; Wakefield, 2014).

The Diversity of the Primary Care Workforce

Health profession education is a common good, so programs should be expected to supply graduates prepared to care for their immediate and regional communities. To the extent that they fail to do this, they are failing their public mission. Health disparities are a long-standing, well-recognized problem in the United States, perpetuated in part by a health care workforce that does not come from, represent, or commit to the populations it purports to serve.

In 2017, men accounted for 55 percent of the total PCP workforce, though that percentage varied widely by discipline. Women were 52 percent of the geriatricians and 64 percent of the pediatricians, while men were 59 percent of the family practitioners, 62 percent of internists, and 75 percent of general practitioners (Petterson et al., 2018). In 2017, more than 25 percent of PCPs were 60 years and older (see Figure 6-2).

A 2017 HRSA report revealed that white workers represent the majority of all 30 health occupations studied and are overrepresented in 23 of the 30 occupations based on their total representation in the U.S. workforce (HRSA, 2017). In comparison, Hispanic, Native Hawaiians, and Other Pacific Islander professionals are significantly under-represented in all the occupations classified as "health diagnosing and treating practitioners," while non-Hispanic Black individuals are under-represented in all of these occupations, except among dieticians and nutritionists (15.0 percent) and respiratory therapists (12.8 percent). American Indians and Alaska Natives are under-represented in all occupations except for PAs and have the lowest representation among physicians and dentists (0.1 percent in each occupation). Asian professionals are well represented as "health diagnosing and treating practitioners" but under-represented among speech–language pathologists (2.2 percent) and advanced practice registered nurses (APRNs) (4.1 percent). Data for allopathic training programs for primary care specialties show a similar story. Among internal medicine residents in 2020, 4.7 percent were Black and 6.7 percent were Hispanic. Among family medicine

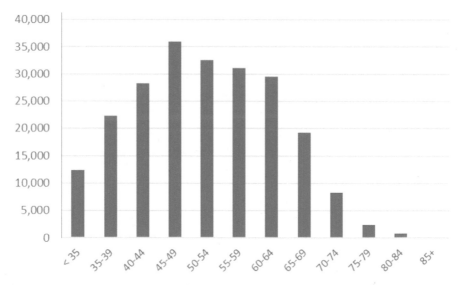

FIGURE 6-2 Age distribution of primary care physicians in 2017.
SOURCE: Petterson et al., 2018.

residents, 9.3 percent were Black and 10.0 percent were Hispanic. American Indians and Alaska Natives, and Native Hawaiians and Other Pacific Islanders are also under-represented and are at or below 1 percent of the total resident population (AAMC, 2020). Black, Indigenous, and people of color are well represented among health care support and personal care and services occupations, whereas whites are under-represented in these. This is a reflection of the systemic discrimination and biases evident in education, housing, finance, and job opportunities that funnel minorities to health care support and personal care service roles as opposed to health diagnosing and treating roles. Approaches such as holistic admissions practices benefit racial, socioeconomic, and perspective diversity of health professions schools, but the work to improve representation in health care extends far beyond admissions processes (Urban Universities for Health, 2014).

AAMC has released two major reports focusing on diversity and equity in the shrinking PCP workforce—*Altering the Course: Black Males in Medicine* (2015) and *Reshaping the Journey: American Indians and Alaska Natives in Medicine* (2018)—to explore and try to answer why diversity efforts have not been more successful in recruiting individuals from under-represented populations. A theme expressed throughout *Altering the Course* was the persistent, structural racism and stereotyping facing Black men and boys that leads to widespread implicit and explicit bias, which can then create exclusionary environments resulting in de facto segregation (AAMC, 2015). For those Black medical students who do make it into the training pipeline, many have cited racial discrimination and prejudice, feelings of isolation, and different cultural expectations as negatively affecting their medical school experience (Dyrbye et al., 2007; Silver et al., 2019). Furthermore, research has documented that minority physicians often confront racism and bias from not only their peers and superiors but also the people and communities they have committed to serve (Acosta and Ackerman-Barger, 2017). What is not clear and needs more study is the number of PCPs from under-represented populations, including Black, Indigenous, and people of color, who leave the field each year, the reasons they may choose to leave (i.e., burnout, discrimination, specialty practice, age), and what impact that may have on the ability of the workforce to achieve health equity and reduce health care disparities.

Although educating and training a more diverse workforce is critical, the education pipeline is complex and lengthy, and the need for more robust community engagement is urgent and cannot wait for a new, diverse generation of clinicians to make their way through that pipeline. One way many communities are bridging this gap is to expand and diversify opportunities for CHWs, care coordinators, health coaches, and health educators (Brownstein et al., 2011; Jackson and Gracia, 2014). For example, CHWs are a diverse reflection of disadvantaged Americans: 65 percent are Black or

Hispanic, 23 percent are white, 10 percent are American Indian or Alaska Native, and 2 percent are Asian or Pacific Islander (Arizona Prevention Research Center, 2015). While CHWs can improve the diversity of the extended primary care team, that should not deter the necessary efforts to diversify the core primary care workforce across professions to create a local workforce that reflects the diversity of the community in which it is practicing, which can lead to a more equitable system for all (Cohen et al., 2002).

Preparing the Diverse Workforce of the Future

Preparing the workforce of the future starts with the characteristics of the students planning to enter primary care. Evidence exists that health profession students who come from underserved communities, whether rural, urban, minority, or other, are far more likely than middle-class white students to work in underserved areas (Cregler et al., 1997; Goodfellow et al., 2016). While recognizing that health profession education programs have diverse missions, such as community health care, training academic leaders, and providing research skills and opportunities, all health profession programs must invest in the common good. If program admission goals and outcomes were public, it would add transparency and accountability that could enable the country to make progress toward eliminating health disparities.

Once programs select appropriate, demographically diverse, primary care–bound health profession students, these programs will have to support their students' values and career goals, which often does not happen. In fact, bright students may be told they are too smart to become primary care clinicians (Marchand and Peckham, 2017; Warm and Goetz, 2013), much like NP students are often asked why, if they are so smart, they do not become doctors. Health professional training programs must ensure that learners do not receive this kind of undermining message and, if they do, they have resources for support and to assist them and their allies in responding. A significant challenge is that many programs, especially research-intensive programs, are not committed to primary care and have different goals for their learners (Bailey, 2016; Frieden, 2009). Holding educational programs to regionally appropriate outcome goals may be a critical element in advancing these programs' mission to address health care disparities through workforce interventions.

Bringing the right students on board is only the first step. Institutions must also ensure that the educational experience provides the opportunity to develop the skills that will enable students to form relationships with their future care-seekers. While disciplinary knowledge and technical skills are critical, the meta-skills of communication, collaboration, leadership, and advocacy are equally essential. In general, health profession students are educated in formal didactic contexts, in a fairly theoretical vein, and in isolation from each other. While theoretical knowledge is important across the health professions, this focus underinvests in the contextual, team-oriented skills that are essential for effective team-based primary care practice. To the extent possible, primary care–bound learners from different disciplines would benefit from learning with each other in classrooms and especially from joint early and sustained experiential learning. In most medical schools, students begin seeing patients in the first or second week of their first year, and they would benefit greatly if these experiences included explicit attention to and work with the full range of members of the primary care interprofessional team.

The ability of a primary care team to address the broad range of population needs, including identifying community expectations, engaging individuals in preventive health care and counseling, and managing simple and moderately complex medical problems, is essential to creating a system in which the requirements of the populations and individuals are addressed efficiently and cost-effectively. Primary care team members should see themselves as the linchpin between communities and link people and families to specialists, acute care hospitals, and chronic care facilities. They need to have a deep grasp of physiology, therapeutics, and technical medicine and also an appreciation of the assets and challenges of the communities they serve, a broad understanding of how the health system is constructed and works, exceptional skills in team-building, communication and collaboration, and oftentimes strong leadership and advocacy skills. The U.S. system of identifying candidates for these roles and preparing learners is often not well designed to accomplish this task.

FUNDING TO SUPPORT THE TRAINING OF THE PRIMARY CARE WORKFORCE

The ability to obtain high-quality primary care depends on the availability of clinicians who are essential members of the primary care core team, including PCPs, NPs, and PAs (Phillips and Bazemore, 2010). Dynamic changes are occurring in the type of primary care clinicians being educated, and access to a robust workforce varies across geographic regions. While the need for the primary care workforce has been well described in this report, the U.S. Department of Health and Human Services (HHS) offers no consistent source of funding that is based on population needs. Additionally, the committee is not aware of federal support for the funding of training non-clinician team members, such as CHWs or medical assistants.

Primary Care Physicians

A substantial body of evidence shows that increasing the proportion of PCPs in the total physician workforce has significant benefits regarding quality of care, access to care, and medical expenditures (Baicker and Chandra, 2004; Basu et al., 2019; Levine et al., 2019; Starfield, 2001; Steinwald, 2008). However, the United States has not seen rapid growth in PCPs over the past three decades (see Chapter 3 for more on the PCP workforce). Current graduate medical education (GME) and Children's Hospitals Graduate Medical Education (CHGME) funding for physician workforce training results in only 24 percent of trainees pursuing primary care, and fewer than 8 percent go to rural practice (Chen et al., 2013a).[4] The IOM has twice recommended that GME policy produce a workforce that is more aligned with population need by increasing the proportion of its funding directed to primary care workforce training (IOM, 1989, 2014). Other federal workforce advisory committees, including the Council on Graduate Medical Education and the Advisory Committee on Training in Primary Care Medicine and Dentistry, have also recommended repeatedly that federal GME funds be directed to increase primary care and rural workforce outputs (COGME, 2010). To date, these evidence-based reports have not resulted in sustained funding directed specifically to primary care.

The root problem may be that the majority of the $15 billion spent on GME by the Centers for Medicare & Medicaid Services (CMS) and the VA is paid to hospitals and does not support primary care practices or pediatric services that are the training centers for primary care (Chen et al., 2013b; Weida et al., 2010). Training pediatricians in children's hospitals is funded under a separate (and precarious) funding stream through the CHGME program (IOM, 2014), administered by the Bureau of Health Workforce, HRSA, and HHS, because GME funding is calculated based largely on the volume of services a hospital provides to Medicare beneficiaries, who are primarily over age 65 and therefore not treated at children's hospitals (HRSA, 2020a). Despite multiple entities petitioning for more GME and CHGME funding to adequately address the nation's shortage of physicians, federal support has remained effectively frozen since 1997.

Given the findings that the location of medical students' schools and training sites affect where they choose to practice (Fagan et al., 2015; Washko et al., 2015), and the shortage of PCPs in rural and other areas, several proposals and policy decisions have aimed to decentralize training (Bennett et al., 2009; Fagan et al., 2015; Whittaker et al., 2019). For example, the University of Toronto established a family medicine residency

---

[4] Training pediatricians in children's hospitals has a separate federal funding stream, through the CHGME payment program.

program in Barrie, Ontario, located approximately 60 miles north of Toronto, to address a shortage of physicians in the region. Nearly two-thirds of the graduates from the first six classes of this program stayed to work in the region and were happy with that decision (Whittaker et al., 2019).

Nurse Practitioners and Physician Assistants

Between 2010 and 2017, the number of full-time NPs in the United States more than doubled, from approximately 91,000 to 190,000, and growth occurred in every region (Auerbach et al., 2020). Similarly, there were about 98,000 PAs in 2007, compared to almost 140,000 in 2019 (He et al., 2009; NCCPA, 2020). NPs and PAs work in multiple settings, including hospitals, physician offices, and clinics, but their rapid growth has transformed many primary care practices. The National Center for Health Workforce Analysis projects that the number of primary care NPs and PAs will outpace demand at the national level if they continue to be used as they are today (HRSA and NCHWA, 2016). In fact, it has been suggested that the growth in non-physician clinicians in primary care could eliminate predicted shortages of physicians (Morgan, 2019; Van Vleet and Paradise, 2015). Current estimates, however, suggest that less than one-third of APRNs spend most of their time in primary care settings (HHS et al., 2020), although separate estimates of NPs only are higher (AANP, 2020b). Among PAs, 25 percent currently practice in primary care, although this number has been decreasing in recent years (NCCPA, 2020). No consistent federal support exists to educate NPs, PAs, and certified nurse-midwives (CNMs), nor do overburdened clinics receive a financial incentive to offer training slots to NP and PA students. The Graduate Nurse Education (GNE) demonstration project, mandated under Section 5509 of the Patient Protection and Affordable Care Act (ACA),[5] was designed to test whether payments for clinical education increased the number of NP graduates, with the aim of increasing the supply of primary care clinicians to meet growing U.S. demand (IMPAQ International, 2019). From 2012 to 2018, CMS paid five eligible hospital awardees for the reasonable costs attributable to providing qualified clinical education to NP students enrolled as a result of the project. Key findings suggest that the GNE project had a positive impact on NP graduate growth and allowed schools of nursing to enhance and formalize clinical placement processes, strengthen relationships with clinical education sites, and increase awareness of the role and value of NPs (IMPAQ International, 2019). This project was notable in that it was the first large

---

[5] Patient Protection and Affordable Care Act, Public Law 111-148, § 5509 (March 23, 2010).

attempt to broaden the scope of CMS funding beyond physician residency training, though it was discontinued despite positive outcomes.

Practice Settings to Support the Preparation of Primary Care Teams

HRSA has played an important role in investing in the education of the primary care workforce through funding the medical education training programs for physicians, PAs, and behavioral health specialists, and dentistry residency programs in rural and underserved areas. Evidence has shown that these investments through Title VII are producing demonstrably better patient outcomes and that such training increases the primary care workforce, but Title VII funding is only a small fraction of the total GME funding—it has been reduced to less than 10 percent of what it was in the late 1960s (Palmer et al., 2008; Phillips and Turner, 2012)—and the repeated calls to action and modest investments by HRSA have not resulted in significant increases in PCP workforce training.

Federal policies to increase the supply of PCPs in shortage areas, including increasing the funding for health centers, rely largely on HRSA shortage designations that assume the availability of primary care is equivalent to its accessibility (Naylor et al., 2019). In the last decade, the number of health centers has increased almost 80 percent, primarily in urban areas (Chang et al., 2019). Rural health clinics (RHCs), which are not subject to the same requirements of HRSA-funded health centers but are federally certified clinics in rural Medically Underserved Areas or Health Professional Shortage Areas, also provide primary care services. There are currently more than 4,500 RHCs across the country (CMS, 2019). Any growth of health centers or RHCs contributes to increasing health care providers serving in the designated medically underserved areas. From 2003 to 2018, employment in health centers increased from 25,780 to 149,755, including physicians, NPs, PAs, CNMs, and other clinicians (NACHC, 2020; Xue et al., 2018a). RHCs, as a condition of their certification, are required to employ at least one physician and one PA, NP, or CNM (CMS, 2019). An analysis of the impact of health centers on the primary care clinician gap indicated that having a greater number of health center sites was associated with a bigger reduction in the gap in under-resourced areas. However, the increase in primary care clinicians over time has largely been attributed to the use of NPs and PAs and not increasing numbers of PCPs (Xue et al., 2018a). These findings are similar to those reported by the National Association of Community Health Centers that health centers are twice as likely as other primary care practices to employ NPs, PAs, and CNMs. It is not known whether this hiring practice is based on the availability of clinicians in an area or a perceived cost savings, given the difference in the salaries of NPs and PAs compared to physicians.

HRSA has also been instrumental in supporting the training of PCP and dental residents through the Teaching Health Center Graduate Medical Education (THCGME) program. The ACA created the THCGME program in 2010 and it is designed to train health professionals at health centers in underserved communities (Chen et al., 2012). It is the only federally funded GME program to have accountability metrics and reporting requirements and the majority of its trainees stay in primary care and in medically underserved communities (AAFP, 2020). It currently produces more than 280 PCPs and dentists annually (HRSA, 2020b). THCGME is a model of training the primary care workforce where the underserved receive care which has been shown to be an effective way to increase this workforce (Phillips et al., 2013).

HRSA Title VIII programs are also a major source of federal funding for primary care services in underserved areas and have a strong focus on training interprofessional care teams in primary care. Primary care medical and oral health training grants are used to develop and test innovative curricula and training methods to transform health care practice and delivery, in areas such as team-based management of chronic disease in primary care and person-centered models of care. HRSA Title VIII programs are community based, provide interprofessional training programs for all health professionals, and are designed to encourage them to return to community settings after graduation. Title VIII also funds special initiatives that help increase the diversity of the workforce and strategies to improve health care access in underserved areas.

The National Health Service Corps (NHSC), part of Title VIII, has played a significant role in supporting the pipeline of primary care in federally designated shortage areas through scholarships to students in training and paying educational loans for current primary care workers (Politzer et al., 2000). Since its inception, NHSC reports that it has funded more than 63,000 primary care medical, nursing, dental, and mental and behavioral health professionals and that it has more than 16,000 scholarship recipients providing care to more than 17 million people. More than 1,500 NHSC scholars are currently in residency or school preparing to work in underserved primary care settings upon graduation. Evaluations of the program have revealed that NHSC clinicians complement rather than compete with non-NHSC clinicians in primary care and mental health care (Han et al., 2019). NHSC clinicians help enhance care delivery in community health centers, particularly for dental and mental health services, which are the two major areas of service gaps. During the period of the American Recovery and Reinvestment Act, the NHSC workforce increased by 156 percent, with the largest increase seen in the number of mental health clinicians (210 percent) (Pathman and Konrad, 2012).

FINDINGS AND CONCLUSIONS

To achieve the goal of high-quality primary care, it is essential that interprofessional teams be designed to meet the needs of individuals, their families, and communities. Teams would benefit from integrating the skills and expertise of the person and their family, primary care clinicians, members of the extended health care team, and community-based personnel and services. When interprofessional teams are used, they are often not optimized, and individual members are often underused and not functioning at the top of their scope of practice. Although evidence exists that integrated, interprofessional, team-based care offers great promise in achieving high-quality primary care outcomes, no standardized or "one-size-fits-all" approach is available to guide the design and composition of interprofessional teams.

Funding for the preparation of the primary care workforce is inconsistent and insufficient. The shrinking physician workforce simply cannot meet the growing needs of high-quality primary care delivery, and the structure of GME funding does not support the training needs of the PCP workforce. Alternative financing sources are needed for community-based training of physicians, NPs, and PAs in primary care. Primary care practices, with high patient volumes and limited time and resources, need financial incentives to support the intensive training of interprofessional primary care teams.

Relatedly, the diversity of the primary care workforce does not match the needs of local communities and society. For primary care teams to address well-documented disparities in treatment based on race and ethnicity, its team members must reflect the lived experiences of the communities they serve. This can be accomplished by increasing the diversity of both the PCP and interprofessional team workforces and matching the needed resources to the populations' economic, health, and social risks.

Finally, payment has to align with and value interprofessional teams that will vary in design, based on the needs of local communities and patient populations. The current payment system for interprofessional primary care is broken and not aligned to enable the delivery of team-based care. Although significant challenges remain to implementing an integrated, interprofessional workforce that delivers high-quality primary care, the opportunity lies with aligning a payment and financial system that incentivizes and rewards effective, integrated *interprofessional* primary care that produces positive outcomes.

REFERENCES

AAFP (American Academy of Family Physicians). 2019. *Scope of practice—physicians assistants*. Leawood, KS: American Academy of Family Physicians.

AAFP. 2020. *Teaching health centers.* https://www.aafp.org/dam/AAFP/documents/advocacy/workforce/gme/BKG-TeachingHealthCenters.pdf (accessed March 2, 2021).

AAMC (Association of American Medical Colleges). 2015. *Altering the course: Black males in medicine.* Washington, DC: Association of American Medical Colleges.

AAMC. 2018. *Reshaping the journey: American Indians and Alaska Natives in medicine.* Washington, DC: Association of American Medical Colleges.

AAMC. 2019. *2019 state physician workforce data report.* Washington, DC: Association of American Medical Colleges.

AAMC. 2020. *2020 report on residents.* https://www.aamc.org/data-reports/students-residents/interactive-data/report-residents/2020/executive-summary (accessed February 22, 2021).

AANP (American Association of Nurse Practitioners). 2020a. *Nurse practitioner COVID-19 survey: August 2020.* https://www.aanp.org/practice/practice-related-research/research-reports/nurse-practitioner-covid-19-survey-2 (accessed December 28, 2020).

AANP. 2020b. *Nurse practitioners in primary care.* https://www.aanp.org/advocacy/advocacy-resource/position-statements/nurse-practitioners-in-primary-care (accessed December 28, 2020).

AANP. 2021. *2021 nurse practitioner state practice environment.* Arlington, VA: American Association of Nurse Practitioners.

AAPA (American Academy of Physician Assistants). 2020. *AAPA calls on governors to empower physician assistants in COVID-19 fight.* https://www.aapa.org/news-central/2020/03/aapa-calls-on-governors-to-empower-physician-assistants-in-covid-19-fight (accessed June 30, 2020).

AARP and NAC (National Alliance for Caregiving). 2020. *Caregiving in the U.S. 2020.* Washington, DC: AARP.

Acosta, D., and K. Ackerman-Barger. 2017. Breaking the silence: Time to talk about race and racism. *Academic Medicine* 92(3):285–288.

ACP (American College of Physicians). 2020. *Patient and interprofessional partnership committee.* https://www.acponline.org/about-acp/who-we-are/leadership/boards-committees-councils/patient-and-interprofessional-partnership-committee (accessed June 6, 2020).

AIR (American Institutes for Research). 2013. *Empanelment implementation guide.* Washington, DC: American Institutes for Research.

Altschuler, J., D. Margolius, T. Bodenheimer, and K. Grumbach. 2012. Estimating a reasonable patient panel size for primary care physicians with team-based task delegation. *Annals of Family Medicine* 10(5):396–400.

Andrades, M., S. Kausar, and A. Ambreen. 2013. Role and influence of the patient's companion in family medicine consultations: "The patient's perspective." *Journal of Family Medicine and Primary Care* 2(3):283–287.

Arizona Prevention Research Center. 2015. *National community health worker advocacy survey.* Tucson, AZ: University of Arizona.

Aruru, M., H. A. Truong, and S. Clark. 2021. Pharmacy Emergency Preparedness and Response (PEPR): A proposed framework for expanding pharmacy professionals' roles and contributions to emergency preparedness and response during the COVID-19 pandemic and beyond. *Research in Social and Administrative Pharmacy* 17(1):1967–1977.

Atchison, K. A., and J. A. Weintraub. 2017. Integrating oral health and primary care in the changing health care landscape. *North Carolina Medical Journal* 78(6):406–409.

Atchison, K. A., J. A. Weintraub, and R. G. Rozier. 2018. Bridging the dental-medical divide: Case studies integrating oral health care and primary health care. *Journal of the American Dental Association* 149(10):850–858.

Auerbach, D. I., P. I. Buerhaus, and D. O. Staiger. 2020. Implications of the rapid growth of the nurse practitioner workforce in the US. *Health Affairs* 39(2):273–279.

Baicker, K., and A. Chandra. 2004. Medicare spending, the physician workforce, and beneficiaries' quality of care. *Health Affairs* 23(Suppl 1):W4–W197.

Bailey, M. 2016. Harvard has one of the best medical schools. Why does it ignore family medicine? *STAT+*. https://www.statnews.com/2016/04/05/harvard-medical-school-family-medicine (accessed November 10, 2020).

Basu, S., S. A. Berkowitz, R. L. Phillips, A. Bitton, B. E. Landon, and R. S. Phillips. 2019. Association of primary care physician supply with population mortality in the United States, 2005–2015. *JAMA Internal Medicine* 179(4):506–514.

Bearden, T., H. Ratcliffe, J. Sugarman, A. Bitton, L. Anaman, G. Buckle, M. Cham, D. Chong Woei Quan, F. Ismail, B. Jargalsaikhan, W. Lim, N. Mohammad, I. Morrison, B. Norov, J. Oh, G. Riimaadai, S. Sararaks, and L. Hirschhorn. 2019. Empanelment: A foundational component of primary health care. *Gates Open Research* 3(1654).

Beck, A. F., M. M. Tschudy, T. R. Coker, K. B. Mistry, J. E. Cox, B. A. Gitterman, L. J. Chamberlain, A. M. Grace, M. K. Hole, P. E. Klass, K. S. Lobach, C. T. Ma, D. Navsaria, K. D. Northrip, M. D. Sadof, A. N. Shah, and A. H. Fierman. 2016. Determinants of health and pediatric primary care practices. *Pediatrics* 137(3):e20153673.

Beck, A. J., R. W. Manderscheid, and P. Buerhaus. 2018. The future of the behavioral health workforce: Optimism and opportunity. *American Journal of Preventive Medicine* 54(6S3):S187–S189.

Bennett, K., J. Phillips, and B. Teevan. 2009. Closing the gap: Finding and encouraging physicians who will care for the underserved. *The Virtual Mentor* 11(5):390–398.

Berenbrok, L. A., N. Gabriel, K. C. Coley, and I. Hernandez. 2020. Evaluation of frequency of encounters with primary care physicians vs. visits to community pharmacies among Medicare beneficiaries. *JAMA Network Open* 3(7):e209132.

Berg, S. 2020. *Physician burnout: Which medical specialties feel the most stress*. https://www.ama-assn.org/practice-management/physician-health/physician-burnout-which-medical-specialties-feel-most-stress (accessed December 28, 2020).

Bidassie, B. 2017. The Veterans Affairs Patient Aligned Care Team (VA PACT), a new benchmark for patient-centered medical home models: A review and discussion. In *Patient centered medicine*, edited by O. Sayligil. London, UK: IntechOpen Ltd. Pp. 139–160.

Billett, S. 2004. Workplace participatory practices: Conceptualising workplaces as learning environments. *Journal of Workplace Learning* 16(6):312–324.

BLS (U.S. Bureau of Labor Statistics). 2020. *Occupational outlook handbook: Medical assistants*. https://www.bls.gov/ooh/healthcare/medical-assistants.htm (accessed October 27, 2020).

Bodenheimer, T. 2019a. Anatomy and physiology of primary care teams. *JAMA Internal Medicine* 179(1):61–62.

Bodenheimer, T. 2019b. Building powerful primary care teams. *Mayo Clinic Proceedings* 94(7):1135–1137.

Bodenheimer, T., and B. Y. Laing. 2007. The teamlet model of primary care. *Annals of Family Medicine* 5(5):457–461.

Bodenheimer, T. S., and M. D. Smith. 2013. Primary care: Proposed solutions to the physician shortage without training more physicians. *Health Affairs* 32(11):1881–1886.

Bohmer, R. M. 2011. The four habits of high-value health care organizations. *New England Journal of Medicine* 365(22):2045–2047.

Bombard, Y., G. R. Baker, E. Orlando, C. Fancott, P. Bhatia, S. Casalino, K. Onate, J.-L. Denis, and M.-P. Pomey. 2018. Engaging patients to improve quality of care: A systematic review. *Implementation Science* 13(1):98.

Borgès Da Silva, R., I. Brault, R. Pineault, M. C. Chouinard, A. Prud'homme, and D. D'Amour. 2018. Nursing practice in primary care and patients' experience of care. *Journal of Primary Care and Community Health* 9:1–7.

Brownlee, B., and N. Van Borkulo. 2013. *Empanelment: Establishing patient–provider relationships.* Seattle, WA: Qualis Health, The MacColl Center for Health Care Innovation at the Group Health Research Institute.

Brownstein, J. N., G. R. Hirsch, E. L. Rosenthal, and C. H. Rush. 2011. Community health workers "101" for primary care providers and other stakeholders in health care systems. *Journal of Ambulatory Care Management* 34(3):210–220.

Bruner, T. 2016. Physician assistants increase care access. *Journal of the Arkansas Medical Society* 112(13):252–253.

Buerhaus, P. 2018. *A solution for America's primary care shortage.* https://www.realclearhealth.com/articles/2018/11/01/a_solution_for_americas_primary_care_shortage_110837.html (accessed December 28, 2020).

Buttorff, C., and M. Bauman. 2017. *Multiple chronic conditions in the United States.* Santa Monica, CA: RAND.

Cadogan, C. A., and C. M. Hughes. 2020. On the frontline against COVID-19: Community pharmacists' contribution during a public health crisis. *Research in Social and Administrative Pharmacy* 17(1):2032–2035.

Campbell, J. D., M. Brooks, P. Hosokawa, J. Robinson, L. Song, and J. Krieger. 2015. Community health worker home visits for Medicaid-enrolled children with asthma: Effects on asthma outcomes and costs. *American Journal of Public Health* 105(11):2366–2372.

Carrasquillo, O., C. Lebron, Y. Alonzo, H. Li, A. Chang, and S. Kenya. 2017. Effect of a community health worker intervention among Latinos with poorly controlled type 2 diabetes: The Miami Healthy Heart Initiative randomized clinical trial. *JAMA Internal Medicine* 177(7):948–954.

Cassel, C. K., and D. B. Reuben. 2011. Specialization, subspecialization, and subsubspecialization in internal medicine. *New England Journal of Medicine* 364(12):1169–1173.

Cawley, J. F., and R. S. Hooker. 2013. Physician assistants in American medicine: The half-century mark. *American Journal of Managed Care* 19(10):e333–e341.

CDC (Centers for Disease Control and Prevention). 2014. *Policy evidence assessment report: Community health worker policy components.* Atlanta, GA: U.S. Department of Health and Human Services, Centers for Disease Control and Prevention.

Cené, C. W., L. B. Haymore, F. C. Lin, J. Laux, C. D. Jones, J. R. Wu, D. DeWalt, M. Pignone, and G. Corbie-Smith. 2015. Family member accompaniment to routine medical visits is associated with better self-care in heart failure patients. *Chronic Illness* 11(1):21–32.

Chang, C. H., J. P. W. Bynum, and J. D. Lurie. 2019. Geographic expansion of federally qualified health centers 2007–2014. *Journal of Rural Health* 35(3):385–394.

Chen, C., F. Chen, and F. Mullan. 2012. Teaching health centers: A new paradigm in graduate medical education. *Academic Medicine* 87(12):1752–1756.

Chen, C., S. Petterson, R. L. Phillips, F. Mullan, A. Bazemore, and S. D. O'Donnell. 2013a. Towards graduate medical education (GME) accountability: Measuring the outcomes of GME institutions. *Academic Medicine* 88(9):1267–1280.

Chen, C., I. Xierali, K. Piwnica-Worms, and R. Phillips. 2013b. The redistribution of graduate medical education positions in 2005 failed to boost primary care or rural training. *Health Affairs* 32(1):102–110.

Cheney, A. M., C. J. Koenig, C. J. Miller, K. Zamora, P. Wright, R. Stanley, J. Fortney, J. F. Burgess, and J. M. Pyne. 2018. Veteran-centered barriers to VA mental healthcare services use. *BMC Health Services Research* 18(1):591.

Chernoff, M., and K. Cueva. 2017. The role of Alaska's tribal health workers in supporting families. *Journal of Community Health* 42(5):1020–1026.

Cigna. 2016. *Clinical insights drive better outcomes: Cigna dental report.* Bloomfield, CT: Cigna Health and Life Insurance.

Clark, M. B., M. A. Keels, and R. L. Slayton. 2020. Fluoride use in caries prevention in the primary care setting. *Pediatrics* 146(6):e2020034637.

CMM in Primary Care Research Team. 2018. *The patient care process for delivering comprehensive medication management (CMM): Optimizing medication use in patient-centered, team-based care settings.* CMM in Primary Care Research Team.

CMS (Centers for Medicare & Medicaid Services). 2019. *Rural health clinic: Medicare learning network fact sheet.* Baltimore, MD: Centers for Medicare & Medicaid Services.

COGME (Council on Graduate Medical Education). 2010. *Advancing primary care.* Rockville, MD: Council on Graduate Medical Education.

COGME. 2016. *Supporting diversity in health professions.* Rockville, MD: Council on Graduate Medical Education.

Cohen, J. J., B. A. Gabriel, and C. Terrell. 2002. The case for diversity in the health care workforce. *Health Affairs* 21(5):90–102.

Coker, T. R., A. Windon, C. Moreno, M. A. Schuster, and P. J. Chung. 2013. Well-child care clinical practice redesign for young children: A systematic review of strategies and tools. *Pediatrics* 131(Suppl 1):S5–S25.

Coker, T. R., S. Chacon, M. N. Elliott, Y. Bruno, T. Chavis, C. Biely, C. D. Bethell, S. Contreras, N. A. Mimila, J. Mercado, and P. J. Chung. 2016. A parent coach model for well-child care among low-income children: A randomized controlled trial. *Pediatrics* 137(3):e20153013.

Cook, B. L., N.-H. Trinh, Z. Li, S. S.-Y. Hou, and A. M. Progovac. 2017. Trends in racial-ethnic disparities in access to mental health care, 2004–2012. *Psychiatric Services* 68(1):9–16.

Cooper, L. A., and N. R. Powe. 2004. *Disparities in patient experiences, health care processes, and outcomes: The role of patient–provider racial, ethnic, and language concordance.* New York: The Commonwealth Fund.

Cornell, P. Y., C. W. Halladay, J. Ader, J. Halaszynski, M. Hogue, C. E. McClain, J. W. Silva, L. D. Taylor, and J. L. Rudolph. 2020. Embedding social workers in Veterans Health Administration primary care teams reduces emergency department visits. *Health Affairs* 39(4):603–612.

Cornwell, B. L., L. M. Brockmann, E. C. Lasky, J. Mach, and J. F. McCarthy. 2018. Primary care-mental health integration in the Veterans Affairs health system: Program characteristics and performance. *Psychiatric Services* 69(6):696–702.

Cothran, T., B. Holderread, M. Abbott, N. Nesser, and S. Keast. 2019. The pharmacist's role in shaping the future of value-based payment models in state Medicaid programs. *Journal of the American Pharmacists Association* 59(1):121–124.

Cowart, K., and K. Olson. 2019. Impact of pharmacist care provision in value-based care settings: How are we measuring value-added services? *Journal of the American Pharmacists Association* 59(1):125–128.

Cox, M., and M. Naylor, eds. 2013. Transforming patient care: Aligning Interprofessional Education with Clinical Practice Redesign, Proceedings of Conference sponsored by the Josiah Macy Jr. Foundation in January 2013. New York: Josiah Macy Jr. Foundation.

Cregler, L. L., M. L. McGanney, S. A. Roman, and D. V. Kagan. 1997. Refining a method of identifying CUNY medical school graduates practicing in underserved areas. *Academic Medicine* 72(9):794–797.

Dyrbye, L. N., M. R. Thomas, A. Eacker, W. Harper, F. S. Massie, Jr., D. V. Power, M. Huschka, P. J. Novotny, J. A. Sloan, and T. D. Shanafelt. 2007. Race, ethnicity, and medical student well-being in the United States. *Archives of Internal Medicine* 167(19):2103–2109.

Ellner, A. L., and R. S. Phillips. 2017. The coming primary care revolution. *Journal of General Internal Medicine* 32(4):380–386.

Fagan, E. B., C. Gibbons, S. C. Finnegan, S. Petterson, L. E. Peterson, R. L. Phillips, and A. W. Bazemore. 2015. Family medicine graduate proximity to their site of training: Policy options for improving the distribution of primary care access. *Family Medicine* 47(2):124–130.

Farrar, B., J. C. Morgan, E. Chuang, and T. R. Konrad. 2011. Growing your own: Community health workers and jobs to careers. *Journal of Ambulatory Care Management* 34(3):234–246.

Feyereisen, S., and N. Puro. 2020. Seventeen states enacted executive orders expanding advanced practice nurses' scopes of practice during the first 21 days of the COVID-19 pandemic. *Rural and Remote Health* 20(4):6068.

Fierman, A. H., A. F. Beck, E. K. Chung, M. M. Tschudy, T. R. Coker, K. B. Mistry, B. Siegel, L. J. Chamberlain, K. Conroy, S. G. Federico, P. J. Flanagan, A. Garg, B. A. Gitterman, A. M. Grace, R. S. Gross, M. K. Hole, P. Klass, C. Kraft, A. Kuo, G. Lewis, K. S. Lobach, D. Long, C. T. Ma, M. Messito, D. Navsaria, K. R. Northrip, C. Osman, M. D. Sadof, A. B. Schickedanz, and J. Cox. 2016. Redesigning health care practices to address childhood poverty. *Academic Pediatrics* 16(Suppl 3):S136–S146.

Frenk, J., L. Chen, Z. A. Bhutta, J. Cohen, N. Crisp, T. Evans, H. Fineberg, P. Garcia, Y. Ke, P. Kelley, B. Kistnasamy, A. Meleis, D. Naylor, A. Pablos-Mendez, S. Reddy, S. Scrimshaw, J. Sepulveda, D. Serwadda, and H. Zurayk. 2010. Health professionals for a new century: Transforming education to strengthen health systems in an interdependent world. *The Lancet* 376(9756):1923–1958.

Frieden, J. 2009. Harvard's primary care division loses funding. *Internal Medicine News.* https://www.mdedge.com/internalmedicine/article/13672/health-policy/harvards-primary-care-division-loses-funding (accessed November 10, 2020).

Friedman, E. M., and P. K. Tong. 2020. *A framework for integrating family caregivers into the health care team.* Santa Monica, CA: RAND Corporation.

Friedman, J. L., and D. Neutze. 2020. The financial cost of medical assistant turnover in an academic family medicine center. *Journal of the American Board of Family Medicine* 33(3):426–430.

Gardner, A. L., R. Shunk, M. Dulay, A. Strewler, and B. O'Brien. 2018. Huddling for high-performing teams. *Federal Practitioner: For the Health Care Professionals of the VA, DoD, and PHS* 35(9):16–22.

Gittell, J. H. 2008. Relationships and resilience: Care provider responses to pressures from managed care. *Journal of Applied Behavioral Science* 44(1):25–47.

Goodfellow, A., J. G. Ulloa, P. T. Dowling, E. Talamantes, S. Chheda, C. Bone, and G. Moreno. 2016. Predictors of primary care physician practice location in underserved urban or rural areas in the United States: A systematic literature review. *Academic Medicine* 91(9):1313–1321.

Gottlieb, K. 2013. The Nuka system of care: Improving health through ownership and relationships. *International Journal of Circumpolar Health* 72.

Grumbach, K., E. Bainbridge, and T. Bodenheimer. 2012. Facilitating improvement in primary care: The promise of practice coaching. *Issue Brief (Commonwealth Fund)* 15:1–14.

Han, X., P. Pittman, C. Erikson, F. Mullan, and L. Ku. 2019. The role of the national health service corps clinicians in enhancing staffing and patient care capacity in community health centers. *Medical Care* 57(12):1002–1007.

Harada, N. D., L. Traylor, K. W. Rugen, J. L. Bowen, C. S. Smith, B. Felker, D. Ludke, I. Tonnu-Mihara, J. L. Ruberg, J. Adler, K. Uhl, A. L. Gardner, and S. C. Gilman. 2018. Interprofessional transformation of clinical education: The first six years of the Veterans Affairs Centers of Excellence in Primary Care Education. *Journal of Interprofessional Care* 1–9.

He, X. Z., E. Cyran, and M. Salling. 2009. National trends in the United States of America physician assistant workforce from 1980 to 2007. *Human Resources for Health* 7:86.

Hebert, P. L., C.-F. Liu, E. S. Wong, S. E. Hernandez, A. Batten, S. Lo, J. M. Lemon, D. A. Conrad, D. Grembowski, K. Nelson, and S. D. Fihn. 2014. Patient-centered medical home initiative produced modest economic results for Veterans Health Administration, 2010–12. *Health Affairs* 33(6):980–987.

Hess, K., A. Bach, K. Won, and S. M. Seed. 2020. Community pharmacists roles during the COVID-19 pandemic. *Journal of Pharmacy Practice* 0897190020980626.

HHS (U.S. Department of Health and Human Services). 2019. *HHS awards over $85 million to help health centers expand access to oral health care.* https://www.hhs.gov/about/news/2019/09/18/hhs-awards-over-85-million-help-health-centers-expand-access-oral-healthcare.html (accessed December 28, 2020).

HHS, HRSA (Health Resources and Services Administration), and NCHWA (National Center for Health Workforce Analysis). 2020. *Characteristics of the U.S. nursing workforce with patient care responsibilities: Resources for epidemic and pandemic response.* Rockville, MD: Health Resources and Services Administration.

Holingue, C., L. G. Kalb, K. E. Riehm, D. Bennett, A. Kapteyn, C. B. Veldhuis, R. M. Johnson, M. D. Fallin, F. Kreuter, E. A. Stuart, and J. Thrul. 2020. Mental distress in the United States at the beginning of the COVID-19 pandemic. *American Journal of Public Health* 110(11):1628–1634.

HPAC (Health Professions Accreditors Collaborative). 2019. *Guidance on developing quality interprofessional education for the health professions.* Chicago, IL: Health Professions Accreditors Collaborative, National Center for Interprofessional Practice and Education.

HRSA (Health Resources and Services Administration). 2006. *The rationale for diversity in the health professions: A review of the evidence.* Rockville, MD: Health Resources and Services Administration.

HRSA. 2015. *National projections of supply and demand for behavioral health practitioners: 2013–2025.* Rockville, MD: Health Resources and Services Administration.

HRSA. 2017. *Sex, race, and ethnic diversity of U.S. health occupations (2011–2015).* Rockville, MD: Health Resources and Services Administration.

HRSA. 2018. *Health center program compliance manual.* https://bphc.hrsa.gov/programrequirements/compliancemanual/introduction.html (accessed August 27, 2020).

HRSA. 2020a. *Children's Hospitals Graduate Medical Education (CHGME) payment program.* https://www.hrsa.gov/grants/find-funding/hrsa-21-012 (accessed December 28, 2020).

HRSA. 2020b. *Teaching Health Center Graduate Medical Education program: Academic year 2019–2020.* Rockville, MD: Health Resources and Services Administration.

HRSA and NCHWA (National Center for Health Workforce Analysis). 2016. *National and regional projections of supply and demand for primary care pratitioners: 2013–2025.* Rockville, MD: U.S. Department of Health and Human Services, Health Resources and Services Administration.

Hummel, J., K. E. Phillips, B. Holt, and C. Hayes. 2015. *Oral health: An essential component of primary care.* Seattle, WA: Qualis Health.

Hysong, S. J., A. B. Amspoker, A. M. Hughes, L. Woodard, F. L. Oswald, L. A. Petersen, and H. F. Lester. 2019. Impact of team configuration and team stability on primary care quality. *Implementation Science* 14(1):22.

IMPAQ International. 2019. *The Graduate Nurse Education demonstration project: Final evaluation report.* Columbia, MD: IMPAQ International.

IOM (Institute of Medicine). 1983. *Community oriented primary care: New directions for health services delivery.* Washington, DC: National Academy Press.

IOM. 1989. *Primary care physicians: Financing their graduate medical education in ambulatory settings.* Washington, DC: National Academy Press.

IOM. 2001. *Crossing the quality chasm: A new health system for the 21st century.* Washington, DC: National Academy Press.

IOM. 2008. *Retooling for an aging America: Building the health care workforce.* Washington, DC: The National Academies Press.

IOM. 2011a. *Allied health workforce and services: Workshop summary.* Washington, DC: The National Academies Press.

IOM. 2011b. *The future of nursing: Leading change, advancing health.* Washington, DC: The National Academies Press.

IOM. 2013a. *Best care at lower cost: The path to continuously learning health care in America.* Washington, DC: The National Academies Press.

IOM. 2013b. *Interprofessional education for collaboration: Learning how to improve health from interprofessional models across the continuum of education to practice: Workshop summary.* Washington, DC: The National Academies Press.

IOM. 2014. *Graduate medical education that meets the nation's health needs.* Washington, DC: The National Academies Press.

IPEC (Interprofessional Education Collaboration). 2020. *About IPEC.* https://www.ipecollaborative.org/about-ipec.html (accessed September 8, 2020).

Jabbarpour, Y., A. Greiner, A. Jetty, M. Coffman, C. Jose, S. Petterson, K. Pivaral, R. Phillips, A. Bazemore, and A. Neumann Kane. 2019. *Investing in primary care: A state-level analysis.* Washington, DC: Patient-Centered Primary Care Collaborative.

Jackson, C. S., and J. N. Gracia. 2014. Addressing health and health-care disparities: The role of a diverse workforce and the social determinants of health. *Public Health Reports* 129(Suppl 2):57–61.

Jeffcoat, M. K., R. L. Jeffcoat, P. A. Gladowski, J. B. Bramson, and J. J. Blum. 2014. Impact of periodontal therapy on general health: Evidence from insurance data for five systemic conditions. *American Journal of Preventive Medicine* 47(2):166–174.

Kangovi, S., N. Mitra, D. Grande, M. L. White, S. McCollum, J. Sellman, R. P. Shannon, and J. A. Long. 2014. Patient-centered community health worker intervention to improve posthospital outcomes: A randomized clinical trial. *JAMA Internal Medicine* 174(4):535–543.

Kangovi, S., D. Grande, and C. Trinh-Shevrin. 2015. From rhetoric to reality—community health workers in post-reform U.S. health care. *New England Journal of Medicine* 372(24):2277–2279.

Kangovi, S., N. Mitra, D. Grande, J. A. Long, and D. A. Asch. 2020. Evidence-based community health worker program addresses unmet social needs and generates positive return on investment. *Health Affairs* 39(2):207–213.

Katkin, J. P., S. J. Kressly, A. R. Edwards, J. M. Perrin, C. A. Kraft, J. E. Richerson, J. S. Tieder, and L. Wall. 2017. Guiding principles for team-based pediatric care. *Pediatrics* 140(2).

Kivlahan, C., and C. A. Sinsky. 2018. *Identifying the optimal panel sizes for primary care physicians.* Chicago, IL: American Medical Association.

Kivlahan, C., K. Pellegrino, K. Grumbach, S. A. Skootsky, N. Raja, R. Gupta, R. Clarke, T. Balsbaugh, T. Ikeda, L. Friedman, L. Gibbs, and E. Todoki. 2017. *Calculating primary care panel size.* Oakland, CA: University of California Health.

Kuo, D. Z., and A. J. Houtrow. 2016. Recognition and management of medical complexity. *Pediatrics* 138(6):e20163021.

Lai, A. Y., S. M. Skillman, and B. K. Frogner. 2020. Is it fair? How to approach professional scope-of-practice policy after the COVID-19 pandemic. *Health Affairs Blog.* https://www.healthaffairs.org/do/10.1377/hblog20200624.983306/full (accessed December 28, 2020).

Lave, J., and E. Wenger. 1991. Situation learning: Legitimate peripheral participation. In *Learning in doing: Social, cognitive and computational perspectives*, edited by J. S. Brown, R. Pea, C. Heath, and L. A. Suchman. Cambridge, UK: Cambridge University Press.

Leung, L. B., L. V. Rubenstein, J. Yoon, E. P. Post, E. Jaske, K. B. Wells, and R. B. Trivedi. 2019. Veterans Health Administration investments in primary care and mental health integration improved care access. *Health Affairs* 38(8):1281–1288.

Levine, D. M., B. E. Landon, and J. A. Linder. 2019. Quality and experience of outpatient care in the United States for adults with or without primary care. *JAMA Internal Medicine* 179(3):363–372.

Lloyd, J., K. Moses, and R. Davis. 2020. *Recognizing and sustaining the value of community health workers and promotores.* Hamilton, NJ: Center For Health Care Strategies.

Marchand, C., and S. Peckham. 2017. Addressing the crisis of GP recruitment and retention: A systematic review. *British Journal of General Practice* 67(657):e227–e237.

Margolius, D., J. Wong, M. L. Goldman, J. Rouse-Iniguez, and T. Bodenheimer. 2012. Delegating responsibility from clinicians to nonprofessional personnel: The example of hypertension control. *Journal of the American Board of Family Medicine* 25(2):209–215.

Mastal, M. F. 2010. Ambulatory care nursing: Growth as a professional specialty. *Nursing Economics* 28(4):267–269, 275.

McDaniel, S. H., C. L. Grus, B. A. Cubic, C. L. Hunter, L. K. Kearney, C. C. Schuman, M. J. Karel, R. S. Kessler, K. T. Larkin, S. McCutcheon, B. F. Miller, J. Nash, S. H. Qualls, K. S. Connolly, T. Stancin, A. L. Stanton, L. A. Sturm, and S. B. Johnson. 2014. Competencies for psychology practice in primary care. *American Psychologist* 69(4):409–429.

McFarland, M. S., and M. Buck. 2020. *The outcomes of implementing and integrating comprehensive medication management in team-based care: A review of the evidence on quality, access and costs, June 2020.* Tysons Corner, VA: GTMRx Institute.

McGough, P., V. Chaudhari, S. El-Attar, and P. Yung. 2018. A health system's journey toward better population health through empanelment and panel management. *Healthcare (Basel)* 6(2):66.

Mendelsohn, A. L., B. P. Dreyer, V. Flynn, S. Tomopoulos, I. Rovira, W. Tineo, C. Pebenito, C. Torres, H. Torres, and A. F. Nixon. 2005. Use of videotaped interactions during pediatric well-child care to promote child development: A randomized, controlled trial. *Journal of Developmental and Behavioral Pediatrics* 26(1):34–41.

Meyers, D., L. LeRoy, M. Bailit, J. Schaefer, E. Wagner, and C. Zhan. 2018. Workforce configurations to provide high-quality, comprehensive primary care: A mixed-method exploration of staffing for four types of primary care practices. *Journal of General Internal Medicine* 33(10):1774–1779.

Meyers, D. J., A. T. Chien, K. H. Nguyen, Z. Li, S. J. Singer, and M. B. Rosenthal. 2019. Association of team-based primary care with health care utilization and costs among chronically ill patients. *JAMA Internal Medicine* 179(1):54–61.

Miller, C. S., R. L. Fogerty, J. Gann, C. P. Bruti, R. Klein, I. Alexandraki, M. Schapira, J. C. Whittle, M. Wei, and the Society of General Internal Medicine Membership Committee. 2017. The growth of hospitalists and the future of the Society of General Internal Medicine: Results from the 2014 membership survey. *Journal of General Internal Medicine* 32(11):1179–1185.

Minkovitz, C. S., D. Strobino, K. B. Mistry, D. O. Scharfstein, H. Grason, W. Hou, N. Ialongo, and B. Guyer. 2007. Healthy Steps for Young Children: Sustained results at 5.5 years. *Pediatrics* 120(3):e658–e668.

Mitchell, J. D., J. D. Haag, E. Klavetter, R. Beldo, N. D. Shah, L. J. Baumbach, G. J. Sobolik, L. J. Rutten, and R. J. Stroebel. 2019. Development and implementation of a team-based, primary care delivery model: Challenges and opportunities. *Mayo Clinic Proceedings* 94(7):1298–1303.

Mitchell, P., M. Wynia, R. Golden, B. McNellis, S. Okun, C. E. Webb, V. Rohrbach, and I. Von Kohorn. 2012. *Core principles & values of effective team-based health care.* NAM *Perspectives.* Discussion Paper, National Academy of Medicine, Washington, DC.

Morgan, P. 2019. Predicted shortages of physicians might even disappear if we fully account for PAs and NPs. *Journal of the American Academy of PAs* 32(10):51–53.

Moyer, V. A. 2014. Prevention of dental caries in children from birth through age 5 years: US Preventive Services Task Force recommendation statement. *Pediatrics* 133(6):1102–1111.

Murray, M., M. Davies, and B. Boushon. 2007. Panel size: How many patients can one doctor manage? *Family Practice Management* 14(4):44–51.

NACHC (National Association of Community Health Centers). 2020. *Community health center chartbook*. Bethesda, MD: National Association of Community Health Centers.

NASEM (National Academies of Sciences, Engineering, and Medicine). 2016. *Assessing progress on the Institute of Medicine report* The Future of Nursing. Washington, DC: The National Academies Press.

NASEM. 2019a. *Integrating oral and general health through health literacy practices: Proceedings of a workshop*. Washington, DC: The National Academies Press.

NASEM. 2019b. *Taking action against clinician burnout: A systems approach to professional well-being*. Washington, DC: The National Academies Press.

NASEM. 2020. *Caring for people with mental health and substance use disorders in primary care settings: Proceedings of a workshop*. Washington, DC: The National Academies Press.

Nasseh, K., M. Vujicic, and C. Yarbrough. 2014. *A ten-year, state-by-state, analysis of Medicaid fee-for-service reimbursement rates for dental care services*. Chicago, IL: American Dental Association.

Nasseh, K., M. Vujicic, and M. Glick. 2017. The relationship between periodontal interventions and healthcare costs and utilization. Evidence from an integrated dental, medical, and pharmacy commercial claims database. *Health Economics* 26(4):519–527.

Naughton, D., A. M. Adelman, P. Bricker, M. Miller-Day, and R. Gabbay. 2013. Envisioning new roles for medical assistants: Strategies from patient-centered medical homes. *Family Practice Management* 20(2):7–12.

Naylor, K. B., J. Tootoo, O. Yakusheva, S. A. Shipman, J. P. W. Bynum, and M. A. Davis. 2019. Geographic variation in spatial accessibility of U.S. healthcare providers. *PLOS ONE* 14(4).

NCCPA (National Commission on Certification of Physician Assistants). 2020. *2019 statistical profile of certified physician assistants: An annual report of the National Commission on Certification of Physician Assistants*. Johns Creek, GA: National Commission on Certification of Physician Assistants.

Neff, D. F., S. H. Yoon, R. L. Steiner, I. Bejleri, M. D. Bumbach, D. Everhart, and J. S. Harman. 2018. The impact of nurse practitioner regulations on population access to care. *Nursing Outlook* 66(4):379–385.

Nelson, K. M., C. Helfrich, H. Sun, P. L. Hebert, C. F. Liu, E. Dolan, L. Taylor, E. Wong, C. Maynard, S. E. Hernandez, W. Sanders, I. Randall, I. Curtis, G. Schectman, R. Stark, and S. D. Fihn. 2014. Implementation of the patient-centered medical home in the Veterans Health Administration: Associations with patient satisfaction, quality of care, staff burnout, and hospital and emergency department use. *JAMA Internal Medicine* 174(8):1350–1358.

Newman, T. V., A. San-Juan-Rodriguez, N. Parekh, E. C. S. Swart, M. Klein-Fedyshin, W. H. Shrank, and I. Hernandez. 2020. Impact of community pharmacist-led interventions in chronic disease management on clinical, utilization, and economic outcomes: An umbrella review. *Research in Social and Administrative Pharmacy* 16(9):1155–1165.

NRC (National Research Council). 2005. *How students learn: History, mathematics, and science in the classroom*. Washington, DC: The National Academies Press.

O'Brien, M. J., C. H. Halbert, R. Bixby, S. Pimentel, and J. A. Shea. 2010. Community health worker intervention to decrease cervical cancer disparities in Hispanic women. *Journal of General Internal Medicine* 25(11):1186–1192.

Okun, S., S. Schoenbaum, D. Andrews, P. Chidambaran, V. Chollette, J. Gruman, S. Leal, B. A. Bown, P. H. Mitchel, C. Parry, W. Prins, R. Ricciardi, M. A. Simon, R. Stock, D. C. Strasser, C. E. Webb, M. K. Wynia, and D. Henderson. 2014. *Patients and health care teams forging effective partnerships. NAM Perspectives.* Discussion Paper, National Academy of Medicine.

O'Malley, A. S., R. Gourevitch, K. Draper, A. Bond, and M. A. Tirodkar. 2015. Overcoming challenges to teamwork in patient-centered medical homes: A qualitative study. *Journal of General Internal Medicine* 30(2):183–192.

Ortiz, J., R. Hofler, A. Bushy, Y. L. Lin, A. Khanijahani, and A. Bitney. 2018. Impact of nurse practitioner practice regulations on rural population health outcomes. *Healthcare* 6(2).

Palazuelos, D., P. E. Farmer, and J. Mukherjee. 2018. Community health and equity of outcomes: The Partners in Health experience. *The Lancet Global Health* 6(5):e491–e493.

Palmer, E. J., P. J. Carek, S. M. Carr-Johnson, and Association of Family Medicine Residency Directors. 2008. Title VII: Revisiting an opportunity. *Annals of Family Medicine* 6(2):180–181.

Pany, M. J., L. Chen, B. Sheridan, and R. S. Huckman. 2021. Provider teams outperform solo providers in managing chronic diseases and could improve the value of care. *Health Affairs* 40(3):435–444.

Park, E. S., and I. Y. Cho. 2018. Shared decision-making in the paediatric field: A literature review and concept analysis. *Scandinavian Journal of Caring Sciences* 32(2):478–489.

Pathman, D. E., and T. R. Konrad. 2012. Growth and changes in the National Health Service Corps (NHSC) workforce with the American Recovery and Reinvestment Act. *Journal of the American Board of Family Practice* 25(5):723–733.

Patwardhan, A., I. Duncan, P. Murphy, and C. Pegus. 2012. The value of pharmacists in health care. *Population Health Management* 15(3):157–162.

PCPCC (Patient-Centered Primary Care Collaborative). 2012. *The patient-centered medical home: Integrating comprehensive medication management to optimize patient outcomes.* Washington, DC: Patient-Centered Primary Care Collaborative.

Peres, M. A., L. M. D. Macpherson, R. J. Weyant, B. Daly, R. Venturelli, M. R. Mathur, S. Listl, R. K. Celeste, C. C. Guarnizo-Herreño, C. Kearns, H. Benzian, P. Allison, and R. G. Watt. 2019. Oral diseases: A global public health challenge. *The Lancet* 394(10194):249–260.

Peretz, P. J., N. Islam, and L. A. Matiz. 2020. Community health workers and COVID-19—addressing social determinants of health in times of crisis and beyond. *New England Journal of Medicine* 383(19):e108.

Pesec, M., H. L. Ratcliffe, A. Karlage, L. R. Hirschhorn, A. Gawande, and A. Bitton. 2017. Primary health care that works: The Costa Rican experience. *Health Affairs* 36(3):531–538.

Peterson, D. 2019. Overview and definition of experiential learning. *ThoughtCo.* https://www. thoughtco.com/what-is-experiential-learning-31324 (accessed November 10, 2020).

Petterson, S. M., W. R. Liaw, R. L. Phillips, Jr., D. L. Rabin, D. S. Meyers, and A. W. Bazemore. 2012. Projecting U.S. primary care physician workforce needs: 2010–2025. *Annals of Family Medicine* 10(6):503–509.

Petterson, S., R. McNellis, K. Klink, D. Meyers, and A. Bazemore. 2018. *The state of primary care in the United States: A chartbook of facts and statistics.* Washington, DC: Robert Graham Center.

PHCPI (Primary Health Care Performance Initiative). 2019. *Population health management: Empanelment.* Primary Care Performance Initiative.

Phillips, R. L., Jr., and A. W. Bazemore. 2010. Primary care and why it matters for U.S. health system reform. *Health Affairs* 29(5):806–810.

Phillips, R. L., Jr., and B. J. Turner. 2012. The next phase of Title VII funding for training primary care physicians for America's health care needs. *Annals of Family Medicine* 10(2):163–168.

Phillips, R. L., Jr., M. Dodoo, S. Petterson, I. Xierali, A. Bazemore, B. Teevan, K. Bennett, C. Legagneur, J. Rudd, and J. Phillips. 2009. *Specialty and geographic distribution of the physician workforce: What influences medical student and resident choices?* Washington, DC: Robert Graham Center.

Phillips, R. L., Jr., S. Petterson, and A. Bazemore. 2013. Do residents who train in safety net settings return for practice? *Academic Medicine* 88(12):1934–1940.

Phillips, R. L., Jr., A. M. Bazemore, and L. E. Peterson. 2014. Effectiveness over efficiency: Underestimating the primary care physician shortage. *Medical Care* 52(2):97–98.

Politzer, R. M., L. Q. Trible, T. D. Robinson, D. Heard, D. L. Weaver, S. M. Reig, and M. Gaston. 2000. The National Health Service Corps for the 21st century. *Journal of Ambulatory Care Management* 23(3):70–85.

Polivka, L. 2001. *Paying family members to provide care: Policy considerations for states.* San Francisco, CA: Family Caregiver Alliance.

Poma, P. A. 2017. Race/ethnicity concordance between patients and physicians. *Journal of the National Medical Association* 109(1):6–8.

Qato, D. M., G. C. Alexander, R. M. Conti, M. Johnson, P. Schumm, and S. T. Lindau. 2008. Use of prescription and over-the-counter medications and dietary supplements among older adults in the United States. *JAMA* 300(24):2867–2878.

Raffoul, M., M. Moore, D. Kamerow, and A. Bazemore. 2016. A primary care panel size of 2500 is neither accurate nor reasonable. *Journal of the American Board of Family Medicine* 29(4):496–499.

Ramalho de Oliveira, D., A. R. Brummel, and D. B. Miller. 2010. Medication therapy management: 10 years of experience in a large integrated health care system. *Journal of Managed Care Pharmacy* 16(3):185–195.

Ramanuj, P., E. Ferenchik, M. Docherty, B. Spaeth-Rublee, and H. A. Pincus. 2019. Evolving models of integrated behavioral health and primary care. *Current Psychiatry Reports* 21(1):4.

Randall, I., D. C. Mohr, and C. Maynard. 2017. VHA patient-centered medical home associated with lower rate of hospitalizations and specialty care among veterans with posttraumatic stress disorder. *Journal for Healthcare Quality* 39(3):168–176.

Regalado, M., and N. Halfon. 2001. Primary care services promoting optimal child development from birth to age 3 years: Review of the literature. *Archives of Pediatrics & Adolescent Medicine* 155(12):1311–1322.

Rehner, T., M. Brazeal, and S. T. Doty. 2017. Embedding a social work-led behavioral health program in a primary care system: A 2012–2018 case study. *Journal of Public Health Management and Practice* 23:S40–S46.

Reinhard, S. C., B. Given, N. H. Petlick, and A. Bemis. 2008. Supporting family caregivers in providing care. In *Patient safety and quality: An evidence-based handbook for nurses*, edited by R. G. Hughes. Rockville, MD: Agency for Healthcare Research and Quality. Pp. 341–404.

Reiss-Brennan, B., K. D. Brunisholz, C. Dredge, P. Briot, K. Grazier, A. Wilcox, L. Savitz, and B. James. 2016. Association of integrated team-based care with health care quality, utilization, and cost. *JAMA* 316(8):826–834.

Rodriguez, H. P., K. F. Giannitrapani, S. Stockdale, A. B. Hamilton, E. M. Yano, and L. V. Rubenstein. 2014. Teamlet structure and early experiences of medical home implementation for veterans. *Journal of General Internal Medicine* 29(Suppl 2):S623–S631.

Rosland, A.-M., J. D. Piette, H. Choi, and M. Heisler. 2011. Family and friend participation in primary care visits of patients with diabetes or heart failure: Patient and physician determinants and experiences. *Medical Care* 49(1):37–45.

Rowan, K., D. D. McAlpine, and L. A. Blewett. 2013. Access and cost barriers to mental health care, by insurance status, 1999–2010. *Health Affairs* 32(10):1723–1730.

Sachs Hills, L. 2004. Special considerations for hiring an office manager. *Journal of Medical Practice Management* 19(4):189–192.

Sanchez, N., and K. Hermis. 2019. Interprofessional collaboration to improve and sustain patient experience outcomes in an ambulatory setting. *Patient Experience Journal* 6(1):149–153.

Sawyer, R. K., ed. 2005. *The Cambridge handbook of the learning sciences, Cambridge handbooks in psychology.* Cambridge, UK: Cambridge University Press.

Schmitt, M., A. Blue, C. A. Aschenbrener, and T. R. Viggiano. 2011. Core competencies for interprofessional collaborative practice: Reforming health care by transforming health professionals' education. *Academic Medicine* 86(11).

Schottenfeld, L., D. Petersen, D. Peikes, R. Ricciardi, H. Burak, R. McNellis, and J. Genevro. 2016. *Creating patient-centered team-based primary care.* Rockville, MD: Agency for Healthcare Research and Quality.

Seid, M., and G. D. Stevens. 2005. Access to care and children's primary care experiences: Results from a prospective cohort study. *Health Services Research* 40(6 Pt 1):1758–1780.

Shi, L. 2012. The impact of primary care: A focused review. *Scientifica* 2012:432892.

Shrader, S., S. Jernigan, N. Nazir, and J. Zaudke. 2018. Determining the impact of an interprofessional learning in practice model on learners and patients. *Journal of Interprofessional Education & Practice* 1–8.

Silver, J. K., A. C. Bean, C. Slocum, J. A. Poorman, A. Tenforde, C. A. Blauwet, R. A. Kirch, R. Parekh, H. L. Amonoo, R. Zafonte, and D. Osterbur. 2019. Physician workforce disparities and patient care: A narrative review. *Health Equity* 3(1):360–377.

Simon, L. 2016. Overcoming historical separation between oral and general health care: Interprofessional collaboration for promoting health equity. *AMA Journal of Ethics* 18(9):941–949.

Sinsky, C. A., and T. Bodenheimer. 2019. Powering-up primary care teams: Advanced team care with in-room support. *Annals of Family Medicine* 17(4):367–371.

Sinsky, C. A., R. Willard-Grace, A. M. Schutzbank, T. A. Sinsky, D. Margolius, and T. Bodenheimer. 2013. In search of joy in practice: A report of 23 high-functioning primary care practices. *Annals of Family Medicine* 11(3):272–278.

Skillman, S. M., C. R. Snyder, B. Frogner, and D. G. Patterson. 2016. *The behavioral health workforce needed for integration with primary care: Information for health workforce planning.* Seattle, WA: Center for Health Workforce Studies, University of Washington.

Skillman, S. M., A. Dahal, B. K. Frogner, and C. H. A. Andrilla. 2020. Frontline workers' career pathways: A detailed look at Washington state's medical assistant workforce. *Medical Care Research and Review* 77(3):285–293.

Starfield, B. 2001. New paradigms for quality in primary care. *British Journal of General Practice* 51(465):303–309.

Starfield, B., L. Shi, and J. Macinko. 2005. Contribution of primary care to health systems and health. *Milbank Quarterly* 83(3):457–502.

Steinwald, A. B. 2008. *Primary care professionals: Recent supply trends, projections, and valuation of services (testimony before the Committee on Health, Education, Labor, and Pensions, U.S. Senate).* Washington, DC: U.S. Government Accountability Office.

Sullivan, E. E., and A. Ellner. 2015. Strong patient–provider relationships drive healthier outcomes. *Harvard Business Review.* https://hbr.org/2015/10/strong-patient-provider-relationships-drive-healthier-outcomes (accessed January 12, 2021).

Swan, B. A., and S. A. Haas. 2011. Health care reform: Current updates and future initiatives for ambulatory care nursing. *Nursing Economics* 29(6):331–334.

Swanberg, S. M. 2016. Resource reviews: MedEdPORTAL. *Journal of the Medical Library Association* 104(3):250–252.

Swanwick, T. 2005. Informal learning in postgraduate medical education: From cognitivism to "culturism." *Medical Education* 39(8):859–865.

The Larry A. Green Center and PCC (Primary Care Collaborative). 2020. *Quick COVID-19 primary care survey: Clinician survey*. https://www.green-center.org/covid-survey (accessed September 15, 2020).

Urban Universities for Health. 2014. *Holistic admissions in the health professions: Findings from a national survey*. Washington, DC: Urban Universities for Health.

VA (U.S. Department of Veterans Affairs). 2016. Final rule with comment period: Advanced practice registered nurses as published on December 14, 2016. *Federal Register* 81(240):90198–90207. https://www.federalregister.gov/documents/2016/12/14/2016-29950/advanced-practice-registered-nurses (accessed December 18, 2020).

VA. 2020. *Veterans affairs program of comprehensive assistance for family caregivers*. Washington, DC: U.S. Department of Veterans Affairs.

Van Vleet, A., and J. Paradise. 2015. *Tapping nurse practitioners to meet rising demand for primary care*. https://www.kff.org/medicaid/issue-brief/tapping-nurse-practitioners-to-meet-rising-demand-for-primary-care (accessed January 26, 2021).

VHA (Veterans Health Administration). 2017. *Audit of management of primary care panels*. Washington, DC: Veterans Health Administration.

Vujicic, M., T. Buchmueller, and R. Klein. 2016. Dental care presents the highest level of financial barriers, compared to other types of health care services. *Health Affairs* 35(12):2176–2182.

Wakefield, M. 2014. Improving the health of the nation: HRSA's mission to achieve health equity. *Public Health Reports* 129(Suppl 2):3–4.

Wang, E. A., C. S. Hong, S. Shavit, R. Sanders, E. Kessell, and M. B. Kushel. 2012. Engaging individuals recently released from prison into primary care: A randomized trial. *American Journal of Public Health* 102(9):e22–e29.

Warm, E. J., and C. Goetz. 2013. Too smart for primary care? *Annals of Internal Medicine* 159(10):709–710.

Washko, M. M., J. E. Snyder, and G. Zangaro. 2015. Where do physicians train? Investigating public and private institutional pipelines. *Health Affairs* 34(5):852–856.

Watanabe, J. H., T. McInnis, and J. D. Hirsch. 2018. Cost of prescription drug-related morbidity and mortality. *Annals of Pharmacotherapy* 52(9):829–837.

Watt, R. G., B. Daly, P. Allison, L. M. D. Macpherson, R. Venturelli, S. Listl, R. J. Weyant, M. R. Mathur, C. C. Guarnizo-Herreño, R. K. Celeste, M. A. Peres, C. Kearns, and H. Benzian. 2019. Ending the neglect of global oral health: Time for radical action. *The Lancet* 394(10194):261–272.

Weida, N. A., R. L. Phillips, Jr., and A. W. Bazemore. 2010. Does graduate medical education also follow green? *Archives of Internal Medicine* 170(4):389–390.

Whitehead, L., E. Jacob, A. Towell, M. Abu-Qamar, and A. Cole-Heath. 2018. The role of the family in supporting the self-management of chronic conditions: A qualitative systematic review. *Journal of Clinical Nursing* 27(1–2):22–30.

Whittaker, M. K., S. Murdoch, L. Rozmovits, C. Abrahams, and R. Freeman. 2019. If you build it they will come...and stay: A community-based family medicine program. *PRiMER* 3:28.

WHO (World Health Organization). 2010. *Framework for action on interprofessional education & collaborative practice*. Geneva, Switzerland: World Health Organization.

WHO. 2018. *WHO guideline on health policy and system supprt to optimize community health worker programmes*. Geneva, Switzerland: World Health Organization.

Willard-Grace, R., D. Hessler, E. Rogers, K. Dubé, T. Bodenheimer, and K. Grumbach. 2014. Team structure and culture are associated with lower burnout in primary care. *Journal of the American Board of Family Medicine* 27(2):229–238.

Wyatt, K. D., B. List, W. B. Brinkman, G. Prutsky Lopez, N. Asi, P. Erwin, Z. Wang, J. P. Domecq Garces, V. M. Montori, and A. LeBlanc. 2015. Shared decision making in pediatrics: A systematic review and meta-analysis. *Academic Pediatrics* 15(6):573–583.

Xue, Y., E. Greener, V. Kannan, J. A. Smith, C. Brewer, and J. Spetz. 2018a. Federally qualified health centers reduce the primary care provider gap in health professional shortage counties. *Nursing Outlook* 66(3):263–272.

Xue, Y., V. Kannan, E. Greener, J. A. Smith, J. Brasch, B. A. Johnson, and J. Spetz. 2018b. Full scope-of-practice regulation is associated with higher supply of nurse practitioners in rural and primary care health professional shortage counties. *Journal of Nursing Regulation* 8(4):5–13.

Zolot, J. 2020. COVID-19 brings changes to NP scope of practice. *American Journal of Nursing* 120(8):14.

7

Digital Health and Primary Care

Digital technology is an essential tool necessary for primary care to carry out its basic functions. Without high-functioning digital technologies, many of the aspirations of this report are not possible. Technology in other sectors outpaces its performance in health care. The financial industry, for example, has free flow of information and complete interoperability between business silos. Smartphones are customizable with robust "app stores" to easily add and remove features. More importantly, people do not need intensive training to learn how to use smartphones, which are intuitive, recognize users' needs, and can prompt support.

For routine use in primary care, technology has not fundamentally expanded beyond electronic health records (EHRs), registration systems, and patient portals created two decades ago. More concerning, technology remains a leading cause of clinician burnout (NASEM, 2019). In an average day, clinicians spend 6 hours documenting care in an EHR (Arndt et al., 2017). EHRs continue to require dozens of clicks, unique to each individual system and far from intuitive, in a structured format designed for meeting billing and coding requirements rather than enhancing clinical care and relationships. These excessive requirements mean that U.S. clinicians spend significantly more time working in an EHR per day than clinicians using the same EHR in other countries (Holmgren et al., 2020). Interoperability requires that the clinician significantly review and correct information from multiple sources (e.g., specialists, hospitals, vaccine registries, pharmacies), or, even worse, call and fax other care team members to find information that is sitting in a silo elsewhere and then decide if it is current and correct. National efforts to make the use of digital health more meaningful put the majority of the burden on end users, requiring health systems and primary care practices to substantially modify and implement rudimentary base systems and adding to their workload.

The experience for people seeking care is no better. They have lost the attention of their personal clinician, who is distracted by a computer screen (O'Malley et al., 2010; Street et al., 2014). Limited interoperability introduces errors as outdated information is populated in systems, which can lead to clinicians refilling or continuing out-of-date medications. Conversely, overuse occurs when information is not transferred, as clinicians may repeat recent tests or procedures from elsewhere. Adding to this, people have limited access to their own health information through patient portals that present information in medical language. In addition, an individual's medical history is not linked to person-centered educational material or more than a few actionable, relevant steps they can take. Finally, the experience is burdened by the very design of systems that are not created with the needs of the most underserved populations in mind. Patients with limited English language proficiency, health and digital literacy, and access to high-speed Internet often cannot gain the full benefit of technology.

This is the lived experience of health information technology (HIT) for clinicians and patients. The real potentials of digital health to aggregate a wide array of medical, environmental, biological, and social data; make meaningful sense of information; automate care; make care proactive and not reactive; enhance health equity; and enable population health monitoring and management have been barely explored. The concept of "digital capitalism" in the health sector creating a dichotomy of public benefit versus private gain offers a compelling explanation for the current lack of innovation, exploration, and interoperability compared to other sectors (Sharon, 2018). Furthermore, the lack of adequate regulation of digital health companies to ensure innovation, interoperability, and support of the functions of high-quality primary care continues to put solutions out of reach for health care organizations and individual clinicians.

The committee broadly refers to digital health as the use of HIT to care for individuals and communities. Digital health has many uses—documenting care, collecting and storing information, understanding information, delivering care, and communicating. At its best, though, digital health should make it easier for people to receive and clinicians to know how to deliver the right care at the right time, while also supporting relationships between individuals, families, clinicians, and communities. In primary care, digital health can include tools such as EHRs, patient portals, mobile applications, telemedicine platforms, electronic registries, analytic systems, remote monitoring, wearable technology, care-seeker and care team communication support, and geographical and population health displays. Digital health tools used for diagnosis and treatment are beyond the scope of this report, which is focused on implementing high-quality primary care.

Over the past 20 years, rapid improvements in computing power, software development, data storage, and Internet bandwidth, as well as smartphone proliferation, have supported the growth of a digital health industry that has developed products and technologies that are ubiquitous in health care delivery today. Undoubtedly, future technology disruption will continue to change health care and improve primary care. This chapter will discuss digital health's role in delivering care in a way that is convenient, accessible, and efficient, the key attributes of a well-functioning digital health infrastructure, and the barriers to fully benefiting primary care. This chapter will also describe how the recent COVID-19 pandemic has forced many primary care practices to rapidly transform their processes to make virtual care and population care a new norm and how the lessons learned from this experience can enhance equity. These lessons need to be applied to future digital health advances and the policies that enable them. Finally, the chapter will present design principles for digital health systems and implementation strategies for different actors to consider in strengthening the role of digital health to support high-quality primary care.

THE GROWTH OF DIGITAL HEALTH

The digital health landscape has advanced dramatically in the years following *Primary Care: America's Health in a New Era* (IOM, 1996a). In 2004, the Office of the National Coordinator for Health Information Technology (ONC) was established, followed by Congress passing the Health Information Technology for Economic and Clinical Health (HITECH)[1] Act (part of the American Recovery and Reinvestment Act) in 2009. The HITECH Act mandated ONC to regulate and create standards for HIT and create incentives for its adoption (Washington et al., 2017). Congress also passed the Health Insurance Portability and Accountability Act (HIPAA)[2] in 1996, to promote and support health information exchange. However, HIPAA has largely been a barrier to information exchange and is badly in need of updating (NCVHS, 2019).

Largely spurred by the HITECH Act, some digital health care applications, specifically EHRs, are commonplace today and have been widely adopted by a vast majority of health care delivery systems, large and small. By 2017, 86 percent of all office-based physicians were using an EHR and

---

[1] American Recovery and Reinvestment Act of 2009, § 13001, Public Law 111-5 (February 17, 2009).

[2] Health Insurance Portability and Accountability Act of 1996, Public Law 104-191 (August 21, 1996).

80 percent were using a certified EHR product[3] (ONC, 2019). Primary care has been an early adopter of HIT, often leading the way in EHRs and advocating for greater functionality (Phillips et al., 2015; Rittenhouse et al., 2017). In a 2019 survey, a majority of physicians across specialties felt that technology enabled them to provide better care. Among primary care physicians, 40 percent reported that technology gave them a "definite" advantage, and 46 percent reported that it gave them "somewhat" of an advantage in providing care (AMA, 2020).

Electronic Health Records and Meaningful Use

The HITECH Act established programs through the Centers for Medicare & Medicaid Services (CMS), known collectively as Meaningful Use, to incentivize EHR adoption with the goal of improving the quality and coordination of care, patient engagement, and population health, while ensuring the privacy of patients and their personal information (CDC, 2019). Meaningful Use awarded financial incentives if practices satisfied a set of core objectives and several optional objectives (Fernald et al., 2013). Meaningful Use stage 1 focused on data capture and sharing, stage 2 on advanced clinical processes, and stage 3 on improved outcomes (Ornstein et al., 2015), but the EHR functionality and use requirements only supported very basic functions of primary care (Krist et al., 2014). For example, one stage 1 objective was to maintain an up-to-date problem list for 80 percent of patients and a stage 2 objective was to use secure messaging for 10 percent of patient communications.

Meaningful Use did catalyze the uptake of HIT in primary care, and it also created burdens for which the incentives only partially compensated. EHRs were and remain expensive, with most practices paying more for one than they were paid through Meaningful Use incentives (Fleming et al., 2011). In addition, clinicians and staff received inadequate training and support to use EHR functionality to its full potential, and the EHRs had many technical limitations that required extra staff work to fulfill the Meaningful Use criteria (Fernald et al., 2013). Meaningful Use did result in some improvements in quality, safety, and outcomes (Kruse and Beane, 2018), but it also contributed to physician burnout, EHR market oversaturation, and data obfuscation (Colicchio et al., 2019). CMS and ONC had limited authority to enforce Meaningful Use standards and primarily acted through incentive and penalty payments to clinicians. It did not provide a way to incentivize or force EHR vendors to change and improve their systems,

---

[3] A certified EHR product has received certification from the Office of the National Coordinator for Health Information Technology that the system supports all of the required Meaningful Use functionalities (2020).

beyond certification. This put the burden to adopt, modify, and implement base EHR products to meet certification standards on clinicians and health systems. In April 2018, CMS renamed this incentive program to "Promoting Interoperability Programs" and shifted priorities to include patient access to information, interoperability, and e-prescribing (CMS, 2020a).

Today, the global EHR market is estimated to be worth $25 billion and projected to reach $37 billion by 2025 (Medgadget, 2020). Three vendors dominate, with Epic, Cerner, and Meditech controlling 75 percent of the U.S. hospital market share (Landi, 2020). Among large health systems, Epic and Cerner dominate (Tate and Warburton, 2020). For such a large market that has such a large influence on health care, the current landscape of a vendor-dominated economy locks customers into systems and stifles innovation while contributing to rising and unsustainable health care costs (Fisher et al., 2009).

Telehealth, mHealth, and Other Patient-Facing Systems

Other types of digital health, such as telemedicine, remote monitoring applications and devices, patient engagement tools, decision support technology, patient portals, data-sharing tools, and chat bots driven by artificial intelligence or ambient computing to automate care, are not used as widely as EHRs, but their adoption has increased significantly in recent years across all specialties, age groups, and genders (AMA, 2020). Today, many patients and clinicians strive for health care to be less transactional and based more on relationships and partnerships (see Chapter 4). More patients now expect to own their health information, be included with their clinicians in the health care decision-making process, and have their care be collaborative, convenient, and accessible (Meskó et al., 2017). Well-designed, person-centered technology, such as patient portals that allow patients and clinicians to communicate via secure messaging, can fill a need by facilitating efficient communication outside of the office setting and giving people easier access to their medical information (Friedberg et al., 2014; Hoonakker et al., 2017; NASEM, 2019). However, current payment systems do not reimburse clinicians for providing this critical service.

Myriad health information resources are easily accessible to the consumer via the Internet, mobile applications, and patient-facing technologies (e.g., patient portals) that allow people to more easily interact directly with their clinicians. In 2018, for example, a nationally representative survey found that 35 percent of respondents reported owning an electronic monitoring device, such as a smart watch or blood glucose monitor, and 84 percent reported owning a smartphone or tablet. Of the latter, 49 percent reported they used a health or wellness application on their device to track health goals (Patel and Johnson, 2019). However, the corresponding change among many clinicians to adopt technologies that could make care more accessible and convenient has lagged because of a combination of factors, such as burdensome regulatory restrictions, resistance to change from a traditional hierarchical model that is less person centered, and technology-related professional burnout (Meskó et al., 2017; NASEM, 2019). For example, in 2018, only about half of patients reported being offered access to their online medical records, the same as in 2017. Of those who were, 30 percent viewed their records at least once in the past year; the impact of viewing the information on their health and engagement is unknown (Patel and Johnson, 2019).

Telemedicine[4] can make care more accessible to people who have access to the required technology, such as a device with broadband Internet connectivity, by sparing them an often time-consuming and burdensome trip to a medical office. One study of telemedicine trends among a large, commercially insured population showed that primary care was the most frequently delivered form (Barnett et al., 2018). Still, the overall percentage of primary care via telemedicine was low, and it was most commonly used by people in urban locations, who typically have greater access in general compared to those in more rural locations (Barnett et al., 2018).

Personal monitoring devices, such as wearable devices (e.g., smart watch), Internet-connected scales, and glucometers, are used by individuals and clinicians to monitor health goals and vital signs between direct encounters. Wearable devices are generally not remotely integrated with an EHR, yet these same devices are widely integrated across a range of smartphone applications (Dinh-Le et al., 2019). The direct integration of glucometers within the EHR is in the early stages of development and can improve monitoring of people with diabetes between encounters (Weatherly et al., 2019). This type of digital health integration can facilitate engagement from people seeking care and make monitoring and care more efficient and less burdensome for clinicians, but only if the information is shared simply and meaningfully.

Population Health

Population health, an essential component of effective primary care that is most enabled by digital health and currently neglected, encompasses strategies to make the delivery of evidence-based care easy. It shifts care from being reactive (e.g., someone has to schedule an appointment) to being proactive (e.g., identify and reach out to those in need); and it expands

---

[4] Telemedicine is "the use of electronic information and communications technologies to provide and support health care when distance separates the participants" usually via video conference, telephone, or mobile application (IOM, 1996b, p. 1).

care beyond individuals to caring for entire communities. For example, alerts, reminders, and quality or health maintenance tabs[5] built into EHRs increase guideline-based care (Alagiakrishnan et al., 2016). Similarly, safety alerts have been shown to decrease prescribing contraindicated medications. Despite a strong evidence base demonstrating the effectiveness of these features (Bright et al., 2012), EHRs are not preprogrammed with functional and up-to-date, evidence-based guidelines, and each health system or practice must create its own quality or health maintenance tabs. Programmed medication safety alerts are more commonplace, but most systems provide too many such alerts that are not prioritized and often clinically inappropriate, resulting in alert fatigue and reducing their effectiveness (Hussain et al., 2019). Community data or "community vital signs" to consider risks for social needs and environmental exposures are emerging as a promising tool that could notify clinicians of care-seekers' needs (Hughes et al., 2016; Liaw et al., 2018). However, all of these types of functions still occur primarily at the point of care, requiring a visit rather than being true proactive population health care features.

Patient registries are more of a true population health tool. Practices can use registries to identify all patients in their panel who have gaps in care, are overdue for care, or have risks and conditions needing additional attention (AMA, 2015, 2016). Care teams can use these tools to develop intervention strategies that target those with a range of needs to prevent negative health events (ONC, 2013). Registries are an essential function for many practices and health systems to participate in Medicare Shared Savings Programs, accountable care organizations, and other value-based programs. Some EHRs allow clinicians to generate patient lists around basic elements, such as everyone with diabetes, those needing an annual wellness visit, children in need of vaccinations, and patients overdue for colon cancer or developmental screening. However, registries are often an optional add-on to EHRs that practices need to purchase, and many are limited to basic functionality and cannot perform more sophisticated population queries or queries on nontraditional medical values. Few EHR-based registries have automated functionality, requiring users to manually create and run queries (Nelson et al., 2016).

Other population health tools can include geographic information systems (GISs) to understand a practice's footprint and the communities that it serves (Rock et al., 2019). GIS tools can support community-based interventions and collaboration building to better care. Alternatively, clinicians can use information about a patient's place of residence to understand

---

[5] Quality or health maintenance tabs are sections of EHRs dedicated to displaying evidence-based alerts about preventive or chronic care recommendations that a patient may or may not need (Schellhase et al., 2003).

environmental factors that may contribute to health or even use place-based data as a surrogate for health risks (DeVoe et al., 2016; Hughes et al., 2016; Liaw et al., 2018; Tong et al., 2019).

Interoperability

Effective, functional, and automated interoperability is an essential lynchpin to ensure the success of digital health. The free flow of health information between settings and systems does not easily occur in today's health care system because of a lack of interoperability between different technologies. This is an issue for all of health care, but it is particularly relevant for primary care, which needs complete data for whole-person care and is currently responsible for curating a person's "complete" health record. The HITECH Act offered grants and incentives to states and municipalities for developing regional health information exchange (HIE) initiatives. These initiatives have met with variable success. Problems included technical, policy, governance, funding, and security and privacy concerns (Adler-Milstein et al., 2013; Vest and Gamm, 2010).

The ONC National Interoperability Roadmap has set 2024 as a goal for universal interoperability (HealthIT, 2020). Yet, *Taking Action Against Clinician Burnout: A Systems Approach to Professional Well-Being* showed that clinicians are "increasingly frustrated that the digital transition in health care has not translated into having the information necessary for patient care when and where patients need it" (NASEM, 2019, p. 207). The 21st Century Cures Act of 2016 (Cures Act)[6] defines an interoperable HIT system as one that

> (a) enables the secure exchange of electronic health information with, and use of electronic health information from, other health information technology without special effort on the part of the user;
> (b) allows for complete access, exchange, and use of all electronically accessible health information for authorized use under applicable State or Federal law; and
> (c) does not constitute information blocking.

However, the ONC Roadmap appears to be off track for achieving its goal for universal interoperability by 2024, and the ONC does not have any authority over EHR vendors to enforce the Cures Act requirements.

Most current EHRs and other IT systems do not meet the interoperability standard of the Cures Act for a variety of reasons (Blumenthal, 2009; NASEM, 2019; Pronovost et al., 2018), such as the proprietary policies of

---

[6] 21st Century Cures Act of 2016, Public Law No. 114-255 (December 13, 2016).

EHR vendors and health care organizations and ineffective incentives (Ratwani et al., 2018a). The lack of interoperability, and the restriction of the flow of information by some vendors, negatively affects care. Even within a single health system, information is often siloed in different HIT systems that may not be interoperable. For example, one specialty may use an EHR that is different from and not interoperable with the EHR used by the rest of the system (Friedberg et al., 2014). As noted in *Taking Action Against Clinician Burnout*, a lack of interoperability "can increase administrative and clerical efforts to ensure that all tests results, scheduling updates, orders, and clinical notes are accurate and consistent across the different systems" (NASEM, 2019, p. 207). Similarly, even if two different health systems use EHRs from the same vendor, they may not be compatible. As a result, when patients move among health systems, transferring their medical information may require manual input, a time-consuming process prone to human error (Smith et al., 2018). Thus, "the lack of interoperability compounds the administrative burden placed on clinical staff, which erodes efficiency and contributes to fatigue and dissatisfaction" (NASEM, 2019, p. 208).

Several efforts are under way to improve interoperability through the Cures Act. For example, Draft 2 of the Trusted Exchange Framework and Common Agreement, released in April 2019, "outlines a common set of principles, terms, and conditions to facilitate interoperability and information exchange across disparate HIE platforms and help enable the nationwide exchange of electronic health information" (NASEM, 2019, p. 208). When fully implemented, the framework should help achieve seamless access to information across different HIT platforms and health care systems (Rucker, 2018).

Recent mandates to use the Substitutable Medical Applications and Reusable Technologies on Fast Health Interoperability Resources platform may help with data sharing. It is designed to enable medical applications to run unmodified across different HIT systems (Mandel et al., 2016), providing a common format for sharing health data in the EHR across applications and facilitating the flow of data across otherwise incompatible systems. Merely adopting these standards will not ensure success. How they are implemented will also be critical. Whether this translates into true interoperability for care-seekers and clinicians remains to be seen.

Usability

While technology can make it easier compared with paper records to review a medical history, make diagnoses, generate orders and prescriptions, and document treatment plans, poorly designed systems may introduce frustrating processes into the care delivery experience and even make the experience more difficult and error prone (NASEM, 2019). *Health IT* and Patient Safety: Building Safer Systems for Better Care describes key attributes of *safe* digital health (IOM, 2011) (see Box 7-1). Most systems today do not meet these basic standards.

Taking Action Against Clinician Burnout documented many of the usability problems of current EHRs, particularly during a clinical encounter (NASEM, 2019). Poorly designed visual displays, for example, may contribute to prescribing errors (Moacdieh and Sarter, 2015; Ratwani et al., 2018a). Part of the reason for poor usability of EHRs is that the initial motivation behind their design and implementation was to help facilitate billing, reporting, and fulfilling regulatory requirements, not necessarily to improve clinical workflow. Thus, the user interface and standard menus often do not accurately reflect the uniqueness of individual clinical situations or allow the flexibility to adapt (NASEM, 2019). This, in turn, forces clinicians to make unnecessary clicks to move through the EHR, which is one factor contributing to clinician dissatisfaction (Friedberg et al., 2014). Primary care teams who care for children face additional challenges in the usability of EHRs (Ratwani et al., 2018b,c). Children require weight-based medication dosing and age-specific screenings and interventions. EHRs are often not designed with child health–focused usability, and thus errors in medication dosing and in missed or inappropriate care have occurred.

Usability may be even more important for patient-facing digital health systems. While it may be feasible to train clinicians to use an EHR or other digital health tool, patient-facing systems need to be "plug and play": easy to access or download, intuitive to use, and understandable even for those with lower health literacies. Adding to this, some health information can be sensitive (e.g., self-reported substance use or sexual history) or

---

BOX 7-1
Features of Safe Health Information Technology

- Easy retrieval of accurate, timely, and reliable native and imported data
- A system the user wants to interact with
- Simple and intuitive data displays
- Easy navigation
- Evidence at the point of care to aid decision making
- Enhancements to workflow, automating mundane tasks, and streamlining work, never increasing physical or cognitive workload
- Easy transfer of information to and from other organizations and clinicians
- No unanticipated downtime

SOURCE: IOM, 2011, p. 78.

worrisome (e.g., a new diagnosis or abnormal results). While vendors for direct-to-consumer digital health products have paid attention to usability, the science around usability for the products that primary care clinicians share with those they serve is limited, with the available evidence focused more on individuals' desired access to health information (Kerns et al., 2013). Studies have shown that people generally have trouble navigating patient portals, frequently make operational errors, and expect nonexistent functionalities (Baldwin et al., 2017; Yen et al., 2018).

Children, adolescents, and their parents are less likely to use patient portals for information or communication, compared to adults, in large part due to the inadequate usability of EHRs for this population (Sharko et al., 2018; Webber et al., 2019). There are no consistent or widely used standards adopted by EHRs for how (e.g., technical design for proxy access) or when (e.g., automated access offered at age 13) to grant adolescents independent access to their own data and an ability to communicate with the care team, and EHRs largely are not designed to allow care teams to filter sensitive versus non-sensitive data to allow both parents and teens to have access to the EHR simultaneously, without jeopardizing either teen confidentiality and privacy or parental access to important, non-sensitive health information (Society for Adolescent Health Medicine et al., 2014). The result is that many care teams are left with only the options of denying portal access to parents at a pre-specified child age or not using the portal at all once children reach adolescence. These challenges were further exposed during the COVID-19 pandemic (The Larry A. Green Center and PCC, 2020). Usability for patients will likely require a significant implementation element, including training on the system, more flexibility in privacy based on age and status (e.g., adolescents whose parents may have primary access to the portal), assistance and support as users encounter difficulties, and personnel and strategies to keep them engaged in meaningfully using the system to improve their health.

Lessons from the COVID-19 Pandemic

The COVID-19 pandemic forced rapid changes in digital health across all primary care throughout the nation. Within the span of weeks, many practices converted from almost all in-person care to near complete telehealth (Wosik et al., 2020), to reduce the spread of COVID-19 and protect care-seekers, staff, and clinicians while remaining connected to people and communities that continued to need medical care (Krist et al., 2020). However, COVID-19 has also revealed and amplified the growing breadth of the digital divide and added to health inequities (Woolf et al., 2020).

Three policy changes enabled this rapid transformation. First, CMS relaxed strict regulations about which telehealth platforms were HIPAA compliant. This change allowed patients and clinicians to easily adopt tools, such as video calling, that they were already using in their work and personal lives, rather than requiring people to download complex applications or clinicians to purchase applications for use within EHRs. Second, CMS relaxed strict regulations regarding documentation of telehealth visits and rules about who could be seen by which doctors. This allowed clinicians to offer a telehealth visit to someone with whom they had an established relationship but who lived in or was traveling to another state. Third, payment for telehealth visits, including audio-only visits via telephone, was made equal to in-person visits—payment parity. Previously, many payers did not reimburse for telehealth visits at all; if they did, it was at a lower rate and excluded some visit types (e.g., wellness) (Verma, 2020). These policy changes have been transformative (Contreras et al., 2020; Mann et al., 2020) and some, but not all, were made permanent in late 2020 (CMS, 2020b). Combined with collective fears of catching and spreading COVID-19 and the need for everyone to practice social distancing, telehealth, which had limited low use, was widely and rapidly implemented. Adding allowances for telephone visits has provided remote access for those without smartphones, tablets, or computers, which are needed for video-based telehealth applications.

The U.S. telehealth COVID-19 experience highlights the demand for digital health innovations, the need for policy changes to better support digital health while ensuring digital health equity, and the potential for advancement if the health care technology marketplace can be more open. Assessing the global perspective in comparison to the U.S. response makes it evident that quick, responsive, and adequately applied digital health technology has enabled multiple countries to contain the spread of COVID-19 while leveraging a robust primary care and public health infrastructure. Many of these same countries continue to be front-runners in surveillance, testing, contract tracing, quarantine, individual clinical management and effectively managing the burden of COVID-19 across their populations (Whitelaw et al., 2020).

DESIGNING DIGITAL HEALTH FOR PRIMARY CARE: WHAT DOES SUCCESS LOOK LIKE?

Useful digital health systems for primary care need to support the core functions of primary care. An overarching principle is that systems should aggregate information and make that information usable by clinicians, patients, families, and community members to carry out the core functions of primary care, including promoting access to care, coordinating care, ensuring care is integrated across settings, and allowing for high-quality population health (see Figure 7-1). Based on the function and design of primary

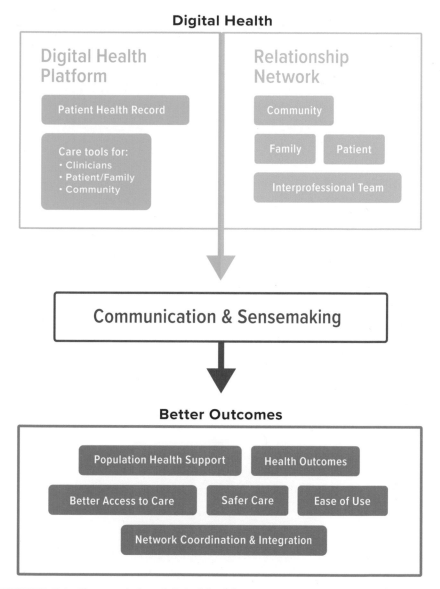

FIGURE 7-1 Characteristics of digital health to support primary care and improve health.

NOTES: Digital health needs to support relationships between members of the care team with patients, families, and the community to improve the essential components of high-quality primary care. These components include care access, coordination, integration, and safety and population health support. Digital health should be easy to use for all team members and care-seekers.

care articulated in this chapter, effective digital health systems will need to (1) support relationships; (2) support high-functioning interprofessional teams to engage in sensemaking, decision making, and action; (3) integrate care delivery across systems and communities; (4) reduce workload; and (5) make care more equitable. Both setting up digital health and using digital health to carry out these functions must occur in a way to reduce workload on primary care and health systems.

Supporting Relationships

Health care is fundamentally relational. This is especially true in primary care, as individuals, families, care teams, and communities collaborate to co-create care plans that evolve over time (Finley et al., 2013). Relationships provide the platform from which all care activities occur, as positive relationships support effective communication. Traditionally, individual–interprofessional team interactions have been episodic and dependent on the person making a burdensome trip to a clinic setting for care and to "engage" in the relationship. Digital health presents an opportunity to increase the frequency and depth of interactions in a manner that is convenient and empowering for the person seeking care and integrates care across health care systems and within communities (Lanham et al., 2016). These increased contacts, in turn, support relationships with patients and care team members across the care and community continuums and improve the quality of care (Lanham et al., 2009). Digital tools are not meant to replace face-to-face visits with a care team but rather to enhance interactions, so that in-person visits become richer in meaning, with deeper interactions resulting from the frequency and level of communication being supported by digital tools. Patient portals, telehealth platforms, health apps, remote monitoring devices, integrated EHRs, and other technologies already exist that can enhance and develop deep interpersonal relationships with the care team.

Person-centered digital health will also enable care to be more transparent, providing information that is understandable and appropriate to the person's unique circumstances. This will promote trust and relationships between patients and their interprofessional care teams, increasing the likelihood of effectively co-created care plans, consistent engagement with the health care system, engagement with community resources, and improvement in health outcomes.

Digital health may also have a unique benefit to adolescents. It provides another avenue for them to build a confidential, trusting relationship with a clinician and care team and a venue in which they can access that team without relying on a parent or guardian to grant access via transportation or even permission. Virtual visits may also be perceived as more confidential than an in-person visit where the parent steps out of the room but is still within earshot.

Supporting High-Functioning Interprofessional Teams

The path from relationships and communication to care plan co-creation and subsequent action requires partnership between interprofessional teams and care-seekers to make sense of information and create mental models that are shared across the relationship network. This process is active—it unfolds over time and is constantly updated (Leykum et al., 2015). Digital health can support the ability of interprofessional teams to make sense of health data. In fact, given the vast amounts of information available about not only each person and their context but an ever-growing evidence base related to health and disease, digital health has become a necessary adjunct and support for teams' effective decision making. The prodigious literature on adverse events, missed diagnoses, and health disparities demonstrates the negative consequences of ineffective sensemaking, and digital health can prevent poor outcomes through several mechanisms (Jordan et al., 2009).

At the individual level, improved safety and harm reduction can happen at the point of care through alerts, reminders, and the prevention of repeat and unnecessary testing, as well as by supporting effective and timely communication among and between care-seekers and the interprofessional team. Digital health provides a common information platform for interprofessional teams, and digital health tools promote effective use of that information by patients and teams to make the most appropriate and effective decisions. At the population level, improved safety and harm reduction can occur by identifying people at risk for poor outcomes. While alerts and registries are already available, the ability to include patients and caregivers, incorporate information across organizational networks, and customize tools to meet local needs and workflows would increase their effectiveness and usefulness.

Digital health tools can also improve health outcomes by promoting prevention, facilitating good health behaviors, improving diagnostic capability, and promoting evidence-based care, again at the individual and population levels. These include the decision support and artificial intelligence tools that are already being implemented to support interprofessional teams and community partners and sometimes also patient monitoring, engagement, and partnership tools that include activity app integration and virtual support communities.

As discussed in *Taking Action Against Clinician Burnout*, HIT (i.e., digital health tools) needs to be optimized to support the clinician (and health team) in providing high-quality care (NASEM, 2019). A properly developed and organized digital health infrastructure will support high-quality care by creating conditions that will nurture deep patient relationships, limit redundant data, optimize data analysis for care and population health, and assist in data interpretation for both the clinician/team and the patient, all while forecasting needs and reducing clinician burnout. Recommendation 4C from *Taking Action Against Clinician Burnout* notes the following:

> This would be an electronic interface that gives the entire care team, including the patient, the ability to collect and use timely and accurate data to achieve high-quality care. A major goal of this new health information system should be to allow clinicians to focus on optimizing patient and population health, while adjuvant processes and technologies derive, to the extent possible, the essential business, administrative, and research data necessary to deliver high-value care efficiently and effectively. (NASEM, 2019, p. 17)

Supporting Integrated Care Delivery

Effective relationships in primary care need to encompass not only the care-seeker, family, and clinician but also potentially other caregivers, the full interprofessional care team, and the community in which care occurs, in an integrated fashion. This integration creates a network around each patient, one that is involved in care plan co-creation and enactment. Integrating care this way occurs in a local context that shapes that care and is shaped by the needs of individuals in the community.

Digital health can support this network by (1) integrating the individuals and organizations in the network and (2) supporting the ties between them. This linkage relies on accurate information transfer and creating a common information platform that enables decision making by the individual and care team. Digital health can ensure that everyone is working with the same set of information to create shared mental models, which requires that information be equally accessible to everyone, when desired by the care-seeker, and it must authentically reflect each patient. Additionally, digital health can support integration across health care systems and communities by facilitating communication that meets a wide spectrum of needs. Some communication, for example, is urgent and requires interpretation, such as that regarding a new, concerning symptom. This scenario requires real-time, person-to-person, direct communication. In other instances, time sensitivity or immediate interpretation may not be necessary, such as notifying about the need for annual preventive care. For this situation, asynchronous distributed information transfer is sufficient. Digital health needs to be nimble enough to support communication and integration across all aspects of the communication spectrum.

Digital health is designed to be person centered and to help individuals get the right care at the right time and can promote integrated care, but only if the systems are easy for people and their families to access and use. A portal that requires downloading software or using specific programs or operating systems will not facilitate information integration. Digital health tools should facilitate the right care at the right time. Tools such as patient portals that help people access integrated information have five essential features. They should (1) link to existing and comprehensive clinical information, (2) allow patients and families to enter information that only they know (values, preferences, behaviors, goals), (3) present content in lay language and the preferred language, (4) interpret content by applying health information to guidelines to say what it means, and (5) make information actionable to allow people to get care and make changes to improve health and well-being (Krist and Woolf, 2011).

There are benefits to standardizing both the function and content of digital health systems to promote integration. For data to be shared across systems, a common data architecture and nomenclature are necessary. Additionally, standardization can help to promote desired care. Alerts, reminders, templates, order entry systems, and educational tools can all be linked to evidence-based guidelines to promote recommended care and deter unnecessary or harmful care.

However, locally tailoring digital health systems is also necessary to support integration in local contexts with the specific interprofessional team and community resources that best partner with each care-seeker. Different populations may have different needs, and different communities may have different resources to deliver care. Each primary care practice will have different workflows depending on staff and skills, and practices engaging in quality improvement will want to use their digital health systems to innovate and redesign care. Having the flexibility to use their systems in novel ways will be essential to continually advance and improve an integrated practice. Finally, digital health provides the means to develop technical support so that someone can take a proactive role in their own health management and care integration, whether this involves medication adherence, preventive screening tests, lifestyle changes, community resources, understanding of chronic conditions and how to manage them, or recognition of when to seek care for a change in their health status.

Making Care More Equitable

As made clear by patients' experiences using telehealth to access care during the COVID-19 pandemic, digital health can increase existing disparities if it is not implemented intentionally to address barriers related to lack of community trust, language needs, Internet access, e-mail use, device capabilities, and an individual's comfort with using digital health and electronic communication platforms (NASEM, 2016; Nouri et al., 2020; Whitelaw et al., 2020). At the same time, digital health represents an opportunity to actively address long-entrenched inequities to assist marginalized populations in achieving more equitable health outcomes. High-quality primary care can use digital health tools to create more equitable care via three main pathways: (1) improved communication, (2) increased access, and (3) reduced disparities in clinical practice.

Improved communication can be achieved through community outreach in conjunction with applying an understanding of local culture to modify digital health interfaces and access points so that digital health can meet the information needs of a marginalized and underserved community (NASEM, 2016). However, simply offering online access to information through a patient portal in a person's native language does nothing to bridge the growing digital divide. Until systemic inequalities and discrimination related to jobs, housing, education, and access to resources are resolved, improving communication with underserved communities will require unique solutions that provide affordable access to high-speed Internet connections and high-impact digital tools. The crux of the problem then becomes how to reduce disparities in digital access and digital health literacy in a manner that will enable culturally appropriate communication, outreach, and education through community partnerships with interprofessional teams to improve access to care for marginalized and underserved communities.

In terms of increased access, a "digital dilemma" now clearly exists in which improved communication and access to digital health resources (i.e., telemedicine) relies on physical access to digital and technological infrastructure. Without that access—whether that involves the Internet, computers, or mobile phone technology—a growing digital divide in access to digital health care and communications will persist. To achieve digital health equity, the "digital dilemma" must be solved. Only then can digital health tools be fully leveraged to improve communications, increase access to care, and reduce health care disparities.

In terms of reducing health care disparities in clinical practice, access to care and culturally appropriate communication are essential starting points. Digital health tools can be used to aggregate and analyze collected information to personalize communication and increase access to care (NASEM, 2016). However, it can also be used to go one step farther—to improve clinical outcomes and reduce health disparities by decreasing implicit bias and improving clinical care (Lau et al., 2015). Theoretically, EHRs and digital health technology can be a great tool for eliminating health care disparities and ensuring equal treatment despite race, gender, or socioeconomic differences. A patient's race, in particular, has been demonstrated as a predictor of health care quality and outcomes in the United States, due to institutional and systemic racism, and ample evidence shows that unconscious or implicit bias among clinicians may influence clinical decision making and lead to disparities in outcomes. Digital health tools represent a unique opportunity to leverage technology to reduce bias, improve clinical decision making, and increase equity in clinical care, if the appropriate policies are implemented to compel stakeholders to leverage digital health tools to reduce health care disparities.

NEEDED FUNCTIONS OF PRIMARY CARE DIGITAL HEALTH SYSTEMS TO ACHIEVE VISION OF SUCCESS

Primary care has a unique need for the most comprehensive access to patients' health information. Starfield and colleagues (2005) described primary care as needing to provide the four Cs—first contact, comprehensive care, coordinated care, and continuous care. Adding to these roles, primary care is the only function in health care responsible for all aspects of a person's health. Succeeding at these tasks depends on comprehensive information. Accordingly, a key responsibility for primary care clinicians is to collect and aggregate health information. Both Meaningful Use certification and the patient-centered medical home recognition mandated them to collect, enter, and manage patient health information within EHR information systems that could then be freely used by all clinicians (Blumenthal and Tavenner, 2010; NCQA, 2020). This is a tremendous burden on primary care that places primary care clinicians in more of an administrative role, detracting from truly helping patients. Additionally, given the volume and breadth of necessary data to inform care, automated tools are needed to make sense of data, identify clinically important data, and improve care. More than any specialty, primary care needs for this information aggregation and analysis to be automated. The current digital health environment makes this an impossible task.

The overarching functions of digital health for primary care include (1) *collecting health information* (creating the platform), (2) *aggregating and making sense of health information* to create a complete health record and highlight critical health information, and (3) *applying health information to improve health* in ways that promote person-centered care, support care teams, span settings of care, and generally make life easier (see Figure 7-2).

Systems that collect health information can be patient facing, clinician facing, automated, or any combination of these. Patient-facing systems allow patients to report information that only they know, such as health behaviors, mood, feelings, quality of life, self-reported outcomes, and goals, and aggregate this information. These systems can include patient portals, smartphone applications, and Web-based surveys. Clinician-facing systems

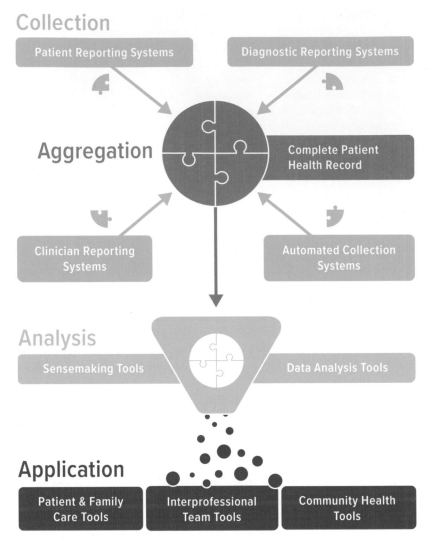

FIGURE 7-2 Functions of digital health for primary care.
NOTES: From a primary care perspective, digital health helps clinicians with collecting information, aggregating and analyzing information, and applying information to decision making and clinical care. Multiple digital health tools can collect information from different audiences (patients, clinicians, diagnostic tests, and automated tools, such as wearables). Once information is aggregated, automated systems are needed to analyze the information to make it usable by patients, families, and care teams.

allow the interprofessional care team to enter information such as medical history, exam findings, diagnoses, treatments, and care plans; the classic such system is the EHR. Automated systems, not currently in routine use, include any system that can collect and aggregate important health-related information, such as about biometrics, behaviors, environment, or exposures, without effort from the clinician, staff, or person seeking care. These automated systems may be important sources of community and contextual information. In the future, automated systems may even act as "scribes," collecting and documenting clinician–patient interactions and allowing clinicians to truly focus on the person. Multiple collection systems can be used simultaneously, and future versions may even replace aspects of existing clinician and patient-facing systems to automate data collection.

Once collected, information needs to be aggregated and analyzed, creating the information platform that patients, families, clinicians, and communities can use to make sense of what is happening and take action. Both functions need to be automated and not dependent on clinicians, staff, or care-seekers to collect, re-enter, or analyze. The information must be comprehensive and not siloed, and while it could be distributed (i.e., stored in multiple systems), it should be connected to yield an immediately comprehensive and complete record when needed. Patients must be in control of who has access to which elements of their information and when. Supporting the comprehensive information, analytics and sensemaking tools are required to sort information in ways that are valuable to users. This is particularly important as these systems incorporate more raw data (e.g., daily weights, smart watch measurements, and environmental data). Tools are needed to identify clinically meaningful data, overdue care, and potential safety issues, aid in diagnosis and care delivery, and even inform population health activities. Existing tools include alerts and reminders, drug interactions, quality measurements, and patient registries, though these are just a starting point if digital health is to truly aid clinicians and individuals in providing and accessing care.

Ultimately, the purpose of digital health is to help patients, families, clinicians, and care teams to improve health. The same tools that collect health information should enable all involved parties to access health information through analytics and tools that promote the ability of patients, families, care teams, and communities to make sense of the available information and take action to improve health. This includes being able to make diagnoses, see what care is needed, deliver care, communicate among team members, coordinate care, and track progress.

To meet these collective needs, the committee has identified the following high-level primary care digital health functions required for success:

Collect Information

- Complete information. Primary care needs systems to collect information from all health care sources (primary care, specialists, community providers, and care-seekers) and non–health care sources that affect health (environmental data, social descriptors) and include all potential settings (inpatient, outpatient, and communities). Nontraditional health care team members will need access to and will generate health information.
- Automate information collection. Information collection should not depend on primary care clinicians entering or reconciling data; it needs intelligent automation.
- Ownership of information. People need to own their health data and be able to grant care team members access to their information. As children age into adolescents, they should become owners of their health information, independent of the parent or guardian. Similarly, if primary care clinicians spend 6 hours per day documenting care, they own those data—not the health system or EHR vendor. Once generated, clinicians should have indefinite access to the data they created.

Aggregate and Analyze Information

- Create a comprehensive record. Primary care needs a comprehensive record that includes all individual health information but is not responsible for creating it; rather, digital health should be a resource that supports primary care. Comprehensive information could exist in distributed sources, simultaneously and seamlessly accessed.
- True interoperability. To aggregate health information and create a comprehensive record, primary care needs digital health systems to be functionally interoperable. The requirements for digital health systems should measure "lived interoperability," not whether systems can theoretically be interoperable. The metric of success for lived interoperability is the daily transfer of health information from one system to another and the amount of data that fails to transfer in a completely automated way.
- Information sensemaking. For a comprehensive health record to be useful, tools such as artificial intelligence are needed to parse relevant data, understand implications and interrelationships of data, and aid decision making and health promotion.

Apply Information

- Engage care-seekers in action. Digital health systems should engage and activate individual patients and populations in their care by translating medical content into lay language, allowing patients to clearly state and communicate their goals of care and providing them with logic, educational support, and tools to facilitate their action. Systems need to work with a broad range of audiences with diverse needs and account for patient confidentiality and privacy.
- Promote evidence-based care and safety. Digital health systems need to promote national quality and safety standards and to include and make usable the most up-to-date national guidelines and quality measures.
- Make care proactive. Registries, alerts, reminders, and other population health tools are needed to identify and target persons who require care.
- Automate more care. Technology disruption is needed to automate some elements of care delivery through artificial intelligence, chat bots and avatars, and ambient computing.
- Coordinate care teams. Integrated communication tools can help teams to better coordinate around care.
- Allow local tailoring. Not all patients, practices, and communities are the same. Local adaptation is necessary to accommodate variations in their needs, workflows, and resources.

Payment and care models also need to change, as described in Chapter 9. Changing digital health without providing resources for primary care to carry out these functions would not result in change and even exacerbate clinician burnout.

HEALTH DISPARITIES AND DIGITAL HEALTH

While digital health is transforming the health care landscape, it is not immune to the pervasive systemic inequalities that have contributed to long-entrenched health care disparities. The COVID-19 pandemic has shed light on these disparities, which have been further amplified by the policy response to the crisis, exacerbating the entrenched inequities in the U.S. health care system, in general, and the primary care system, in particular. The pandemic also showcased how digital health initiatives can further escalate socioeconomic, racial, and geographic inequalities that directly influence health care disparities (Nouri et al., 2020; Woolf et al., 2020). As telehealth rapidly expands and ensures access to care even when primary care practices are closed and people are self-isolating, many older Americans, low-income families, rural communities, and racial and ethnic minorities are unable to access care and suffering from the consequences of delayed treatment (Hirko et al., 2020; Kim et al., 2020; Nouri et al., 2020; Verma, 2020).

In October 2014, the National Academies of Sciences, Engineering, and Medicine held a workshop (Promotion of Health Equity and the Elimination of Health Disparities) (NASEM, 2016) focused on reviewing examples and models of digital health technologies to improve health outcomes for underserved populations. Key themes that emerged include the importance of community engagement to adopt digital health tools; leveraging mobile technology to reach underserved populations; the impact of infrastructure and systemic inequities on the access to these technologies; and the marginalization of minority communities by the current market forces driving digital health innovation. Box 7-2 shows one example of the type of local approach and resources needed to operationalize these themes.

If policies impacting digital health are not changed to create equitable access and outcomes, the nation will be left facing unnecessary and

---

BOX 7-2
Reducing Digital and Health Inequities in Latina
Immigrant Communities (NASEM, 2016)

A partnership between the University of New Mexico (UNM) and La Comunidad Habla (Spanish for "the community speaks") provides one example of how to improve the use of digital health and reduce health disparities in a Latina immigrant community (NASEM, 2016; Young et al., 2018). La Comunidad Habla works predominantly in Southeast Albuquerque, which is the most ethnically diverse area in the state. While the area has relatively affordable housing, most properties are rentals, making it difficult to build social capital as people move in and out of the area. Despite increases in online access, this community experiences the digital divide, which has marginalizing health, social, and economic effects. La Comunidad Habla and UNM sought to not only provide online access to digitally marginalized communities but also field a series of culturally appropriate interventions to ensure uptake and engagement. In one initiative through a pediatric clinic, La Comunidad Habla provided women with technological and health advocacy and leadership opportunities in the community (Ginossar and Nelson, 2010a,b). This initiative began with evening computer classes in Spanish for women, with childcare provided. The project then provided opportunities for community members to access health information and technology, in part through a bilingual online health care resource directory with low literacy and culturally appropriate content. With only limited resources, the program reached and trained more than 1,000 community members and providers.

premature deaths within its most vulnerable populations. Additionally, without stronger accountability and oversight, the U.S. health care system will continue to provide the most expensive and advanced digital health technology to those who can afford it rather than to those who would most benefit.

DIGITAL HEALTH IMPLEMENTATION NEEDS

This chapter presents a bold future vision for how digital health can support primary care. Achieving this vision requires (1) buy-in from clinicians and care-seekers who use digital health systems, (2) support from practice and health system informaticists who field these systems, (3) a willingness on the part of digital health vendors to transform their systems, (4) disruption of the existing centralized marketplace to allow for innovation, (5) new authorities and policies to enforce digital health meets standards, and (6) policy makers' commitment to implement rules, regulations, and metrics that assess the lived experiences of digital health users. For successful implementation, all requirements must be satisfied concurrently and satisfying requirements cannot add burden to primary care. Failure from any sector will result in continuing with the status quo.

As the end users, clinicians and those seeking care need to demand digital health tools that meet their needs. While they have the least power to effect change, they suffer the most when digital health fails to meet their needs and bear the greatest burden when changing from one digital health system to another. Accordingly, they must be protected throughout the transformation process. Practice and health system informaticists often decide about digital health systems to adopt; many of them are not clinicians, and few are routine end users. These decision makers need to understand the lived experience of those they serve.

While Meaningful Use incentives stimulated the national adoption of EHRs, it also consolidated the market, creating powerful, resourced, and established vendors. Rather than merely adding code or database architecture to their existing systems or acquiring and integrating a new system, vendors need to move past the 1990s and 2000s and create new systems. To support this, the digital health marketplace needs to be a free marketplace that supports innovation. Clinicians and health systems should not be bound to existing systems because transitioning is prohibitively labor intensive, resulting in losing data that they spent years entering. The linchpin to transforming the marketplace and promoting innovation will be true interoperability, not the checkbox interoperability that exists today.

To achieve true interoperability, there must be a common health information database available to all health care clinicians to support data sharing while ensuring local control of the data to ensure security and meet privacy requirements. One option is a centralized national medical database. This model has been successfully deployed in other countries, as exemplified by the Historia Clínica Digital del Sistema Nacional de Salud (the National Health System Electronic Health Records Project) in Spain (Huerta et al., n.d.). Another option that would optimally support high-quality primary care is a distributed data network capable of transferring information between EHR databases in response to health information queries that can provide aggregated data to the end user or data requestor. In 2010, the Agency for Healthcare Research and Quality published a report providing a blueprint for a distributed research network to conduct population studies and safety surveillance (Brown et al., 2010). The report highlighted a distributed architecture, scalability, query distribution, data holder autonomy, and privacy protection as key attributes that would be needed to successfully implement a centralized distributed data network to support health information. This model can be adapted nationwide to create a digital health backbone that supports delivering high-quality primary care to people, families, and communities who ultimately retain control of their own data. An obvious first step would be to create a digitally encoded card with individual health data for those with state and federally funded health insurance coverage that would allow secure transfer, queries, and analysis. If successful, the concept can be expanded broadly to all people regardless of insurance type. However, to build the distributed database of the future, federal government support is required, including new legislation authorizing its creation, regulatory oversight, and funding to design and support the system.

Policy makers are well positioned to catalyze and ensure that the needed transformation of digital health occurs, although they need greater authority over digital health vendors to ensure their systems meet requirements. Doing so requires fundamentally prioritizing patients and clinicians over existing businesses and focusing on creating the next generation of measures and standards that track and assess users' lived experience, not merely digital health's potential to meet standards in an ideal and even theoretical way. The next phase of digital health standards should focus on measuring in real time the transfer of data, the integrity of data, how often data need manual reconciliation, the number of clicks to perform tasks, data entry time, and use of the system by clinicians and patients that can be directly linked to improved health and well-being.

DIGITAL HEALTH RESEARCH NEEDS

Evidence should guide digital health development and use for primary care. Both digital health functionality and implementation need to be studied using improvements in the quadruple aim as the desired outcome

(Bodenheimer and Sinsky, 2014). Digital health applications need to show they enhance the care experience, improve population health, reduce costs, achieve equitable outcomes, and improve the work life of clinicians and staff.

While relationships, interprofessional care teams, comprehensive care, and health equity are critical elements of effective primary care, the direct evidence about how digital health can best support these functions is still evolving. This understanding will require work that goes beyond the current examination of clinician use of features or decision support tools, or individual logins to health portals or use of secure messages, and a rich, mixed methods, ethnographic research agenda that engages patients, families, interprofessional care teams, and community partners to understand optimal use over time. This work needs to be in partnership with groups engaged in developing digital health tools to ensure that they create the most effective tools.

Disruptive digital health advances that transform aspects of future health care delivery are inevitable. Innovations using artificial intelligence and avatars can automate care. Ambient computing can collect, aggregate, and analyze information. New unforeseen technologies will bring advances to diagnosis, treatment, and delivery of care. Research is needed to develop these disruptive technologies, to assess their impact on health outcomes, to evaluate them for unforeseen complications, and to determine how to implement and integrate them into future care delivery models.

FINDINGS AND CONCLUSIONS

Digital health, particularly EHRs that serve as the hub of patient information, is an essential tool to improve systems of care. It is also the major source of professional dissatisfaction and clinician burnout (NASEM, 2019). The committee supports three major informatics changes needed to advance digital health for primary care—changes to the marketplace, aggregated comprehensive patient data, and new federal standards to drive meaningful change. This chapter describes the principles needed for these changes.

The current dominance of the market by a few informatics vendors coupled with limited interoperability has locked clinicians and practices into existing systems and stifled innovation. Switching from one EHR to another is a tremendous effort and sacrifices essential data. While many EHRs technically meet interoperability standards, they are not functionally interoperable. Because the privatization and monetization of health information is how vendors maintain the market share of their products, they are not incented to be truly interoperable. Vendor policies, inconsistent data storage and architecture, and limited mechanisms for efficient data transfer all contribute to limited interoperability.

A key action that will change the marketplace, catalyze innovation, and advance care is to create a national comprehensive and aggregated patient data system, which would enable primary care clinicians, interprofessional teams, patients, and families to easily access the comprehensive data needed to provide whole-person care. It could be used by any certified digital health vendor to create innovations, and patients could control who has access to their health information. There are several ways this could be achieved. It could be set up as either a centralized data warehouse or individual health card or distributed sources connected by a real-time functional HIE. Access to centralized comprehensive data would represent an essential innovation for primary care teams responsible for whole-person care. It shifts the burden that national quality metrics and performance payments currently impose on primary care clinicians to manually enter patient information to create a comprehensive record, placing it on an automated system that would allow clinicians and teams to focus on care. The committee recognizes that these changes will require innovation from vendors and state and national support agencies and that accomplishing these goals will not be easy to ascertain. However, this is an essential need.

The committee supports federal standards setting for this field but has determined that the past Meaningful Use requirements inadequately met the needs of primary care and unacceptably put the burden of meeting the requirements onto primary care. A new phase of federal standards is needed to ensure that HIT aligns with primary care functions, makes it easy to deliver the right care at the right time, is designed to support equitable access, can help clinicians make sense of complex information, and fundamentally reduces clinician and patient workload. The lived experience of clinicians and care-seekers should be measured and used to assess whether HIT is meeting expected standards, not the theoretical ability of systems, as previously done. Vendors and state and national support agencies should be charged with designing base digital health systems to meet these requirements, and should be held accountable when systems fail to meet benchmarks.

REFERENCES

Adler-Milstein, J., D. W. Bates, and A. K. Jha. 2013. Operational health information exchanges show substantial growth, but long-term funding remains a concern. *Health Affairs* 32(8):1486–1492.

Alagiakrishnan, K., P. Wilson, C. A. Sadowski, D. Rolfson, M. Ballermann, A. Ausford, K. Vermeer, K. Mohindra, J. Romney, and R. S. Hayward. 2016. Physicians' use of computerized clinical decision supports to improve medication management in the elderly—the Seniors Medication Alert and Review technology intervention. *Clinical Interventions in Aging* 11(1):73–81.

AMA (American Medical Association). 2015. *Panel management: Provide preventative care and improve patient health.* https://edhub.ama-assn.org/steps-forward/module/2702192 (accessed May 6, 2020).

AMA. 2016. *Point-of care registries: Proactively manage chronic care conditions.* https://edhub.ama-assn.org/steps-forward/module/2702745 (accessed May 6, 2020).

AMA. 2020. *AMA digital health research: Physicians' motivations and requirements for adopting digital health and attitudinal shifts from 2016–2019.* Chicago, IL: American Medical Association.

Arndt, B. G., J. W. Beasley, M. D. Watkinson, J. L. Temte, W. J. Tuan, C. A. Sinsky, and V. J. Gilchrist. 2017. Tethered to the EHR: Primary care physician workload assessment using EHR event log data and time-motion observations. *Annals of Family Medicine* 15(5):419–426.

Baldwin, J. L., H. Singh, D. F. Sittig, and T. D. Giardina. 2017. Patient portals and health apps: Pitfalls, promises, and what one might learn from the other symptoms. *Healthcare* 5(3):81–85.

Barnett, M. L., K. N. Ray, J. Souza, and A. Mehrotra. 2018. Trends in telemedicine use in a large commercially insured population, 2005–2017. *JAMA* 320(20):2147–2149.

Blumenthal, D. 2009. Stimulating the adoption of health information technology. *New England Journal of Medicine* 360(15):1477–1479.

Blumenthal, D., and M. Tavenner. 2010. The "Meaningful Use" regulation for electronic health records. *New England Journal of Medicine* 363(6):501–504.

Bodenheimer, T., and C. Sinsky. 2014. From triple to quadruple aim: Care of the patient requires care of the provider. *Annals of Family Medicine* 12(6):573–576.

Bright, T. J., A. Wong, R. Dhurjati, E. Bristow, L. Bastian, R. R. Coeytaux, G. Samsa, V. Hasselblad, J. W. Williams, M. D. Musty, L. Wing, A. S. Kendrick, G. D. Sanders, and D. Lobach. 2012. Effect of clinical decision-support systems: A systematic review. *Annals of Internal Medicine* 157(1):29–43.

Brown, J., B. Syat, K. Lane, and R. Platt. 2010. *Blueprint for a distributed research network to conduct population studies and safety surveillance.* Rockville, MD: Agency for Healthcare Research and Quality.

CDC (Centers for Disease Control and Prevention). 2019. *Public health and promoting interoperability programs.* https://www.cdc.gov/ehrmeaningfuluse/introduction.html (accessed May 7, 2020).

CMS (Centers for Medicare & Medicaid Services). 2020a. *Promoting interoperability.* https://www.cms.gov/Regulations-and-Guidance/Legislation/EHRIncentivePrograms/Stage3Medicaid_Require (accessed May 6, 2020).

CMS. 2020b. *Trump administration finalizes permanent expansion of Medicare telehealth services and improved payment for time doctors spend with patients.* https://www.cms.gov/newsroom/press-releases/trump-administration-finalizes-permanent-expansion-medicare-telehealth-services-and-improved-payment (accessed January 27, 2021).

Colicchio, T. K., J. J. Cimino, and G. Del Fiol. 2019. Unintended consequences of nationwide electronic health record adoption: Challenges and opportunities in the post-Meaningful Use era. *Journal of Medical Internet Research* 21(6):e13313.

Contreras, C. M., G. A. Metzger, J. D. Beane, P. H. Dedhia, A. Ejaz, and T. M. Pawlik. 2020. Telemedicine: Patient–provider clinical engagement during the COVID-19 pandemic and beyond. *Journal of Gastrointestinal Surgery* 24(7):1692–1697.

DeVoe, J. E., A. W. Bazemore, E. K. Cottrell, S. Likumahuwa-Ackman, J. Grandmont, N. Spach, and R. Gold. 2016. Perspectives in primary care: A conceptual framework and path for integrating social determinants of health into primary care practice. *Annals of Family Medicine* 14(2):104–108.

Dinh-Le, C., R. Chuang, S. Chokshi, and D. Mann. 2019. Wearable health technology and electronic health record integration: Scoping review and future directions. *JMIR mHealth uHealth* 7(9):e12861.

Fernald, D. H., R. Wearner, and W. P. Dickinson. 2013. The journey of primary care practices to Meaningful Use: A Colorado Beacon Consortium study. *Journal of the American Board of Family Medicine* 26(5):603–611.

Finley, E. P., J. A. Pugh, H. J. Lanham, L. K. Leykum, J. Cornell, P. Veerapaneni, and M. L. Parchman. 2013. Relationship quality and patient-assessed quality of care in VA primary care clinics: Development and validation of the work relationships scale. *Annals of Family Medicine* 11(6):543–549.

Fisher, E. S., J. P. Bynum, and J. S. Skinner. 2009. Slowing the growth of health care costs—lessons from regional variation. *New England Journal of Medicine* 360(9):849–852.

Fleming, N. S., S. D. Culler, R. McCorkle, E. R. Becker, and D. J. Ballard. 2011. The financial and nonfinancial costs of implementing electronic health records in primary care practices. *Health Affairs* 30(3):481–489.

Friedberg, M. W., P. G. Chen, K. R. Van Busum, F. Aunon, C. Pham, J. Caloyeras, S. Mattke, E. Pitchforth, D. D. Quigley, R. H. Brook, F. J. Crosson, and M. Tutty. 2014. Factors affecting physician professional satisfaction and their implications for patient care, health systems, and health policy. *RAND Health Quarterly* 3(4):1.

Ginossar, T., and S. Nelson. 2010a. La Comunidad Habla: Using internet community-based information interventions to increase empowerment and access to health care of low income Latino/a immigrants. *Communication Education* 59(3):328–343.

Ginossar, T., and S. Nelson. 2010b. Reducing the health and digital divides: A model for using community-based participatory research approach to e-health interventions in low-income Hispanic communities. *Journal of Computer-Mediated Communication* 15(4):530–551.

HealthIT. 2020. *Interoperability*. https://www.healthit.gov/topic/interoperability (accessed January, 26 2020).

Hirko, K. A., J. M. Kerver, S. Ford, C. Szafranski, J. Beckett, C. Kitchen, and A. L. Wendling. 2020. Telehealth in response to the COVID-19 pandemic: Implications for rural health disparities. *Journal of the American Medical Informatics Association* 27(11):1816–1818.

Holmgren, A. J., N. L. Downing, D. W. Bates, T. D. Shanafelt, A. Milstein, C. D. Sharp, D. M. Cutler, R. S. Huckman, and K. A. Schulman. 2020. Assessment of electronic health record use between U.S. and non-U.S. health systems. *JAMA Internal Medicine*. https://doi.org/10.1001/jamainternmed.2020.7071 (accessed December 29, 2020).

Hoonakker, P. L. T., P. Carayon, and R. S. Cartmill. 2017. The impact of secure messaging on workflow in primary care: Results of a multiple-case, multiple-method study. *International Journal of Medical Informatics* 100:63–76.

Huerta, J. E., C. A. Villar, M. C. Fernández, G. M. Cuenca, and I. A. Acebedo. n.d. *NHS electronic health record system*. Madrid: Health Information Institute.

Hughes, L. S., R. L. Phillips, Jr., J. E. DeVoe, and A. W. Bazemore. 2016. Community vital signs: Taking the pulse of the community while caring for patients. *Journal of the American Board of Family Practice* 29(3):419–422.

Hussain, M. I., T. L. Reynolds, and K. Zheng. 2019. Medication safety alert fatigue may be reduced via interaction design and clinical role tailoring: A systematic review. *Journal of the American Medical Informatics Association* 26(10):1141–1149.

IOM (Institue of Medicine). 1996a. *Primary care: America's health in a new era*. Washington, DC: National Academy Press.

IOM. 1996b. *Telemedicine: A guide to assessing telecommunications in health care*. Washington, DC: National Academy Press.

IOM. 2011. *Health IT and patient safety: Building safer systems for better care*. Washington, DC: The National Academies Press.

Jordan, M. E., H. J. Lanham, B. F. Crabtree, P. A. Nutting, W. L. Miller, K. C. Stange, and R. R. McDaniel, Jr. 2009. The role of conversation in health care interventions: Enabling sensemaking and learning. *Implementation Science* 4:15.

Kerns, J. W., A. H. Krist, D. R. Longo, A. J. Kuzel, and S. H. Woolf. 2013. How patients want to engage with their personal health record: A qualitative study. *BMJ Open* 3(7):e002931.

Kim, J. H., E. Desai, and M. B. Cole. 2020. *How the rapid shift to telehealth leaves many community health centers behind during the COVID-19 pandemic.* https://www.healthaffairs.org/do/10.1377/hblog20200529.449762/full (accessed December 2, 2020).

Krist, A. H., and S. H. Woolf. 2011. A vision for patient-centered health information systems. *JAMA* 305(3):300–301.

Krist, A. H., J. W. Beasley, J. C. Crosson, D. C. Kibbe, M. S. Klinkman, C. U. Lehmann, C. H. Fox, J. M. Mitchell, J. W. Mold, W. D. Pace, K. A. Peterson, R. L. Phillips, R. Post, J. Puro, M. Raddock, R. Simkus, and S. E. Waldren. 2014. Electronic health record functionality needed to better support primary care. *Journal of the American Medical Informatics Association* 21(5):764–771.

Krist, A. H., J. E. DeVoe, A. Cheng, T. Ehrlich, and S. M. Jones. 2020. Redesigning primary care to address the COVID-19 pandemic in the midst of the pandemic. *Annals of Family Medicine* 18(4):349–354.

Kruse, C. S., and A. Beane. 2018. Health information technology continues to show positive effect on medical outcomes: Systematic review. *Journal of Medical Internet Research* 20(2):e41.

Landi, H. 2020. *Epic, meditech gain U.S. hospital market share as other EHR vendors lose ground.* https://www.fiercehealthcare.com/tech/epic-meditech-gain-u-s-hospital-market-share-as-other-ehr-vendors-lose-ground (accessed December 2, 2020).

Lanham, H. J., R. R. McDaniel, Jr., B. F. Crabtree, W. L. Miller, K. C. Stange, A. F. Tallia, and P. Nutting. 2009. How improving practice relationships among clinicians and nonclinicians can improve quality in primary care. *Joint Commission Journal on Quality and Patient Safety* 35(9):457–466.

Lanham, H. J., R. F. Palmer, L. K. Leykum, R. R. McDaniel, Jr., P. A. Nutting, K. C. Stange, B. F. Crabtree, W. L. Miller, and C. R. Jaen. 2016. Trust and reflection in primary care practice redesign. *Health Services Research* 51(4):1489–1514.

Lau, B. D., A. H. Haider, M. B. Streiff, C. U. Lehmann, P. S. Kraus, D. B. Hobson, F. S. Kraenzlin, A. M. Zeidan, P. J. Pronovost, and E. R. Haut. 2015. Eliminating health care disparities with mandatory clinical decision support: The Venous Thromboembolism (VTE) example. *Medical Care* 53(1):18–24.

Leykum, L. K., H. Chesser, H. J. Lanham, P. Carla, R. Palmer, T. Ratcliffe, H. Reisinger, M. Agar, and J. Pugh. 2015. The association between sensemaking during physician team rounds and hospitalized patients' outcomes. *Journal of General Internal Medicine* 30(12):1821–1827.

Liaw, W., A. H. Krist, S. T. Tong, R. Sabo, C. Hochheimer, J. Rankin, D. Grolling, J. Grandmont, and A. W. Bazemore. 2018. Living in "cold spot" communities is associated with poor health and health quality. *Journal of the American Board of Family Practice* 31(3):342–350.

Mandel, J. C., D. A. Kreda, K. D. Mandl, I. S. Kohane, and R. B. Ramoni. 2016. Smart on FHIR: A standards-based, interoperable apps platform for electronic health records. *Journal of the American Medical Informatics Association* 23(5):899–908.

Mann, D. M., J. Chen, R. Chunara, P. A. Testa, and O. Nov. 2020. COVID-19 transforms health care through telemedicine: Evidence from the field. *Journal of the American Medical Informatics Association* 27(7):1132–1135.

Medgadget. 2020. *Electronic health records market size 2020 industry analysis, share, growth, upcoming trends, segmentation and forecast by 2025.* https://www.medgadget.com/2020/02/electronic-health-records-market-size-2020-industry-analysis-share-growth-upcoming-trends-segmentation-and-forecast-by-2025.html (accessed December 2, 2020).

Meskó, B., Z. Drobni, É. Bényei, B. Gergely, and Z. Győrffy. 2017. Digital health is a cultural transformation of traditional healthcare. *mHealth* 3:38.

Moacdieh, N., and N. Sarter. 2015. Clutter in electronic medical records: Examining its performance and attentional costs using eye tracking. *Human Factors* 57(4):591–606.

NASEM (National Academies of Sciences, Engineering, and Medicine). 2016. *The promises and perils of digital strategies in achieving health equity: Workshop summary.* Washington, DC: The National Academies Press.

NASEM. 2019. *Taking action against clinician burnout: A systems approach to professional well-being.* Washington, DC: The National Academies Press.

NCQA (National Committee for Quality Assurance). 2020. *Patient-centered medical home (PCMH).* https://www.ncqa.org/programs/health-care-providers-practices/patient-centered-medical-home-pcmh (accessed June 2, 2020).

NCVHS (National Committee on Vital and Health Statistics). 2019. *Additional recommendations for HHS actions to improve the adoption of standards under the Health Insurance Portability and Accountability Act (HIPAA) of 1996.* Hyattsville, MD: National Committee on Vital and Health Statistics.

Nelson, E. C., M. Dixon-Woods, P. B. Batalden, K. Homa, A. D. Van Citters, T. S. Morgan, E. Eftimovska, E. S. Fisher, J. Ovretveit, W. Harrison, C. Lind, and S. Lindblad. 2016. Patient focused registries can improve health, care, and science. *BMJ* 354:i3319.

Nouri, S., E. C. Khoong, C. R. Lyles, and L. Karliner. 2020. Addressing equity in telemedicine for chronic disease management during the COVID-19 pandemic. *NEJM Catalyst.* https://catalyst.nejm.org/doi/full/10.1056/CAT.20.0123 (accessed January 8, 2021).

O'Malley, A. S., J. M. Grossman, G. R. Cohen, N. M. Kemper, and H. H. Pham. 2010. Are electronic medical records helpful for care coordination? Experiences of physician practices. *Journal of General Internal Medicine* 25(3):177–185.

ONC (Office of the National Coordinator for Health Information Technology). 2013. *Building technology capabilities to aggregate clinical data and enable population health measurement.* Washington, DC: Office of the National Coordinator for Health Information Technology.

ONC. 2019. *Office-based physician electronic health record adoption.* dashboard.healthit.gov/quickstats/pages/physician-ehr-adoption-trends.php (accessed December 8, 2020).

Ornstein, S. M., L. S. Nemeth, P. J. Nietert, R. G. Jenkins, A. M. Wessell, and C. B. Litvin. 2015. Learning from primary care meaningful use exemplars. *Journal of the American Board of Family Practice* 28(3):360–370.

Patel, V., and C. Johnson. 2019. *Trends in individuals' access, viewing and use of online medical records and other technology for health needs: 2017–2018.* Washington, DC: Office of the National Coordinator for Health Information Technology.

Phillips, R. L., Jr., A. W. Bazemore, J. E. DeVoe, T. J. Weida, A. H. Krist, M. F. Dulin, and F. E. Biagioli. 2015. A family medicine health technology strategy for achieving the triple aim for us health care. *Family Medicine* 47(8):628–635.

Pronovost, P., M. M. E. Johns, S. Palmer, R. C. Bono, D. B. Fridsma, A. Gettinger, J. Goldman, W. Johnson, M. Karney, C. Samitt, R. D. Sriram, A. Zenooz, and Y. C. Wang, eds. 2018. *Procuring interoperability: Achieving high-quality, connected, and person-centered care.* Washington, DC: National Academy of Medicine.

Ratwani, R. M., M. Hodgkins, and D. W. Bates. 2018a. Improving electronic health record usability and safety requires transparency. *JAMA* 320(24):2533–2534.

Ratwani, R. M., B. Moscovitch, and J. P. Rising. 2018b. Improving pediatric electronic health record usability and safety through certification: Seize the day. *JAMA Pediatrics* 172(11):1007–1008.

Ratwani, R. M., E. Savage, A. Will, A. Fong, D. Karavite, N. Muthu, A. J. Rivera, C. Gibson, D. Asmonga, B. Moscovitch, R. Grundmeier, and J. Rising. 2018c. Identifying electronic health record usability and safety challenges in pediatric settings. *Health Affairs* 37(11):1752–1759.

Rittenhouse, D. R., P. P. Ramsay, L. P. Casalino, S. McClellan, Z. K. Kandel, and S. M. Shortell. 2017. Increased health information technology adoption and use among small primary care physician practices over time: A national cohort study. *Annals of Family Medicine* 15(1):56–62.

Rock, R. M., W. R. Liaw, A. H. Krist, S. Tong, D. Grolling, J. Rankin, and A. W. Bazemore. 2019. Clinicians' overestimation of their geographic service area. *Annals of Family Medicine* 17(Suppl 1):S63–S66.

Rucker, D. 2018. *Achieving the interoperability promise of 21st Century Cures*. https://www.healthaffairs.org/do/10.1377/hblog20180618.138568/full (accessed May 6, 2020).

Schellhase, K. G., T. D. Koepsell, and T. E. Norris. 2003. Providers' reactions to an automated health maintenance reminder system incorporated into the patient's electronic medical record. *Journal of the American Board of Family Practice* 16(4):312–317.

Sharko, M., L. Wilcox, M. K. Hong, and J. S. Ancker. 2018. Variability in adolescent portal privacy features: How the unique privacy needs of the adolescent patient create a complex decision-making process. *Journal of the American Medical Informatics Association* 25(8):1008–1017.

Sharon, T. 2018. When digital health meets digital capitalism, how many common goods are at stake? *Big Data & Society* 5(2):1–12.

Smith, C., C. Balatbat, S. Corbridge, A. Dopp, J. Fried, R. Harter, S. Landefeld, C. Martin, F. Opelka, L. Sandy, L. Sato, and C. Sinsky. 2018. *Implementing optimal team-based care to reduce clinician burnout*. Washington, DC: National Academy of Medicine.

Society for Adolescent Health Medicine, S. H. Gray, R. H. Pasternak, H. C. Gooding, K. Woodward, K. Hawkins, S. Sawyer, and A. Anoshiravani. 2014. Recommendations for electronic health record use for delivery of adolescent health care. *Journal of Adolescent Health* 54(4):487–490.

Starfield, B., L. Shi, and J. Macinko. 2005. Contribution of primary care to health systems and health. *Milbank Quarterly* 83(3):457–502.

Street, R. L., Jr., L. Liu, N. J. Farber, Y. Chen, A. Calvitti, D. Zuest, M. T. Gabuzda, K. Bell, B. Gray, S. Rick, S. Ashfaq, and Z. Agha. 2014. Provider interaction with the electronic health record: The effects on patient-centered communication in medical encounters. *Patient Education and Counseling* 96(3):315–319.

Tate, C., and P. Warburton. 2020. *U.S. hospital EMR market share 2020 report*. https://klasresearch.com/resources/blogs/2020/06/15/us-hospital-emr-market-share-2020-report (accessed January 26, 2021).

The Larry A. Green Center and PCC (Primary Care Collaborative). 2020. *Quick COVID-19 primary care survey: Clinician survey*. https://www.green-center.org/covid-survey (accessed September 15, 2020).

Tong, S., R. A. Mullen, C. J. Hochheimer, R. T. Sabo, W. R. Liaw, D. E. Nease, Jr., A. H. Krist, and J. J. Frey, 3rd. 2019. Geographic characteristics of loneliness in primary care. *Annals of Family Medicine* 17(2):158–160.

Verma, S. 2020. *Early impact of CMS expansion of Medicare telehealth during COVID-19*. https://www.healthaffairs.org/do/10.1377/hblog20200715.454789/full (accessed December 2, 2020).

Vest, J. R., and L. D. Gamm. 2010. Health information exchange: Persistent challenges and new strategies. *Journal of the American Medical Informatics Association* 17(3):288–294.

Washington, V., K. DeSalvo, F. Mostashari, and D. Blumenthal. 2017. The HITECH era and the path forward. *New England Journal of Medicine* 377(10):904–906.

Weatherly, J., S. Kishnani, and T. Aye. 2019. Challenges with patient adoption of automated integration of blood glucose meter data in the electronic health record. *Diabetes Technology & Therapeutics* 21(11):671–674.

Webber, E. C., D. Brick, J. P. Scibilia, P. Dehnel, Council on Clinical Information Technology, Committee on Medical Liability and Risk Management, and Section on Telehealth Care. 2019. Electronic communication of the health record and information with pediatric patients and their guardians. *Pediatrics* 144(1).

Whitelaw, S., M. S. Mamas, E. J. Topol, and H. G. C. Van Spall. 2020. Applications of digital technology in COVID-19 pandemic planning and response. *The Lancet.* https://www.thelancet.com/action/showPdf?pii=S2589-7500%2820%2930142-4 (accessed December 2, 2020).

Woolf, S. H., D. A. Chapman, R. T. Sabo, D. M. Weinberger, and L. Hill. 2020. Excess deaths from COVID-19 and other causes, March–April 2020. *JAMA* 324(5):510–513.

Wosik, J., M. Fudim, B. Cameron, Z. F. Gellad, A. Cho, D. Phinney, S. Curtis, M. Roman, E. G. Poon, J. Ferranti, J. N. Katz, and J. Tcheng. 2020. Telehealth transformation: COVID-19 and the rise of virtual care. *Journal of the American Medical Informatics Association* 27(6):957–962.

Yen, P. Y., D. M. Walker, J. M. G. Smith, M. P. Zhou, T. L. Menser, and A. S. McAlearney. 2018. Usability evaluation of a commercial inpatient portal. *International Journal of Medical Informatics* 110:10–18.

Young, R. A., S. K. Burge, K. A. Kumar, J. M. Wilson, and D. F. Ortiz. 2018. A time-motion study of primary care physicians' work in the electronic health record era. *Family Medicine* 50(2):91–99.

8

Primary Care Measures and Use: Powerful, Simple, Accountable

There will always be a need for primary care: a place where people can work together with a clinician or clinical team to advance their health and address the majority of their concerns in the context of a trusted relationship. Ensuring that the nation's primary care system can deliver this basic common good requires the ability to monitor quality and accountability. Two reports, *To Err Is Human* (IOM, 2000) and *Crossing the Quality Chasm* (IOM, 2001a), catalyzed a quality movement that led to developing quality metrics that have improved the performance of the U.S. health care system (IOM, 2015). However, these metrics tend to focus on individual components of health care, such as diabetes risk and control, cancer screening and prevention, and blood pressure monitoring and management, and are not well suited for measuring the quality of a primary care system that integrates multiple components of care.

This chapter calls attention to the need to align primary care measures with its definition and high-value functions to support the implementation of high-quality primary care. It does not set forth a standard set of superior measures for primary care. Such a set would need to be established through a coordinated process involving key stakeholders and a systematic review of current measures used with consideration both for a reduction in the number of measures employed and an addition of measures able to cover critical gaps in the scope of primary care assessment. This is beyond the scope of this report. Instead, this chapter provides important guidance to support that task.

Advancing meaningful quality assessment, performance standards, and accountability for primary care in the United States requires both *identification* and *implementation* of a parsimonious set of measures. In this chapter, the committee focuses on approaches to build and choose a parsimonious set of measures that are "fit for purpose" (Duffy and Irvine, 2004) in the U.S. primary care environment and that reduce administrative burdens and increase overall systemic value (MacLean et al., 2018). This chapter also highlights the need to change the process for assessing primary care performance and accountability using a simple core set of measures, similar to the strategy promoted in the *Vital Signs* report regarding how best to design a core set of population-based health measures (IOM, 2015). The committee first establishes a common understanding of key terms. Next, it discusses how the use to which measures are put also shapes their meaning and purpose. In explaining the challenges and tensions of primary care assessment, the committee outlines why current measures, though numerous, are insufficient, and even harmful, to what the nation needs primary care to do. The committee then provides pragmatic guidance to allow development of a more effective slate of primary care measures. The challenge is not necessarily creating new measures but rather measuring key functions of primary care whose value is well established by more than 50 years of research. The chapter concludes with a discussion of possible systems of accountability within the federal government.

The discussion builds on a shared understanding regarding the following key terms:

- **A measure**—*a unit or degree of something at a static point*. A measure is typically a unit of something larger and often cannot be understood without that larger context.
- **Quality**—*a standard created by comparing measures of similar things*. Quality is the degree to which something meets expectations, allowing for assessing comparative performance among groups/individuals.
- **Performance**—*how well a task is accomplished*. Measuring performance is about assessing how well something is done.
- **Value**—*what is thought to be beneficial*. It is a judgment based on shared agreement regarding social norms and expectations.
- **Accountability**—*a measure of how well actions are aligned with shared expectations*. Accountability measures a subset of activities for which a person or organization has responsibility. It assesses actions that, through shared agreement, align with expectations, values, and professional norms in ways that enable the wider scope of responsibility.

When applied to health care, the Institute of Medicine (IOM) defined quality, and therefore the expectations inherent to assessment, as "the degree to which health services for individuals and populations increase the likelihood of desired health outcomes and are consistent with current professional knowledge" (IOM, 1990, p. 4). The IOM further distilled these expectations with frameworks of quality measure domains for relevant to health care systems and consumers (IOM, 2001a,b) (see Box 8-1).

QUALITY, MEASURES, AND ACCOUNTABILITY IN PRIMARY CARE

The process of enabling high-quality primary care is governed by the combination of (1) measures aligned with purpose and value and (2) the use to which those measures are put. Combined, these form the *ecology of primary care measures*. A high-performing ecology of primary care measures facilitates patient care team relationships, integrated health care delivery, design of care teams as best fits health stewardship, and the ability of primary care to mitigate social inequities that may prevent optimal health attainment. This type of dynamic enables primary care settings to provide elements of high-quality care as identified in Box 8-1: safe, effective,

---

BOX 8-1
Domains for Assessing Quality

Health Care System–Based Quality Domains
1. Safety. Relates to actual or potential bodily harm.
2. Timeliness. Relates to obtaining needed care while minimizing delays.
3. Effectiveness. Relates to providing care processes and achieving outcomes as supported by scientific evidence.
4. Efficiency. Relates to maximizing the quality of a comparable unit of health care delivered or unit of health benefit achieved for a given unit of health care resources used.
5. Equity. Relates to providing health care of equal quality to those who may differ in personal characteristics other than their clinical condition or preferences for care.
6. Patient-centeredness. Relates to meeting patients' needs and preferences and providing education and support (IOM, 2001a).

Consumer-Based Quality Domains
1. Staying healthy. Getting help to avoid illness and remain well.
2. Getting better. Getting help to recover from an illness or injury.
3. Living with illness or disability. Getting help with managing an ongoing, chronic condition or dealing with a disability that affects function.
4. Coping with the end of life. Getting help to deal with a terminal illness (IOM, 2001b).

equitable, and both population focused and person centered. The current measures environment pollutes the ecology of primary care measures by overemphasizing external motivations, such as those created by payment systems or productivity requirements, disease-specific measures, and even measures that compete with one another, while underemphasizing patient expectations and known social drivers of health.

Creating an environment that can foster and sustain high-quality primary care requires that the measurement enterprise reorient itself to support primary care quality and accountability aligned with expectations, values, and professional norms as shared across stakeholders. Previous studies, such as *To Err Is Human* (IOM, 2000), *Crossing the Quality Chasm* (IOM, 2001a), and *Vital Signs* (IOM, 2015), focused on quality measures as instruments for corrective action. Those efforts were important and necessary to institute national corrections in overuse, underuse, and misuse of health services. However, they also had the unintended consequence of harming assessment of primary care function and value by focusing on disease-specific particulars—hundreds of them—rather than core, meaningful functions (Stange et al., 2014). Moreover, primary care quality improvement often entails checking boxes for external assessment and payment while trying to deliver good care that is not currently well measured. This is a recipe for burnout, as it pits professional motivation against financial reality and time pressures (Berenson, 2016; McWilliams, 2020; NASEM, 2019; Phillips, 2020; Phillips et al., 2019). Measures specific for primary care, however, can improve performance, support beneficial systems of accountability, and foster professional behaviors and fulfillment while reducing burnout.

Within a high-functioning ecology, measures that assess quality, measures that assess accountability, and measures that inform clinical decision making are best understood as distinct. Many primary care measures subsumed under current mandates for accountability are tangential to the purpose of primary care, such as those related to proof of service delivery or primarily used to differentiate practice settings. Such measures can be useful; however, some measures can do harm if they compete with or crowd out high-value functions. For example, creating a time window target for access to care may encourage behaviors to improve access that inadvertently discourage behaviors to maintain continuity, when both access *and* continuity are foundational to high-quality care (Campbell et al., 2009; Casalino and Khullar, 2019). Additionally, while many measures, informed by clinical guidelines, are critical to clinical decision making and good care, these can also compete with each other in people with multi-morbid conditions. Variations in these measures may be required for good care and would not necessarily indicate poor quality. For instance, the guidelines that suggest optimal blood pressure control for individuals with diabetes must often be adapted when that individual suffers more than one condition (as is common) or is over the age of 65, because optimal blood pressure control for that age is at odds with optimal blood pressure control for diabetes.

Assessing Quality

In primary care, quality is governed by the shared norms and expectations among patients, clinicians, care teams, and systems, as well as by *medical professionalism*, defined as "an active, ongoing, and iterative process that involves debate, advocacy, leadership, education, study, enforcement, and continuous transformation" (Byyny et al., 2017, p. 4; Phillips et al., 2019, p. 2). Quality assessment is most effective when aligned with professionalism and the agreed-upon principles and actions that guide professional behavior. Unfortunately, most of the hundreds of measures currently applied to primary care settings are based on confirmed diagnoses, disease-specific clinical decision making, and the ability to isolate and treat specific diseases, organs, or parts, without considering an individual's total health profile or the social milieu in which they live (Stange et al., 2014). One unintended result of this misalignment between the content of quality measures used and the clinical reality of primary care is that an approach to measure implementation by practices and systems often focuses on administrative behaviors, rather than shared norms of professional behaviors and expectations.

The challenge, then, is to unhitch primary care from a subspecialty model that uses measures derived from partial representations or pieces of patients and instead link it to measures appropriate for its generalist, whole-person approach to medicine. Such measures actually have a rich evidence base, and they better align with patients' perspectives on quality. Moreover, current metrics do not measure the ability of primary care clinicians to help people assess and understand ambiguous, sometimes undifferentiated symptoms that may or may not be a threat to their health but often reduce their well-being. Primary care provides this key diagnostic triage and anxiety-allaying function, which delivers great value to people seeking care but is often overlooked. Within primary care, this sorting, triage, and reassurance are framed by a clinical approach that differs from emergency room and subspecialist care. It involves *recognizing* the full range of health problems and/or opportunities present in any interaction, *prioritizing* which problems/opportunities should receive attention and action above others in order to promote health and healing, and *personalizing* the care plan or approach in ways informed by the person's social and environmental context. When this occurs in primary care, as opposed to emergency rooms or after multiple subspecialist visits, it creates value for both individuals and the health care system (Ellner and Phillips, 2017).

Measures

Measures are the means of conveying an assessment of quality. Whereas quality is the degree to which care meets expectations, measures are tools that highlight the behaviors or aspects of care that most contribute to those expectations. Measures used in primary care will only be effective if they align with what it aims for (its purpose) and what it does (its function). Meaningful measures best serve efforts to implement high-quality primary care when they connect to its purpose, function, and definition (see Chapter 2).

Meaningful primary care measures should support accountability, be flexible to patient need, and assess value at multiple levels. Such measures enable shared and commonly held expectations of primary care, such as the following (Green and the Starfield Writing Team, 2017):

- Primary care is a function, not a specific discipline, specialty, or service line. It is vital to all people of any age, background, and socioeconomic circumstance (Starfield et al., 2005).
- Primary care accomplishes its desirable results by creating a place for people to address a wide range of health problems. It helps people with most of their concerns, promotes health, guides people through health care systems, and facilitates ongoing relationships with clinicians in which people participate in decision making about their health and health care (Phillips and Bazemore, 2010a).
- Primary care reduces undesired variability in health care services while assuring desired variation to personalize and customize care in the context of family and community (IOM, 1996; Stange et al., 2014).
- Primary care clinicians partner with patients in ways that minimize fear, locate hope, translate symptoms and diagnoses, witness courage and endurance, and comfort suffering (Heath, 2016).
- The key elements of primary care do not operate independently. They exist in common as a whole and must be measured simultaneously (Bell et al., 2019; Etz et al., 2019).

Accountability

Accountability should be based on shared expectations of professionalism, quality, and performance. However, in the United States, accountability has come to be associated with financial rewards or penalties tied to outcomes. For example, the Quality Payment Program created by the Medicare Access and CHIP (Children's Health Insurance Program) Reauthorization

Act (MACRA)[1] scores clinicians on four measures—quality, cost, promoting interoperability, and improvement activities—and then modifies Medicare Part B payments based on those scores so that total payment adjustments are budget neutral (AAFP, 2020). Emerging evidence indicates that schemes such as this systematically disadvantage smaller practices and those that care for more disadvantaged patients (Colla et al., 2020).

Poorly designed measures and incentives place accountability at odds with the valuable functions of primary care. They corrupt quality and reduce it to target attainment above all else, regardless of shared expectations and professional behavior, which has the unintended consequence of confining professional responsibility and limiting professionalism (IOM, 2001a; Phillips et al., 2019). Rather than incentivizing physicians to work harder, value-based payment programs should support physician professionalism (Casalino and Khullar, 2019).

With each patient, primary care assumes professional responsibility for an integrated understanding of the fullness of an individual's experiences, through which they gain or lose health. This understanding and capacity to improve health comes from relationships over time. Narratives framed around proof of activity and proof of desired outcomes are counterproductive to therapeutic relationships and addressing patient priorities. Linking payment and accountability targets compounds these negative consequences by promoting behaviors aimed at meeting those targets rather than those actions that reflect professionalism and value (Gillam et al., 2012). Instead, meaningful accountability is based on the principles of professionalism and value that lead to quality and its associated outcomes, and these are measurable (Bovens and Schillemans, 2014; Kanter et al., 2013).

THE BENEFITS OF AN IMPROVED MEASUREMENT ECOSYSTEM

Several systemic weaknesses in U.S. measurement systems have resulted in the failed national assessment of primary care quality and performance and under-reported the benefits of primary care to populations and health systems. These include a lack of national agreement regarding which parsimonious set of measures should be applied to primary care and how to specify them (Cook et al., 2015; Phillips and Bazemore, 2010b), which often leads to inaccurate assessment of core primary care functions, unclear objectives to guide quality improvements initiatives, and a proliferation of measures (Berenson and Rich, 2010; O'Malley et al., 2015). The sheer number of measures creates a large administrative burden (IOM, 2015),

---

[1] Medicare Access and CHIP Reauthorization Act of 2015, Public Law 114-10 (April 16, 2015).

made worse by the number that are of questionable significance to clinicians (Mutter, 2019; Petterson et al., 2011; Raffoul et al., 2015). The result is poorly supported clinical decisions, minimal gains in person or population health, and competing time commitments for clinicians, who struggle to meet measure requirements while also providing the unmeasured work that helps patients. The environment in which measures are put to use is healthiest when measures are meaningful and purposeful.

The needed shift in thinking about quality measurement is to consider alignment between external and internal motivations and embracing both patient- and person-centeredness[2] in order to promote health equity.

Prevent Waste, Create a Unified Vision, and Divorce Measures from a Myopic Focus on External Motivations

Achieving value in health care requires a refinement of how quality is measured, starting with reduced inefficiencies and redundancies. Current measurement activities require health systems to devote an average of 50–100 full-time equivalent employees at a cost of $3.5 to $12 million per year (IOM, 2015). The Quality Payment Program in MACRA reflects federal investment in payment models and measures that shift the focus from volume of care to value (CMS, 2017) (see Chapter 9 for more on payment models). The move from volume to value holds great promise if aligned with purpose, given that systems emphasizing primary care purpose and function have lower per capita costs and better health outcomes (Starfield et al., 2005). However, the administrative burden related to the high number of misaligned and non-meaningful quality measures on which primary care is required to report undermines effective use of primary care resources (Casalino et al., 2016; Dean and Adashi, 2015). Primary care reports on dozens of measures from different sources that are not always in agreement. For example, the Centers for Medicare & Medicaid Services (CMS) inventory includes 70 measures, whereas the National Quality Forum (NQF) Quality Positioning System has 126 (CMS, 2020c; NQF, 2021). Additional research shows that primary care physicians spend an average of 3.9 hours per week on measurement reporting, at a national average cost of $40,000 per physician per year (Casalino et al., 2016). Reducing the measures used, beginning with those only tangentially related to the function and purpose, can represent a first important step in correcting the dysfunction of the current primary care measure use environment.

MACRA has created a federal mandate to assess and pay primary care practices based on quality outcomes, yet no national agreement exists

---

[2] As discussed in Chapter 4, the concept of person-centeredness takes into account the family and community contexts that affect a person's health and the need to learn about and address problems in these contexts.

regarding what outcomes best match with primary care quality (CMS, 2016). A unified vision within primary care will be critical to enabling a high-function measures use environment. In addition, attention to full scope primary care requires measures that extend beyond the scope of clinical processes and outcomes (Stange, 2002; Stange et al., 2014; Starfield, 2011b). For 15 years, primary care in the United Kingdom employed a unified vision for primary care measures. The Quality Outcomes Framework relied heavily on external motivations, and it specifically targeted predictable clinical outcomes associated with primary care. In 2017, the United Kingdom changed use of the Quality Outcomes Framework when it found that the framework caused physicians to focus on process activities unrelated to care quality to hit outcome targets. In addition, it failed to support functions that were not clinically defined, such as problem recognition (Starfield, 2009), relationship-based care (McDonald and Roland, 2009), and patient goal–oriented care (Campbell et al., 2009; Gillam et al., 2012).

Balance Patient-Centered Care with Person-Centered, Team-Based Care to Promote Health Equity

High-quality primary care cannot be supported by payment models that divorce accountability from shared agreement about primary care values and professional norms among stakeholders. Payment and systemic forms of accountability are important, but they too often reduce measures' function to target attainment, as achieved through the actions of a single clinician rather than a care team and as evidenced by outcomes assumed to result mainly from the actions of that person. This cuts out any reasonable focus on other non-physician care team leaders or important team members and contributes to structural obstacles that can prevent attention paid to the social drivers of health. Health and illness both result from a complex variety of factors, which is why primary care is deeply invested in both horizontal and vertical integration that helps individuals gain optimal health through a variety of interrelated strategies and partnerships between medical and social systems of support while guided by a clinician and care team best matched to individual needs and resources.

Primary care is not limited to diagnosing and treating illness, but as previous chapters have explained, it includes the full lifespan, individuals' long-term goals, and opportunities for health promotion, preventive care, and relief of suffering of both mind and body. Measurement of patient-centered care alone is insufficient to this mission. Assessment of primary care must include both patient- and person-centered measures (Starfield, 2011b), and embracing both types of measures requires balance (see Chapter 4 for more on person-centered primary care). Measures able to assess the personalizing function of primary care can enable adopting measures generated from disease-specific guidelines and combining them with the many other biological and biographical particulars of an individual, such as adapting suggested guidance for blood pressure control in a person with diabetes, over the age of 65, and with other comorbidities.

High-quality primary care includes the ability of the clinician and/or care team to prioritize individuals' needs by combining expertise based on their experiential, social, and scientific profile and navigating a series of competing needs and demands as best fits the whole person. It recognizes those persons' accumulated knowledge and understands person-based needs as nested within population-based needs. The same high-quality care, delivered in the same relational and purpose-driven way, may result in different timelines for health goal attainment or clinical improvement based on many factors, such as a lack of trust in the health care system, challenges in health literacy, or social inequities, such as limited access to healthy foods, insecure housing, or limited access to education. Measurement systems based solely on patient-centered rather than person-centered care fail to account for such things.

Rather than allow measurement to be dominated by diseases, organs, life expectancies, and what is easily counted, there should be a balance between the easily counted and measures that also reflect how individuals live, their experiences in life, and what they find valuable about primary care. This can be accomplished by adopting meaningful primary care measures, aligned with primary care purpose and function, and making greater use of patient-reported assessments of care.

GUIDANCE FOR SELECTING PRIMARY CARE MEASURES

Primary care measures enable clinicians and care teams to achieve the purpose of primary care by providing actionable markers for improvement of the relationship with the patient and the coordination of care beyond episodic interactions. A reasonable goal for primary care measures is that all stakeholders can easily understand what good care is and how it is effectively assessed. The need for quality and performance assessment will also need to be balanced with the purpose, burden, and use environment for the information or measures collected. A national Starfield Summit of 70 national and international experts in primary care that included patients, insurers, employers, and clinicians of all primary care disciplines established that superior primary care measures are ones that (Etz and the Starfield Writing Team, 2017):

1. Are meaningful—to patients, families, health systems, policy makers, and clinicians;

2. Assess primary care as defined, practiced, experienced, and co-created between patients, clinicians, and teams;
3. Assess the intended outcomes of primary care (e.g., achievement of health and health goals, illness prevention and health promotion, healing, avoidance of unnecessary pain and suffering, and equity);
4. Balance the tensions endemic to primary health care: standardization alongside customization, predictability alongside ambiguity;
5. Are flexible—adaptive to setting (from the individual to national levels), lifespan (infant to elderly), health state (changing health status), and individual differences (context, family, and preferences);
6. Provide evaluation and improvement information actionable at the local, regional, and national levels;
7. Support self-assessment, self-learning, and aspiration;
8. Are feasible, reliable, and without undo data collection burden;
9. Point out and establish the importance of things that cannot yet be counted;
10. Inform evaluation of a broad vision that understands health and illness exist within a social and cultural framework; and
11. Reflect the complexity of the discipline—the whole is more than an additive sum of parts. Embrace interconnectivity, reject reduction to cause and effect of individual elements, assess and support emergence—where just adding up what happens to parts (diseases, individuals) does not equal the whole (people, populations).

Achieving parsimony is one goal of effective and efficient measurement of primary care, because a core set of measures increases focus, reduces burden, and is an opportunity to increase alignment across payers, patients, health systems, and clinicians. Current low-value care measures do little to advance high-quality primary care, even while they may be appropriate in other settings (Barreto et al., 2019). It is more likely that research on known core aspects of primary care, including care coordination, comprehensiveness, relationships, and trust, and how they interrelate with each other and with health outcomes, may explain more about reducing low-value downstream costs associated with hospitalizations and subspecialty services.

The American Board of Internal Medicine Foundation has a renewed focus on trust as a measure (Lynch, 2020), which has been used in the past; research has shown it to be significantly associated with patient satisfaction, though it is not clear how it is related to other outcomes (Safran et al., 1998). Trust may also be a function of continuity and comprehensiveness or be best captured by self-reported outcomes. Investigators have developed several tools to assess team-based care, but a systematic review concluded that setting-specific team effectiveness measurement tools need further development (Kash et al., 2018).

Equity is increasingly important as an outcome goal for all of health care, and yet a ready-for-use measure of equity in primary care does not yet exist. Equally important, primary care lacks evidence regarding how the critical functions of prioritizing, integrating, and personalizing care work to inform better outcomes (Stange et al., 2014). Such evidence is required to create meaningful primary care measures that are able to support high-quality care and advance the knowledge base in primary care–related professions.

Pediatrics, as a subspecialty of primary care, has had a shortage of appropriate measures. The Children's Health Insurance Program Reauthorization Act of 2009 (CHIPRA) accelerated interest in pediatric quality measurement and created the opportunity to improve the quality of health care delivered to the nation's children, including the almost 40 million enrolled in Medicaid or CHIP (CMS, 2020c; NQF, 2017). When CHIPRA was enacted, the Agency for Healthcare Research and Quality (AHRQ) and CMS began working together to implement selected provisions of the related legislation, and NQF launched its Pediatric Measures project in 2015 to evaluate the measures that AHRQ and CMS develop.

COVID-19, Health Equity, and Measures

The COVID-19 pandemic has provided an unprecedented opportunity to reevaluate the capabilities of the nation's medical and public health systems and the means by which the quality of care delivery is assessed. The weaknesses of a health care system designed primarily as a reactive and financially driven enterprise are clear. As communities reel with overcrowded inpatient and intensive care unit beds, inadequate testing infrastructure, and increasing mortality, the reality of the inequities that leave the most disadvantaged and underserved communities, especially Black, Indigenous, and Hispanic groups, at high risk for exposure, infection, and death raises sincere questions about a reactionary health system's ability to provide equitable care. Race and racism are social drivers of health (Gee and Ford, 2011; NASEM, 2017; Walker et al., 2016), and despite evidence of their impact on medical decision making and patient outcomes (Dovidio and Fiske, 2012; van Ryn et al., 2011), there are currently no measures tailored to achieve the desired outcome—removing bias and eradicating health disparities based on race, ethnicity, and other socially defined markers of inequity.

During the pandemic, many insurers and health systems temporarily suspended the need to systematically report current primary care quality measures (CMS, 2020b). The shifts in care delivery required to meet the unique, pandemic-related challenges exposed both the amount of time current measures require and the disconnect between those measures and care quality. In addition to being disease centric, most measures focus on in-office, predictable, and algorithmic work processes and commonly known intermediate health outcomes, as surrogates for care quality. These methods were not adequate to capture care delivery and quality during the pandemic. Improvement might require a change in emphasis from interventions developed to achieve improvements on a specific measure to those intended to support the elements of high-quality care and evaluated using a core set of high-value measures. This would represent a paradigm shift from seeking successful measures to seeking measurable success (McWilliams, 2020).

IMPLEMENTATION NEEDS

The U.S. health care system needs quality measures adequate to the task of assessing, valuing, and fostering continuous improvement within the fields of primary care (Appleby et al., 2016; Epstein and Street, 2011; IOM, 2001a; O'Malley et al., 2015; Stange, 2002, 2010). The shift in national conversations from "volume to value" (HHS, 2015; Saver et al., 2015) within health services delivery has gained significant traction, as signaled by two publications: *Vital Signs: Core Measures for Health and Healthcare Progress* (IOM, 2015) and MACRA (CMS, 2016). *Vital Signs* outlined the cost and waste associated with current performance measurement systems, and it set the tone for future work by recommending a relatively small, parsimonious set of measures able to assess U.S. population health. The authors of *Vital Signs* advised that key stakeholders at every level, rather than the usual content "experts," must be central to any effort focused on generating meaningful health care measures. This is true now more than ever. The shift from volume to value relies on the ability to recognize and assess value through performance measurement. MACRA legislation makes this point and recognizes that current quality measures, particularly those for primary health care, are not up to the task. The central messages of *Vital Signs*, MACRA, and primary care leadership are aligned: quality measures are necessary to achieve national health objectives, yet current measurement systems are costly and provide limited return.

Policy makers and health care leaders have called for reducing the number of quality measures applied to primary health care (Berwick, 2016; Casalino et al., 2016; IOM, 2015; O'Malley et al., 2015). Hundreds of measures are in use (Conway, 2015), and yet most of these are not aligned with its purpose or function, for either adult or pediatric populations (CMS, 2020a; Rich and O'Malley, 2015). The work of NQF helps to reduce the number of measures most often applied, yet that number still remains in the hundreds (Conway, 2015; Dunlap et al., 2016; Roski and McClellan, 2011). Reducing it will decrease the administrative burden associated with measurement reporting. However, with a focus on adapting current measures rather than redesigning them, these efforts fail to address the challenges endemic to the current system (Meltzer and Chung, 2014; O'Malley et al., 2015; Rollow and Cucchiara, 2016; Stange, 2002; Stange et al., 2014), including the following:

- a myopic focus on disease-specific clinical processes and outcomes (Campbell et al., 2009; McDonald and Roland, 2009; Stange, 2002; Starfield, 2011b);
- measures reactive to the needs of policy and payment rather than proactively informed by health and healing (Epstein et al., 2010; O'Malley and Rich, 2015; Reuben and Tinetti, 2012);
- misrepresentation and under-representation of primary health care's contributions (Baicker and Chandra, 2004; Epstein et al., 2010);
- a disconnect between health outcomes important to care-seekers and those items being measured (Epstein and Street, 2011; Stange, 2013; Starfield, 2011b); and
- the absence of a unified vision regarding what should be measured and why (Mold et al., 1991; O'Malley and Rich, 2015; O'Malley et al., 2015; Stange et al., 2014; Starfield, 1979).

Evidence shows that the United States lacks a quality measurement system able to assess key aspects of primary care, such as problem recognition (Starfield, 2009), patient-centered care (Etz et al., 2019), patient-reported outcomes (Mold et al., 1991; Weiner et al., 2010), or healing relationships (Epstein et al., 2010). The measurement atlases compiled by AHRQ and the core set of quality measures recently proposed by CMS and America's Health Insurance Plans are important steps (Conway, 2015), yet strategies that rely on revising and centralizing current measures fail to address the gap between the work of primary care, as defined in this report, and the ways in which that work is assessed (Appleby et al., 2016; O'Malley et al., 2015; Rollow and Cucchiara, 2016; Starfield, 2011a).

ACCOUNTABILITY

As this report argues, relying on market mechanisms to shore up the glaring shortcomings of policy and payment design will not produce the high-quality primary care system required to improve population health and slow the rise of health care spending. Rebalancing a system that is off kilter will require seeing primary care as a common good, worthy of societal investment, and being a state and federal policy priority. The investments and actions needed are of sufficient magnitude as to require mechanisms that will ensure that policy and fiscal allocations are coordinated throughout the various layers of government and the private sector. The nation may have failed to adopt the recommendations in *Primary Care: America's Health in a New Era* because no entity was accountable for implementing them (IOM, 1996). That report did call for creating a public–private consortium to lead the implementation, but the report lacked detail on which actor(s) would organize or participate in the proposed consortium. With no one organization or agency tasked explicitly to do so, key stakeholders looked to each other, and ultimately no one entity stepped up to lead the work.

This committee is charged specifically with creating an implementation plan that builds on the 1996 recommendations (see Chapter 12 for the plan). It agrees with the 1996 study committee that an accountability mechanism is needed, and it offers more specifics and a clearer path to create that mechanism. Critically, a responsible and clearly identified entity is needed to oversee accountability for policy goals, coordinate disparate research and policy efforts, establish a standard and parsimonious set of measures, synchronize training and workforce initiatives, and align efforts for payment reform. Private-sector stakeholders are disparate and have demonstrated that they largely cannot overcome competitive self-interest and fiduciary duty to investors or stakeholders to come together effectively on their own. As a result, this committee believes that the primary account-ability mechanism must ultimately rest within a federal government entity, as it does for other areas of health sector activity.

Currently, the federal government plays an active, albeit uncoordinated, role in primary care. For example, through CMS, the federal government directly pays for close to 40 percent of all health care and influences com-mercial payers (CMS, 2018) (see Chapter 9 for more detail). It also can convene private-sector payers with appropriate safe harbors and hold them accountable to major new policy initiatives (Peikes, 2019). While this mandate is regionally effective, states alone cannot carry it out, and other market actors, such as clinician groups, can participate but are not in posi-tion to advance the whole of the necessary work.

Given the rationale for a central federal entity to advance the work of aligning existing primary care activities and implementing primary care pol-icy and workforce recommendations, it is then important to consider which entity or entities within the federal government might be able to carry out these tasks in a coordinated manner. CMS is the major payer in the United States, but its purview is technically limited to the over age 65 and disabled population, individuals with end-stage renal disease or amyotrophic lateral sclerosis, and state Medicaid programs. These are important large groups, but they leave many areas uncovered. The Health Resources and Services Administration (HRSA) is responsible for improving health care among geographically isolated or economically or medically vulnerable people. However, it does not generally focus on the insured or providing primary care for populations not defined as vulnerable or underserved. AHRQ works to improve the quality of care in the United States through research and implementation grants, and it has a National Center for Excellence in Primary Care Research (NCEPCR) that notably remains unfunded (AHRQ, 2019). AHRQ does not generally coordinate policy and has historically been under fiscal threat of defunding at the agency level (McCann, 2012; Sheber, 2018). In fact, the 2021 President's Budget proposed to consolidate AHRQ into the National Institutes of Health (NIH) (AHRQ, 2020; Bindman, 2017). No clear private-sector entities are available to coordinate necessary public–private policy research, workforce, and payment alignment.

Several possible entities could contribute to or lead the implementation of this committee's recommendations. The first option could be for HRSA's Bureau of Primary Health Care (BPHC) to lead on the workforce-related recommendations. Currently, BPHC has oversight of safety net systems and shortage areas through its Health Center Program that serves only approximately 8 percent of people in the United States (NACHC, 2020). Moreover, despite its name, its purview is not limited to primary care. Expanding its remit beyond its current form requires an act of Congress, and it does not have capacity or ownership over a broad research program, nor has it coordinated workforce or quality efforts outside of safety net systems and federally qualified health centers. If strengthened and broadened, it could coordinate key workforce priorities and align with other entities below to carry out these recommendations. This would still leave payment policy out of its reach since this responsibility sits within CMS.

A second option would be to fund the AHRQ NCEPCR to implement the research-related recommendations in this report. It is currently directed to lead research on primary care but has never received direct funding for it. It is also required to align what research it supports with a definition of primary care that is not consistent with this report. NCEPCR could coordinate practice-related primary care research (PCR) and basic science and expand the field of inquiry and implementation. However, if funded, it would still be separate from NIH-related PCR that would either need to be aligned, at minimum, or perhaps encompassed partly within this AHRQ research center. It is unlikely that NCEPCR could have purview outside of research, given AHRQ's limited scope and chronic funding and authorization challenges. Nonetheless, it is an established entity with a mandate for PCR that could accomplish much more, if fully funded, than it currently does (see Chapter 9 for more on PCR).

These options, while not mutually exclusive, do little to coordinate primary care activities across the government and would require congressional action. Another, and likely the most effective, option to coordinate primary care activities across government and centrally hold the different actors accountable for implementing changes would be to establish a Secretary's council on primary care within the U.S. Department of Health and Human Services (HHS) that would expressly be charged with carrying out the recommendations in this report through interagency coordination. One advantage to this option would be that it could be established relatively quickly, coordinate and hold the individual agencies accountable, oversee the implementation of the recommendations, and fill gaps as they arise. Creating such a council would not need legislative approval and likely not entail a major outlay of resources. To help guide its work and ensure that diverse stakeholder voices and interests are included, the council could further be informed by regular guidance and recommendations from an advisory committee, established under the Federal Advisory Committee Act,[3] with membership from national organizations that represent significant primary care stakeholder groups, such as patients, certifying boards, professional organizations, health care worker organizations, payers, and employers. The committee recognizes that establishing this council (and advisory committee) would require political capital and buy-in at high levels of federal government policy making. However, the scale of the task ahead to implement high-quality primary care would likely require this level of commitment to investing in primary care to see it through to success.

FINDINGS AND CONCLUSIONS

Current measures applied to primary care are not aligned with its purpose and function and therefore fail to adequately assess its quality and accountability. Effective primary care measurement relies on appropriate design of the use environment and should align both external and internal motivations of actors. It should do so in ways that embrace both patient- and person-centeredness in order to promote health equity.

Primary care also currently suffers from a dual challenge of having too many measures (many of questionable benefit) and an absence of measures fit to the purpose of assessing primary care's value, added benefit, and functions. The number of measures that exists should be reduced and new measures created that appropriately support primary care.

No single entity is yet working to ensure that the field of primary care writ large is held to account for its performance. The private sector has demonstrated that it cannot effectively assume this role. No single agency or function is equipped to coordinate the various activities related to primary care across government, and existing agencies are not equipped, in their current form, to take on this role. Such an entity could ensure that

---

[3] Federal Advisory Committee Act, Public Law 92-463 (October 6, 1972).

the various government primary care activities are coordinated and held to account. It could also coordinate the implementation of this report's recommendations attributable to government and increase the chances of implementation of recommendations by private-sector actors. To be effective, such an entity should have adequate authority and influence to be an effective agent for change.

REFERENCES

AAFP (American Academy of Family Physicians). 2020. *Merit-based incentive payment system (MIPS)*. https://www.aafp.org/family-physician/practice-and-career/getting-paid/mips. html (accessed November 3, 2020).

AHRQ (Agency for Healthcare Research and Quality). 2019. *Operating plan for FY 2020*. Washington, DC: U.S. Department of Health and Human Services.

AHRQ. 2020. *Budget estimates for appropriations committees, fiscal year 2021*. https://www. ahrq.gov/cpi/about/mission/budget/2021/index.html (accessed November 5, 2020).

Appleby, J., V. Raleigh, F. Frosini, G. Bevan, H. Gao, and T. Lyscom. 2016. *Variations in health care: The good, the bad, and the inexplicable*. London: The King's Fund.

Baicker, K., and A. Chandra. 2004. Medicare spending, the physician workforce, and beneficiaries' quality of care. *Health Affairs* 23(Suppl 1):W184–W197.

Barreto, T. W., Y. Chung, P. Wingrove, R. A. Young, S. Petterson, A. Bazemore, and W. Liaw. 2019. Primary care physician characteristics associated with low value care spending. *Journal of the American Board of Family Practice* 32(2):218–225.

Bell, N. R., G. Thériault, H. Singh, and R. Grad. 2019. Measuring what really matters: Screening in primary care. *Canadian Family Physician* 65(11):790–795.

Berenson, R. A. 2016. If you can't measure performance, can you improve it? *JAMA* 315(7):645–646.

Berenson, R. A., and E. C. Rich. 2010. U.S. approaches to physician payment: The deconstruction of primary care. *Journal of General Internal Medicine* 25(6):613–618.

Berwick, D. M. 2016. Era 3 for medicine and health care. *JAMA* 315(13):1329–1330.

Bindman, A. 2017. Moving AHRQ into the NIH: New beginning or beginning of the end? *Health Affairs Blog* (November 6). https://www.healthaffairs.org/do/10.1377/ hblog20170327.059384/full (accessed March 27, 2020).

Bovens, M., and T. Schillemans. 2014. Meaningful accountability. In *The Oxford handbook of public accountability*, edited by M. Bovens, R. E. Goodin, and T. Schillemans. Oxford, UK: Oxford University Press. Pp. 673–682.

Byyny, R. L., M. A. Papadakis, D. S. Paauw, and S. A. Pfeil. 2017. *Medical professionalism best practices: Professionalism in the modern era*. Aurora, CO: Alpha Omega Alpha Honor Medical Society.

Campbell, S. M., D. Reeves, E. Kontopantelis, B. Sibbald, and M. Roland. 2009. Effects of pay for performance on the quality of primary care in England. *New England Journal of Medicine* 361(4):368–378.

Casalino, L. P., and D. Khullar. 2019. Value-based purchasing and physician professionalism. *JAMA* 322(17):1647–1648.

Casalino, L. P., D. Gans, R. Weber, M. Cea, A. Tuchovsky, T. F. Bishop, Y. Miranda, B. A. Frankel, K. B. Ziehler, M. M. Wong, and T. B. Evenson. 2016. U.S. physician practices spend more than $15.4 billion annually to report quality measures. *Health Affairs* 35(3):401–406.

CMS (Centers for Medicare & Medicaid Services). 2016. *CMS quality measure development plan: Supporting the transition to the merit-based incentive payment system (MIPS) and alternative payment models (APMs).* Baltimore, MD: Centers for Medicare & Medicaid Services.

CMS. 2017. *CMS quality measure development plan: Supporting the transition to the quality payment program 2017 annual report.* Baltimore, MD: Centers for Medicare & Medicaid Services.

CMS. 2018. *NHE fact sheet.* https://www.cms.gov/Research-Statistics-Data-and-Systems/Statistics-Trends-and-Reports/NationalHealthExpendData/NHE-Fact-Sheet (accessed July 20, 2020).

CMS. 2020a. *Children's health care quality measures.* https://www.medicaid.gov/medicaid/quality-of-care/performance-measurement/adult-and-child-health-care-quality-measures/childrens-health-care-quality-measures/index.html (accessed November 4, 2020).

CMS. 2020b. *Exceptions and extensions for quality reporting requirements for acute care hospitals, PPS-exempt cancer hospitals, inpatient psychiatric facilities, skilled nursing facilities, home health agencies, hospices, inpatient rehabilitation facilities, long-term care hospitals, ambulatory surgical centers, renal dialysis facilities, and MIPS eligible clinicians affected by COVID-19.* Baltimore, MD: Centers for Medicare & Medicaid Services.

CMS. 2020c. *Measures inventory tool.* https://cmit.cms.gov/CMIT_public/ListMeasures (accessed January 15, 2021).

Colla, C. H., T. Ajayi, and A. Bitton. 2020. Potential adverse financial implications of the merit-based incentive payment system for independent and safety net practices. *JAMA* 324(10):948–950.

Conway, P. H. 2015. The core quality measures collaborative: A rationale and framework for public–private quality measure alignment. *Health Affairs Blog* (June 23). https://www.healthaffairs.org/do/10.1377/hblog20150623.048730/full (accessed December 7, 2020).

Cook, D. A., E. S. Holmboe, K. J. Sorensen, R. A. Berger, and J. M. Wilkinson. 2015. Getting maintenance of certification to work: A grounded theory study of physicians' perceptions. *JAMA Internal Medicine* 175(1):35–42.

Dean, L. A., and E. Y. Adashi. 2015. Repealed and replaced: SGR gives way to value-based Medicare payment reform. *American Journal of Medicine* 128(10):1052–1053.

Dovidio, J. F., and S. T. Fiske. 2012. Under the radar: How unexamined biases in decision-making processes in clinical interactions can contribute to health care disparities. *American Journal of Public Health* 102(5):945–952.

Duffy, J. A., and E. A. Irvine. 2004. Clinical governance: The role of measures. *Quality in Primary Care* 12:283–288.

Dunlap, N. E., D. J. Ballard, R. A. Cherry, W. C. Dunagan, W. Ferniany, A. C. Hamilton, T. A. Owens, T. Rusconi, S. M. Safyer, P. J. Santrach, A. Sears, M. R. Waldrum, and K. E. Walsh. 2016. *Observations from the field: Reporting quality metrics in health care.* NAM Perspectives. Discussion Paper, National Academy of Medicine, Washington, DC.

Ellner, A. L., and R. S. Phillips. 2017. The coming primary care revolution. *Journal of General Internal Medicine* 32(4):380–386.

Epstein, R. M., and R. L. Street, Jr. 2011. The values and value of patient-centered care. *Annals of Family Medicine* 9(2):100–103.

Epstein, R. M., K. Fiscella, C. S. Lesser, and K. C. Stange. 2010. Why the nation needs a policy push on patient-centered health care. *Health Affairs* 29(8):1489–1495.

Etz, R. S., and the Starfield Writing Team. 2017. *Guidance for developing primary care measures.* Washington, DC: Starfield Summit III.

Etz, R. S., S. J. Zyzanski, M. M. Gonzalez, S. R. Reves, J. P. O'Neal, and K. C. Stange. 2019. A new comprehensive measure of high-value aspects of primary care. *Annals of Family Medicine* 17(3):221–230.

Gee, G. C., and C. L. Ford. 2011. Structural racism and health inequities: Old issues, new directions. *Du Bois Review* 8(1):115–132.

Gillam, S. J., A. N. Siriwardena, and N. Steel. 2012. Pay-for-performance in the United Kingdom: Impact of the quality and outcomes framework: A systematic review. *Annals of Family Medicine* 10(5):461–468.

Green, L., and the Starfield Writing Team. 2017. *What matters in primary care: Back to basics.* https://static1.squarespace.com/static/5d7ff8184cf0e01e4566cb02/t/5f326bb0bec49413e0af1 0da/1597139889272/SIII+Brief-+What+Matters+in+Primary+Care.pdf (accessed November 19, 2020).

Heath, I. 2016. How medicine has exploited rationality at the expense of humanity: An essay by Iona Heath. *BMJ* 355:i5705.

HHS (U.S. Department of Health and Human Services). 2015. *Better, smarter, healthier: In historic announcement, HHS sets clear goals and timeline for shifting Medicare reimbursements from volume to value.* Washington, DC: U.S. Department of Health and Human Services.

IOM (Institute of Medicine). 1990. *Medicare: A strategy for quality assurance, Volume I.* Washington, DC: National Academy Press.

IOM. 1996. *Primary care: America's health in a new era.* Washington, DC: National Academy Press.

IOM. 2000. *To err is human: Building a safer health system.* Washington, DC: National Academy Press.

IOM. 2001a. *Crossing the quality chasm: A new health system for the 21st century.* Washington, DC: National Academy Press.

IOM. 2001b. *Envisioning the national health care quality report.* Washington, DC: National Academy Press.

IOM. 2015. *Vital signs: Core metrics for health and health care progress.* Washington, DC: The National Academies Press.

Kanter, M. H., M. Nguyen, M. H. Klau, N. H. Spiegel, and V. L. Ambrosini. 2013. What does professionalism mean to the physician? *The Permanente Journal* 17(3):87–90.

Kash, B. A., O. Cheon, N. M. Halzack, and T. R. Miller. 2018. Measuring team effectiveness in the health care setting: An inventory of survey tools. *Health Services Insights* 11:1178632918796230.

Lynch, T. 2020. *Building trust and health equity during COVID-19: Background paper.* Philadelphia, PA: American Board of Internal Medicine Foundation.

MacLean, C. H., E. A. Kerr, and A. Qaseem. 2018. Time out—charting a path for improving performance measurement. *New England Journal of Medicine* 378(19):1757–1761.

McCann, E. 2012. AHRQ funding eliminated in house subcommittee vote. *Healthcare Finance* (July 19). https://www.healthcarefinancenews.com/news/ahrq-funding-eliminated-house-subcommittee-vote (accessed December 10, 2020).

McDonald, R., and M. Roland. 2009. Pay for performance in primary care in England and California: Comparison of unintended consequences. *Annals of Family Medicine* 7(2):121–127.

McWilliams, J. M. 2020. Professionalism revealed: Rethinking quality improvement in the wake of a pandemic. *NEJM Catalyst* 1(5).

Meltzer, D. O., and J. W. Chung. 2014. The population value of quality indicator reporting: A framework for prioritizing health care performance measures. *Health Affairs* 33(1):132–139.

Mold, J. W., G. H. Blake, and L. A. Becker. 1991. Goal-oriented medical care. *Family Medicine* 23(1):46–51.

Mutter, J. B. 2019. A new stranger at the bedside: Industrial quality management and the erosion of clinical judgment in American medicine. *Social Research: An International Quarterly* 86(4):931–954.

NACHC (National Association of Community Health Centers). 2020. *Community health center chartbook*. Bethesda, MD: National Association of Community Health Centers.

NASEM (National Academies of Sciences, Engineering, and Medicine). 2017. *Communities in action: Pathways to health equity*. Washington, DC: The National Academies Press.

NASEM. 2019. *Taking action against clinician burnout: A systems approach to professional well-being*. Washington, DC: The National Academies Press.

NQF (National Quality Forum). 2017. *Pediatric performance measures 2017: Final technical report*. Washington, DC: National Quality Forum.

NQF. 2021. *Primary care measures (generated interactively via the Quality Positioning System tool)*. https://www.qualityforum.org/QPS/QPSTool.aspx (accessed January 15, 2021).

O'Malley, A. S., and E. C. Rich. 2015. Measuring comprehensiveness of primary care: Challenges and opportunities. *Journal of General Internal Medicine* 30(Suppl 3):S568–S575.

O'Malley, A. S., E. C. Rich, A. Maccarone, C. M. DesRoches, and R. J. Reid. 2015. Disentangling the linkage of primary care features to patient outcomes: A review of current literature, data sources, and measurement needs. *Journal of General Internal Medicine* 30(Suppl 3):S576–S585.

Peikes, D. 2019. *Independent evaluation of Comprehensive Primary Care Plus (CPC+): First annual report*. Princeton, NJ: Mathematica Policy Research.

Petterson, S., A. W. Bazemore, R. L. Phillips, I. M. Xierali, J. Rinaldo, L. A. Green, and J. C. Puffer. 2011. Rewarding family medicine while penalizing comprehensiveness? Primary care payment incentives and health reform: The Patient Protection and Affordable Care Act (PPACA). *Journal of the American Board of Family Practice* 24(6):637–638.

Phillips, R. L., Jr. 2020. The built environment for professionalism. *Journal of the American Board of Family Medicine* 33(Suppl):S57–S61.

Phillips, R. L., Jr., and A. Bazemore. 2010a. The nature of primary care. In *Who will provide primary care and how will they be trained?* edited by L. Cronenwett and V. Dzau. Durham, NC: Josiah Macy, Jr. Foundation. Pp. 43–57.

Phillips, R. L., Jr., and A. W. Bazemore. 2010b. Primary care and why it matters for U.S. health system reform. *Health Affairs* 29(5):806–810.

Phillips, R. L., Jr., A. Bazemore, and W. P. Newton. 2019. Medical professionalism: A contract with society. *The Pharos* Autumn:2–7.

Raffoul, M., S. Petterson, M. Moore, A. Bazemore, and L. Peterson. 2015. Smaller practices are less likely to report PCMH certification. *American Family Physician* 91(7):440.

Reuben, D. B., and M. E. Tinetti. 2012. Goal-oriented patient care—an alternative health outcomes paradigm. *New England Journal of Medicine* 366(9):777–779.

Rich, E., and A. O'Malley. 2015. Measuring what matters in primary care. *Health Affairs Blog* (October 6). https://www.healthaffairs.org/do/10.1377/hblog20151006.051032/full (accessed December 18, 2020).

Rollow, W., and P. Cucchiara. 2016. Achieving value in primary care: The primary care value model. *Annals of Family Medicine* 14(2):159–165.

Roski, J., and M. McClellan. 2011. Measuring health care performance now, not tomorrow: Essential steps to support effective health reform. *Health Affairs* 30(4):682–689.

Safran, D. G., D. A. Taira, W. H. Rogers, M. Kosinski, J. E. Ware, and A. R. Tarlov. 1998. Linking primary care performance to outcomes of care. *Journal of Family Practice* 47(3):213–220.

Saver, B. G., S. A. Martin, R. N. Adler, L. M. Candib, K. E. Deligiannidis, J. Golding, D. J. Mullin, M. Roberts, and S. Topolski. 2015. Care that matters: Quality measurement and health care. *PLOS Medicine* 12(11):e1001902.

Sheber, S. 2018. Trump's proposed budget seeks to eliminate AHRQ, slash OCR and ONC funding. *Journal of AHIMA* (February 16). https://journal.ahima.org/trumps-proposed-budget-seeks-to-eliminate-ahrq-slash-ocr-and-onc-funding (accessed December 10, 2020).

Stange, K. C. 2002. The paradox of the parts and the whole in understanding and improving general practice. *International Journal for Quality in Health Care* 14(4):267–268.

Stange, K. C. 2010. Ways of knowing, learning, and developing. *Annals of Family Medicine* 8(1):4–10.

Stange, K. C. 2013. In this issue: Mindfulness in practice and policy. *Annals of Family Medicine* 11(5):398–399.

Stange, K. C., R. S. Etz, H. Gullett, S. A. Sweeney, W. L. Miller, C. R. Jaen, B. F. Crabtree, P. A. Nutting, and R. E. Glasgow. 2014. Metrics for assessing improvements in primary health care. *Annual Review of Public Health* 35:423–442.

Starfield, B. 1979. Measuring the attainment of primary care. *Journal of Medical Education* 54(5):361–369.

Starfield, B. 2009. Primary care and equity in health: The importance to effectiveness and equity of responsiveness to peoples' needs. *Humanity & Society* 33(1–2):56–73.

Starfield, B. 2011a. The hidden inequity in health care. *International Journal for Equity in Health* 10(1):15.

Starfield, B. 2011b. Is patient-centered care the same as person-focused care? *The Permanente Journal* 15:63–69.

Starfield, B., L. Shi, and J. Macinko. 2005. Contribution of primary care to health systems and health. *Milbank Quarterly* 83(3):457–502.

van Ryn, M., D. J. Burgess, J. F. Dovidio, S. M. Phelan, S. Saha, J. Malat, J. M. Griffin, S. S. Fu, and S. Perry. 2011. The impact of racism on clinician cognition, behavior, and clinical decision making. *Du Bois Review* 8(1):199–218.

Walker, R. J., J. Strom Williams, and L. E. Egede. 2016. Influence of race, ethnicity and social determinants of health on diabetes outcomes. *The American Journal of the Medical Sciences* 351(4):366–373.

Weiner, S. J., A. Schwartz, F. Weaver, J. Goldberg, R. Yudkowsky, G. Sharma, A. Binns-Calvey, B. Preyss, M. M. Schapira, S. D. Persell, E. Jacobs, and R. I. Abrams. 2010. Contextual errors and failures in individualizing patient care: A multicenter study. *Annals of Internal Medicine* 153(2):69–75.

9

Payment to Support High-Quality Primary Care

The committee supports a low-burden payment model that enables sustainable, team- and relationship-based, high-quality, integrated primary care; allows all people to have ready access to primary care teams across modalities; and assists people in addressing social determinants of health (SDOH). Payment should be adequate to support high-quality, independent primary care practices and flexible enough to support an emerging array of new delivery models. Payment reform should not, however, be a mechanism for reducing U.S. health care costs significantly in the short term but rather represent an investment for improving the health of the population.

WHY MONEY MATTERS

A fundamental assumption in the vision above is that money matters for achieving policy priorities. Payment models create the fiscal space in which care delivery can either flourish or be constrained. Vision statements, research evidence, leadership, and well-intentioned policy will not change the structure and performance of a system if they are not supported by adequate, goal-aligned resources. While a broad range of personal and social values motivate maintaining health and providing health care, an element of health care is transactional, with payment rendered for services provided. During the committee's information-gathering activities, patients underscored the difficulty and burdensome nature of navigating the health system and payment for services, highlighting that the fragmented and fee-for-service (FFS) U.S. payment system has observable effects on patient care and outcomes. How much payment is rendered and how significantly affect the volume and nature of primary care services available to a population (Quinn, 2015).

Primary care clinicians work in many organizational contexts, as discussed throughout this report. This chapter briefly touches upon income but does not focus on how clinicians are compensated within their organization or how funds flow from payers through organizations to clinicians; rather, it addresses how their organizations are paid by governments, insurers, and people seeking care. Although compensation plays an important role in individual behavior, the extent and methods of payment from third parties to the organization have more fundamental effects on the extent and nature of primary care in the United States, the focus of the committee's work. However, how primary care payments flow through organizations to reach and influence primary care delivery, and whether they are aligned with overall intent, remains a critical issue.

For the purposes of this chapter and the committee's report, the committee assumes that the current multi-payer, largely employment-based system will implement its recommendations. Changes to this assumption would affect the committee's recommendations significantly but are outside of its scope of work. Please see other work from the Institute of Medicine and the National Academies of Sciences, Engineering, and Medicine for discussions on financing insurance in the United States (IOM, 2004, 2009; NASEM, 2019b).

How Much Payment Is Rendered

How much payment is rendered for a service confers social value. In the United States, primary care physicians (PCPs), while well compensated relative to average overall wages, are poorly compensated relative to their peers in specialty services. The ratio of average annual income for a specialty physician compared to a PCP in the United States was 1.6 in 2003–2004 (Fujisawa and Lafortune, 2008). By 2017, the median compensation in radiology, procedural, and surgical specialties had an almost twofold difference compared with primary care (Doximity, 2019; MedPAC, 2019). While the difference is less, primary care nurses and physician assistants also make less than those in other specialties (AAPA, 2020; Nurse.org, 2020).

As this chapter will describe, this valuation is not derived from market-based negotiations governed by the laws of supply and demand. Rather, it starts with the idiosyncratic process by which Medicare values services, which attempts to account for training, operational costs, and professional risks. This approach, however, places little intrinsic value on promoting health or keeping people healthy. Rather, it is skewed toward procedures, tests, and specialists over relationships, holistic consideration of the individual and their diagnoses, and population health. Usually, the sicker the patient and the more technical care they receive, the more clinicians are paid. In addition, the U.S. health care system is focused, and paid, on the notion of treating illness rather than on maintaining health. Technology-enabled services oriented primarily to diagnosing and treating advanced disease draw higher prices than reimbursement for clinician time spent with patients and their families.

Money is but one factor affecting clinicians' decisions, yet payment methods clearly affect whether, how, and how much care they provide (Quinn, 2015). Because they are more likely to provide services with greater returns, relative prices affect use and the mix of services provided. Indeed, when prices change, this has measurable effects on the number and mix of services provided to patients (Clemens and Gottlieb, 2014; Cromwell and Mitchell, 1986; Gruber et al., 1998; Hadley, 2003; Rice, 1983). Examples include hospital length of stay, diagnostic imaging in physician offices, home health care visits, coordination between physicians and hospitals, the volume and mix of services delivered, and which drugs are used for treatment (Bodenheimer, 2008; Coulam and Gaumer, 1991; GAO, 2012; Jacobson et al., 2010; Schlenker et al., 2005; Schroeder and Frist, 2013).

The results of primary care's devaluation are not surprising. The portion of total health care expenses devoted to primary care in the United States is at or lower than most other countries (Koller and Khullar, 2017; Phillips and Bazemore, 2010), and evidence suggests that it is declining (The Larry A. Green Center and PCC, 2020). One result is that retaining seasoned primary care clinicians has become challenging. Moreover, when faced with the prospect of medical education debt, more limited future financial remuneration, and lower perceived social and professional status, many medical students opt for specialty professions over primary care. The COVID-19 pandemic has further distressed the primary care profession by limiting in-person visits, driving a significant number of practices to close (Basu et al., 2020; Phillips et al., 2020).

A health care system oriented more to primary care would result in a healthier population (Basu et al., 2019) with more consistent access to primary care and potentially a more equitable distribution of health care (Dwyer-Lindgren et al., 2017; Friedberg et al., 2010; Macinko et al., 2007). As recently reiterated by The Commonwealth Fund's 2020 Task Force on Payment and Delivery System Reform (2020), the nation will only achieve these goals with changes in how and how much primary care is paid (Zabar et al., 2019).

How Payment Is Rendered

How payment is rendered influences the behavior of both clinicians and care-seekers in primary care. Payment methods matter because of the incentives they create and the actions they reward. The historically dominant method of FFS payment encourages a focus on providing and receiving individual, billable services. Generally, the unit of service and analysis is the short office visit. While FFS is considered to promote access and accountability (Dowd and Laugesen, 2020; Kern et al., 2020), it discourages other team members who may not be able to bill for their services from providing care. It also disincentivizes the primary care team from focusing on non-billable services, outside of a brief office visit, that may have beneficial effects on the health of individuals or a population, such as identifying and educating people with chronic disease (Berenson and Goodson, 2016).

The Spectrum of Physician Payment Models

Theory and evidence show that payment methods have distinctive effects on clinician behavior. Generally, the models fall along a spectrum according to the unit of payment, such as FFS (which pays for each individual service provided) or a bundled payment (which pays for a group of services or a specific period) (see Figure 9-1). On the one hand, concerns about stinting in providing care dominate when clinicians bear financial risk in a bundled payment model, because health care use can be unpredictable. On the other hand, concerns about overtreatment dominate when the financial risk is on payers, such as in FFS, where the insurer pays a given fee for each service. Most research shows empirical results in parallel with theory: FFS encourages use, and capitation—a payment model that provides a fixed amount of money per patient per unit of time paid in advance to the physician for the delivery of health care services, whether or not that patient seeks care and how much it costs—discourages resource consumption; productivity-based pay encourages and capitated payments undermine productivity (Berenson et al., 2020; Hellinger, 1996; Kralewski et al., 2000).

All payment methods have inherent incentives, both good and bad, that cannot be eliminated even with optimal design (Robinson, 2001). Their perverse effects can be attenuated to some extent through design, but even the most sophisticated mechanisms merely diminish the incentives for overtreatment, undertreatment, and other undesirable behaviors. Blended methods, using the best attributes of each, outperform pure FFS and pure capitation in supporting primary care (Berenson et al., 2020; Ellis and McGuire, 1990; Robinson, 2001).

Simplicity is a virtue for several reasons when it comes to designing and implementing payment models. The administrative costs of designing, negotiating, implementing, disbursing, disputing, and adjudicating complex payment methods are high. Simplicity is especially important in the multi-payer U.S. context because adoption of payment models is undermined when physicians face different policies and incentives from multiple

Spectrum of Physician Payment Models
ACTIVITY-BASED VS FIXED PAYMENT MODELS

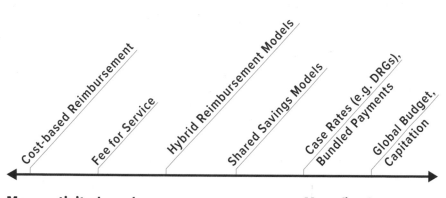

FIGURE 9-1 Payment models fall along a spectrum according to the unit of payment. NOTE: DRG = diagnosis-related group.

insurers. Simplicity also supports transparency for all stakeholders, including clinicians, patients, and policy makers.

HISTORY OF PRIMARY CARE PAYMENT

As part of an effort to manage the rising costs of health care and ensure the solvency of Medicare, Congress enacted the Medicare prospective payment system for hospitals in 1983 (Altman, 2012). Instead of paying hospitals for each service delivered, Medicare pays a set fee per stay based on the diagnosis and treatment path. This change incentivized hospitals to reduce length of stay and shift more care to outpatient settings. Although it was not intended to impact primary care, it had many downstream consequences.

In the late 1980s, rising and varied physician-set prices and the widening gap between generalist and specialist incomes led Congress to establish the resource-based relative value scale to set prices for physician services, which account for about 20 percent of Medicare spending (CMS, 2019b). The Physician Fee Schedule (PFS), implemented in 1992, was designed to be built around a scientific measurement of work and practice expenses (Hsiao et al., 1993), with physician work accounting for around 50 percent of the total relative value unit. Changes to the original measures during the implementation process resulted in a fee redistribution to PCPs about half as large as that projected by the original estimates (Berenson, 1989).

The Patient Protection and Affordable Care Act (ACA),[1] passed in 2010, included two provisions to adjust payments to PCPs upward: (a) a 10 percent incentive payment under the Medicare primary care incentive payment (PCIP) for 5 years and (b) raising the Medicaid primary care payment rates up to at least 100 percent of the Medicare rate for 2 years (Davis et al., 2011; Mulcahy et al., 2018). Federal funding for this Medicaid increase expired in 2014, but as of 2016, 19 states had continued this "fee bump" in whole or in part (Zuckerman et al., 2017) and some have called for payment equity between Medicaid and Medicare to be a permanent strategy to improve access and equity for children (Perrin et al., 2020). Not all PCPs were eligible for the PCIP because the criteria were based on meeting a 60 percent threshold of allowed charges for specific ambulatory evaluation and management codes. Some family physicians, particularly in rural areas, perform procedures and provide care in hospitals such that they did not meet the threshold (The Lewin Group, 2015).

The PCIP program had a modestly positive impact on the availability and use of primary care services in Medicare. An early analysis found the almost 75 percent Medicaid rate increase improved primary care appointment availability for enrollees with participating clinicians without generating longer wait times (Polsky et al., 2015; Zuckerman and Goin, 2012). However, a recent analysis concluded the payment increase had no association with PCP participation in Medicaid or on Medicaid service volume (Mulcahy et al., 2020).

Medicare has also added supplemental primary care services to the PFS to improve quality (Berenson et al., 2020).[2] An additional focus in the 2019 and 2020 PFS updates was liberalizing payment for a variety of relatively new telehealth codes. Given these codes' complexity and stringent requirements, uptake has been inconsistent, particularly by small practices (Carlo et al., 2020; Dewar et al., 2020; Reddy et al., 2020). Despite barriers to adoption, including billing and workflow adjustments, uptake is increasing,

---

[1] Patient Protection and Affordable Care Act, Public Law 111-148 (March 23, 2010).

[2] These include covering certification of home health and hospice services, managing care transitions from hospital to the community, managing care for patients with chronic conditions, advance care planning, managing care for patients with cognitive impairment and behavioral health conditions in collaborative arrangements with behavioral health professionals, and providing add-on payments for visits that last at least 31 minutes or prolonged management services conducted before and/or after direct care.

improving value to beneficiaries and the program while increasing revenue to practices (Berenson et al., 2020).

In 2019, the Centers for Medicare & Medicaid Services (CMS) implemented the Merit-Based Incentive Payment System, providing additional payments to organizations participating in alternative payment models and financially rewarding or penalizing clinicians based on quality measures, promoting interoperability, and improvement activities (PAI, 2020). In this zero-sum game, where bonuses for the highest performers come from penalties of lower-performing practices, research has shown that independent practices—those that are not part of a larger system—and safety net practices are more likely to have lower performance and suffer financially (Colla et al., 2020).

PRIMARY CARE PAYMENT TODAY

Financing health care in the United States is complex, with health care organizations receiving revenue from multiple sources: public payers (directly and also indirectly through contracted insurers), commercial insurers, self-insured employers (directly and also through their administrators), and directly from patients. In addition, separate systems exist for veterans and active-duty military families. Oversight authority is divided between private and public payers and between state and federal regulators. This complexity is a contributing factor to the fragmentation of care and why implementing changes to payment models is difficult. In 2017, family physicians reported that their patient panel was 41 percent private insurance, 28 percent Medicare, 18 percent Medicaid, and 7 percent uninsured. Since 2012, notable shifts have taken place in the payer mix for family physicians, with Medicare and Medicaid comprising a greater percentage (AAFP, 2017a). Among pediatricians, that payer mix looks different, at 49 percent Medicaid, 46 percent private insurance, and about 4 percent uninsured (AAP, 2019).

Primary care spending accounted for 6.5 percent of total U.S. health care expenditures in 2002 and 5.4 percent in 2016 (Martin et al., 2020). The proportion was even lower among Medicare FFS beneficiaries, with primary care representing 2.12–4.88 percent of total medical and prescription spending in 2015 (Reid et al., 2019). Medicare Advantage beneficiaries had higher rates of primary care visits and lower costs for these services, but the differences were not substantial (Park et al., 2020). Among commercially insured groups, children had the highest primary care spending as a share of their total health care spending, with 20.33 percent in 2013 and 19.54 percent in 2017, and individuals aged 55–64 years had the lowest, with 7.25 percent in 2013 and 6.33 percent in 2017 (Reiff et al., 2019).

Across payers in 2013, FFS was the dominant method: nearly 95 percent of all physician office visits, with the remaining 5 percent via capitation. The exact numbers varied by geography and payer (Zuvekas and Cohen, 2016). In 2016, 83.6 percent of practice revenue was FFS, while bundled payments accounted for almost 9 percent, pay-for-performance and capitation made up close to 7 percent, and shared shavings made up only 2 percent (Rama, 2017).

The traditional Medicare program still mainly pays primary care through FFS, with modest adjustments for quality and efficiency (MedPAC, 2020a). A quarter of beneficiaries fall under an alternative payment model (such as an accountable care organization [ACO], described below). In 2019, 34 percent of beneficiaries were enrolled in a Medicare Advantage plan (MedPAC, 2020b), where payment for primary care services varies by plan but is generally FFS and anchored to the Medicare fee schedule (Trish et al., 2017). About 10 percent of beneficiaries in Medicare Advantage are in a plan that passes on global financial risk to clinician teams (Galewitz, 2018).

In Medicaid, states have broad flexibility to determine payments for physician services. While 81 percent of enrollees are in managed care plans, the majority of Medicaid spending occurs under direct state FFS arrangements (MACPAC, 2020). Medicaid physician fees are well below that of fees for Medicare and private payers: only roughly 54 percent of Medicare rates for primary care services (MACPAC, 2013). These lower rates are thought to negatively impact physician participation in Medicaid (Cunningham and May, 2006; Decker, 2012; Holgash and Heberlein, 2019).

State Medicaid programs use different types of managed care arrangements: comprehensive risk-based managed care (35 states), primary care case management (7 states), or a combination of the two (5 states). Some states carve out specific services from their managed care arrangements such as oral health, institutional care, or transportation (Hinton et al., 2019; MACPAC, 2011). Sixty-nine percent of Medicaid enrollees in 2018 received their benefits though a comprehensive risk-based arrangement (KFF, 2020). In primary care case management, enrollees have a designated primary care team paid a monthly case management fee to assume responsibility for care management and coordination. Individual clinicians are not at financial risk; they continue to be paid on an FFS basis for providing covered services. In some cases, financial incentives for both primary care teams and the care management entity are added.

In risk-based arrangements, Medicaid managed care organizations (MCOs) are paid a capitation rate that is calculated based on the state's FFS rates. The MCO, in turn, contracts with health care organizations through a series of privately negotiated, proprietary arrangements. The MCO is responsible for assembling a network of clinicians that meets state access requirements based on minimum standards set by CMS, which also maintains separate network access standards for Medicaid FFS programs.

The access standards for Medicaid MCOs were promulgated by CMS under its Medicaid Managed Care Rule in 2016, but none are specific to primary care. Prior to the 2016 rule, inadequate enforcement of Medicaid access policies was the source of dozens of suits against states (Rosenbaum, 2009, 2020). In 2020, CMS eliminated an access standard for the time and distance traveled to access a clinician, only requiring states to set a quantitative minimum access standard, such as minimum clinician-to-enrollee ratios; a minimum percentage of contracted clinicians that are accepting new patients; maximum wait times for an appointment; or hours of operation requirements (BPC, 2020; CMS, 2020e).

More than half of managed care states (21 of 40) set a target percentage in their contracts for the percentage of payments, network clinicians, or plan members that must be paid via alternative payment models in fiscal year 2019 (Hinton et al., 2019). Most plans use FFS with incentives or bonus payments tied to performance measures. Fewer plans reported using bundled or episode-based payments or shared savings and risk arrangements.

Commercial health insurance consists of employer-sponsored coverage and individual insurance. Insurers and administrators assemble provider networks through proprietary confidential contracts. Analysis of multiple sources indicates that commercial insurers pay on average 143 percent of Medicare rates for physician services, with considerable variation by specialty type (Lopez et al., 2020). Codes most frequently billed by PCPs were paid at 107 percent of Medicare (Trish et al., 2017). This disparity in payments relative to Medicare likely reflects greater negotiating leverage for specialty physicians. More than half of commercial contract payments use FFS without any quality or performance bonuses (HCPLAN, 2019).

Findings for Primary Care Today

- Primary care makes up a small and declining proportion of medical spending.
- FFS is the dominant payment mechanism for primary care clinicians.
- Compared to Medicare, Medicaid pays substantially less for primary care services and commercial insurers slightly more.
- Medicaid determines payment sufficiency through the ability of states and managed care contractors to maintain adequate networks of clinicians. Federal oversight of these standards is not specific to primary care, and, while they were already inadequate, they have recently been further relaxed.
- Commercial insurers pay specialty physicians more relative to Medicare than they pay PCPs.

REFORMING PAYMENT TO PRIMARY CARE

In this section, the committee presents a spectrum of options for improving payment for primary care to better meet people's needs. These options are not mutually exclusive, and it will likely be necessary to employ multiple levers to produce the changes necessary to support primary care.

- Option 1 builds incrementally on the existing PFS to value primary care services more accurately.
- Option 2 discusses overarching models to blend FFS and fixed payments.
- Option 3 discusses global payment models for practices prepared to take on further financial risk.
- Option 4 discusses creating a societal goal for the proportion of health care spending that goes to primary care.

Option 1: The Medicare Physician Fee Schedule and the Relative Value Scale Update Committee

While Medicare accounts for 20 percent of national health spending (KFF, 2019), the relative prices set by the PFS have a profound effect on professional prices beyond Medicare beneficiaries. Three-quarters of the services physicians billed to commercial insurers are pegged to Medicare's relative prices (Clemens et al., 2015), and TRICARE, the health care program for uniformed service members, also uses the Medicare PFS. Many state Medicaid and state workers compensation programs use the Medicare rates as a benchmark. In addition, many alternative payment models are based on spending projections that use the PFS, and payers use shadow prices from the PFS to calculate capitation rates.

The Role of the Relative Value Scale Update Committee (RUC)

Shortly after CMS implemented the Medicare PFS, the American Medical Association created the RUC and offered the committee's expertise to the Health Care Financing Administration, CMS's predecessor. The RUC selects physician procedures for review and determines the value of services relative to other physician services for three categories of activity: physician work, practice expense, and malpractice risk. The RUC passes the resulting numerical assessments on to CMS, which can accept or modify recommendations and then convert them into an entry on the PFS using a geographic adjustment and inflation multiplier. Historically, CMS has deferred to nearly all the RUC's recommendations, accepting them unaltered 87.4 percent of the time between 1994 and 2010. On average, RUC-recommended work values were higher than final CMS values (Laugesen et al., 2012).

Today, the RUC comprises 31 physicians and 300 advisors representing medical specialties. Primary care has one rotating seat and three seats appointed by the American Academy of Family Physicians (AAFP), the American College of Physicians (representing internal medicine), and the American Academy of Pediatrics. Two seats also rotate between internal medicine subspecialties. Of the 31 physician seats, only one each is dedicated to child health and geriatrics (AMA, 2016).

There are reasons to question the accuracy and independence of the RUC process, including documented voting alliances in the RUC among proceduralists that often distort the equitable allocation of valuing work (Laugesen, 2016). Researchers working with CMS and the Assistant Secretary for Planning and Evaluation have gathered evidence that the PFS's time estimates for clinician work are inflated (MedPAC, 2018b; Merrell et al., 2014; Zuckerman et al., 2016), suggesting a bigger gap between estimated and actual times for surgical and procedural services than office visits, especially those occurring in primary care (McCall et al., 2006; MedPAC, 2018b). The available evidence suggests that surgical services are overvalued, while primary care visits and services are largely undervalued (CMS, 2019a; Reid et al., 2019).

Inaccuracies in relative pricing along with CMS acceptance of most RUC recommendations have contributed to the differences in compensation across specialties, the distribution of physicians across specialties, inefficient distortions in use, and inadequate beneficiary access to undervalued services, as described above (MedPAC, 2018b; Nicholson and Souleles, 2001). These deficiencies in the RUC process compound over time because changes to Medicare's fee schedule must be budget neutral. As a result, primary care services generally, and evaluation and management codes specifically, have become passively devalued in the PFS as their relative prices fall as a result of other service prices (including new technologies) increasing. A variety of factors interplay to cause this devaluation:

- For procedure-based services, work time often falls as physicians become familiar with the service and technology improves. However, work relative value units (RVUs) for these services often are not re-evaluated (MedPAC, 2006). Evaluation and management services consist largely of activities that require specified clinician time.
- Requests for new codes or refinement are initiated by specialty societies, and refinement generally results in increases (Laugesen, 2016). New technologies and methods of diagnosis and treatment

can create pathways to higher relative values, compared to visits, which have few new technologies (Zuckerman et al., 2015).

- Procedural, task-driven work may lend itself more easily to judgments of physician work units, which are composites of time, mental effort, judgment, technical skill, physical effort, and psychological stress. Measurement may be harder in evaluation and management services with a broad range of clinical issues, less defined temporal sequences, and a more nonlinear workflow, as found in the management of chronic conditions in primary care (Katz and Melmed, 2016; Laugesen, 2016). Furthermore, primary care has involved increasing complexity over time, at the level of different organ systems, individual factors, societal variables, and population dynamics. It is difficult to measure the continuity, comprehensiveness, coordination, trust, personal connection, and personal accessibility necessary to provide high-quality primary care (Shi, 2012).

- Under budget neutrality, an increase in units for the large number of evaluation and management visits would mean relative prices fall for everything else, making the RUC less likely to recommend these changes. Most evaluation and management codes are passed in the RUC below the 25th percentile of the range of clinician responses regarding work time, whereas procedures typically end up between the 25th and 50th percentile of survey responses (Laugesen, 2016).

- Documented voting alliances in the RUC among proceduralists often distort the equitable allocation of valuing work (Laugesen, 2016).

Thus, because the fee schedule is budget neutral and the phenomena described above are routine, primary care services have become passively devalued. For example, the total RVUs for a Level III office or outpatient visit for an established patient (HCPCS 99213), the most frequently billed office or outpatient visit, declined slightly from 2.14 in 2013 to 2.06 in 2018 (MedPAC, 2018b). This devaluation is reflected in a widening gap in pay between primary care and specialists. Data from the Medical Group Management Association indicate that from 1995 to 2004, the median income for PCPs increased by 21.4 percent, while that for specialists increased by 37.5 percent (Bodenheimer, 2006). In 2017, median compensation for nonsurgical, procedural specialists, surgical specialties, and primary care was $426,000, $420,000, and $242,000 (MedPAC, 2019), respectively. This compensation gap is associated with reduction in medical student choice of primary care careers and with shifting hospital graduate medical education priorities away from primary care (COGME, 2010; Phillips et al., 2009; Weida et al., 2010).

Recent Reforms

Several effective steps have been taken in the last decade, including revising misvalued codes, temporarily increasing the primary care fee, and adding new primary care codes. Nonetheless, the definition and conceptualization of physician work inherent in the PFS do not support the committee's conceptualization of high-quality primary care.

For the last decade, CMS and the RUC have identified and reviewed "potentially misvalued services," including codes associated with fast use growth or services that have not been reviewed since the PFS was implemented. The Protecting Access to Medicare Act of 2014[3] and Medicare Access and CHIP (Children's Health Insurance Program) Reauthorization Act of 2015[4] provided CMS with new powers to change misvalued codes and collect data to evaluate the PFS. The law expanded the number of codes that would potentially be evaluated, creating a new target for relative value adjustments, with a savings target of 0.5 percent of expenditure every year between 2017 and 2020 (Laugesen, 2016). A recent survey of the RUC process resulted in a major upward revision in the 2021 Medicare PFS for fees for office visits (CMS, 2020d). CMS endorsed the RUC recommendation for the two most commonly billed office visit codes: a 34 percent increase for code 99213 and a 28 percent increase for 99214.

CMS remains limited, however, by the lack of current, accurate, and objective data on clinician work time and practice expenses (GAO, 2015; Mulcahy et al., 2020; Wynn et al., 2015; Zuckerman et al., 2016). As a result, CMS continues to depend on a RUC process that has drifted away from science-based estimates toward interest group input. This drift is facilitated because complexity and lack of transparency effectively mask payment policy. The complexity of the PFS and its determinants, paired with the lack of resources at CMS, has led to a situation where physician societies have informational advantages and leverage them to achieve higher valuations (Laugesen, 2016; McCarty, 2013; Shapiro, 2008).

CMS and other policy makers have little recourse to change the RUC structure or processes. As a private organization, the RUC has an important voice in the policy process and substantial autonomy to determine how it chooses its valuation practices. Many have noted that without more oversight or coordination of a fair arbitration process, the relative value scale

---

[3] Protecting Access to Medicare Act of 2014, Public Law 113-93 (April 1, 2014).

[4] Medicare Access and CHIP Reauthorization Act of 2015, Public Law 114-10 (April 16, 2015).

was bound to be biased toward specialty care (Berenson and Goodson, 2016; Laugesen et al., 2012).

However, the committee sees no regulatory or institutional barrier to CMS establishing its own parallel capacity to independently value physician services that aligns better with its stated organizational goals to move toward value-based, accountable payment and away from the misvalued PFS. In fact, it is hard to imagine that it could do so in the absence of an independent valuing mechanism within or external to the agency, such as the Medicare Payment Advisory Commission (MedPAC).[5] Establishing such a capacity will require allocating a relatively modest level of resources and staff and would not prevent the RUC from continuing to make its recommendations to CMS and other entities. However, by having an additional resource to evaluate and compare its own estimates with that of the RUC and others, CMS would be able to more adequately and fairly price primary care services in a way that accounts for their complexity and value to patients and society.

Altering the Fee Schedule to Accomplish Policy Objectives

Direct changes to relative prices could include a payment increase for ambulatory evaluation and management services, such as the change implemented in January 2021, or freezing rates for these services while reducing others. In 2015, MedPAC recommended establishing per-beneficiary payments for primary care clinicians to encourage care coordination, including the non-face-to-face activities that are a critical component of care coordination. MedPAC recommended setting the per-beneficiary payment at 10 percent of primary care spending, which at that time would have meant an annual payment of $28 per patient with no beneficiary cost sharing. To be budget neutral, this funding level would have required reducing fees for non–primary care services in the PFS by 1.4 percent (MedPAC, 2015). A hybrid reimbursement approach such as this is discussed more below.

In its June 2018 report, MedPAC modeled a 10 percent payment rate increase for evaluation and management services. In 2019, a 10 percent increase would have raised annual spending for ambulatory evaluation and management services by $2.4 billion. To maintain budget neutrality, payment rates for all other PFS services would be reduced by 3.8 percent (MedPAC, 2018b). Other options to offset a payment increase for ambulatory evaluation and management codes include automatic reductions to

---

[5] MedPAC is a non-partisan legislative branch agency that provides the U.S. Congress with analysis and policy advice on the Medicare program. Additional information is available at www.medpac.gov (accessed February 27, 2021).

prices of new services after their introduction or automatic reductions in services with high growth rates (MedPAC, 2018b).

In summary, the Medicare PFS is not well designed to support primary care. It is oriented toward discrete, often procedural, technical services with defined beginnings and ends, the antithesis of high-quality continuous primary care. Some have gone so far as to say that the RUC and the PFS have led to more procedures, the recruitment of more physicians into the procedure-oriented specialties, the underrepresentation of primary care in the workforce, the under-provision of primary care, and the consolidation of primary care practices into larger delivery systems (Berenson and Goodson, 2016; Calsyn and Twomey, 2018; Laugesen, 2016).

Findings for Option 1

- The relative prices set by the Medicare PFS have profound effects on prices paid by Medicaid, commercial payers, and others. The RUC exerts significant influence on the relative prices assigned by CMS.
- The RUC, together with the structure of the PFS, have resulted in systematically devaluing primary care services relative to other services and its population health benefit, reflected in large and widening gaps between primary care and specialty compensation.
- The widening compensation gap between primary care and other physician specialties is associated with reductions in medical trainees' likelihood of choosing primary care careers and with hospitals' graduate medical education training priorities.
- With adequate resources and leadership, CMS has the authority to address these weaknesses and internalize the functions of the RUC (data collection and valuation tools) to generate payment levels aligned with high-quality primary care.

Option 2: Hybrid Reimbursement Models

A second option for increasing and reforming payment to primary care is to mix FFS payment mechanisms with lump-sum or per-person payments to encourage team-based, technology-enabled advanced primary care.

Patient-Centered Medical Home Model

Over the past 15 years, implementation of advanced primary care in the United States has focused largely on the hybrid patient-centered medical home (PCMH) model. Early PCMH models showed promising results in terms of reducing spending and avoidable use, especially among the chronically ill (Maeng et al., 2016).

Commercial payers began to sponsor limited tests of these models within their care networks, usually with small care management fees on top of FFS. By 2010, these tests encompassed more than 14,000 physicians in 18 states caring for almost 5 million patients (Bitton et al., 2010), but they were hampered by the low levels of care management fees, often under $5 per patient per month, and a lack of multi-payer participation. The early results of studies on PCMH effects on total spending were mixed (Jackson et al., 2013; Sinaiko et al., 2017). These evaluations rarely factored the cost of practice transformation or the provision of care management fees into the analysis.

As the PCMH model spread, payers provided more substantial care management fees, multi-payer participation increased somewhat, and payer-initiated PCMH models began to include shared savings incentives (Edwards et al., 2014). The total amount of money, and transformation resources in the form of facilitation, generally increased. Nonetheless, FFS continued to be the mainstay of payment, and robust multi-payer involvement was the exception, not the norm. The cost effects of these PCMH initiatives continued to be mixed, though quality and patient experience were more often improved (Jackson et al., 2013; Kern et al., 2016; Lebrun-Harris et al., 2013; Sinaiko et al., 2017).

However, more recent research on PCMH outcomes from nearly 6,000 practices in 14 states found reductions in total expenditures of more than 8 percent after up to 9 years of implementation, as well as significant decreases in emergency department utilization and outpatient care (Saynisch et al., 2021). Emergency department reductions were highest among practices that offered electronic access, suggesting that the choice of adopted capabilities is important.

The PCMH model has also been implemented for pediatric populations. Integrated Care for Kids, a child- and family-centered integrated delivery care model, is one example with a matched state payment model for children insured by Medicaid or CHIP (see Chapter 5 for more detail).

Comprehensive Primary Care Model

To test a multi-payer approach to primary care transformation at scale, the Center for Medicare & Medicaid Innovation (CMMI) launched the Comprehensive Primary Care (CPC) model as a 4-year, multi-payer demonstration in 2012. CPC provided population-based care management fees and shared savings opportunities, on top of standard FFS, to nearly 500 participating primary care practices in seven regions as a means of supporting the provision of a core set of five "comprehensive" primary care functions (CMS, 2020a). Regions were selected based on the ability of their payer partners to provide participating practices with at least 60 percent of combined revenue. CPC showed mixed results on the cost and quality outcomes assessed in its evaluation. The growth rate in overall FFS expenditures was reduced for attributed beneficiaries, though the decrease was not enough to offset the care management fees (Peikes et al., 2018). In addition, those fees were not sufficient to enable upfront and long-term investments in staff. Though practice quality improvements as measured through claims were modest, an analysis of electronic clinical quality measures (used by practices themselves to measure improvement) showed significant gains compared to benchmarks established during the initiative (LaBonte et al., 2019).

Comprehensive Primary Care Plus Program

CPC was a precursor to the CPC+ program launched in 2017. CPC+ is a national multi-payer advanced primary care model that aims to strengthen primary care through regionally based, multi-payer payment reform and care delivery transformation (Burton et al., 2017). It is active in 18 regions, with more than 50 payers and more than 3,000 participating practices serving more than 3 million Medicare beneficiaries and an estimated 15 million people overall (CMS, 2020b). CPC+ includes two practice tracks with incrementally advanced care delivery requirements and payment options and has three major payment elements: (1) a risk-adjusted care management fee per beneficiary that is paid quarterly and not visit based; (2) performance-based incentives paid prospectively with retrospective reconciliation, with performance measures that include patient experience, clinical quality, and use; and (3) payment under the PFS. In Track 1, PFS payment continues as usual along with the care management fees and performance-based payments, but in Track 2, PFS payments are reduced and shifted into a CPC payment.

CPC+'s first evaluation[6] focused on Medicare FFS enrollees in 2,905 practices that started CPC+ in 2017. The median care management fees per practitioner in the first year equaled $32,000 in Track 1 and $53,000 in Track 2, with CMS providing the most fees relative to other participating payers. Other payers were slower to adopt the reduced PFS payments and partially capitated payments in Track 2. In the first year, 71 percent of Track 2 practices opted for the lowest FFS reduction of 10 percent in exchange for capitated payments; only 16 percent of CPC+ Track 2 practices,

---

[6] This reflects available evaluations at the time of writing. The reader should refer to https://innovation.cms.gov/innovation-models/comprehensive-primary-care-plus (accessed February 27, 2021) for updated evaluations.

or roughly 8 percent of all participants, opted for a 40 or 65 percent reduction in FFS in exchange for larger capitated payments. As expected, CPC+ in its first year had small effects on quality of care and health care spending, and the care management investments were larger than any cost savings.

Despite the investments in care management, data feedback, and learning support, participating practices also expressed challenges implementing care delivery requirements, though system-owned practices and those with a robust health information technology infrastructure found it easier to identify the resources for practice transformation and manage reporting requirements. Commercial insurer participation in the CPC+ model has persisted, indicating they perceive value in the model. There are also non-peer-reviewed analyses of multi-payer projects in Arkansas, Ohio, and Oregon that show more promising performance for commercially insured people and improvements over time (Bianco et al., 2020; Brown and Tilford, 2020; Dulsky Watkins, 2019).

Challenges to Implementing Hybrid Reimbursement Models

Most PCMH-like primary care transformation efforts implemented by individual payers have used hybrid payment methods largely based on FFS and struggled to provide the financial resources to cover transformation costs or the ongoing cost of maintaining integrated team-based care. Some commercial payers, such as the Capital District Physicians' Health Plan (CDPHP) in New York and the Hawaii Medical Service Association, have moved further to structure payments for primary care practices around a risk-adjusted primary care capitation model. An evaluation of the CDPHP model showed some pharmacy cost savings and use declines in people with chronic conditions but no overall cost savings (Salzberg et al., 2017). An initial assessment of the Hawaii program found improvements in quality but did not assess cost or use changes (Navathe et al., 2019).

As with payer-specific hybrid payment models, it was likely difficult for practices to change their overall structure when one payer offered risk-adjusted capitation for 10 to 20 percent of patients but FFS contracts constituted the rest. With the advent of large multi-payer initiatives, such as CPC+, this dynamic is changing, as payers in some regions are starting to increase available capital to practices and change payment for a plurality, if not majority, of patients in a practice. Nonetheless, most U.S. primary care practices, even those involved in PCMH efforts, are not paid substantially extra for these efforts.

Poorly funded incremental PCMH efforts across practices have diluted the effects of the limited capital invested in them, and until recently, this capital has not been explicitly tied to reductions in total cost of care. The majority of payer-initiated PCMH and advanced primary care demonstrations have shown mixed or no effects on total cost. The lack of spending reductions has limited further investment in augmented PCMH or advanced primary care models, whose high ongoing staff and transformation costs are well documented. Without a substantial source of new, predictable, and sustainable revenue from multiple payers to maintain and expand new services, practices find it difficult to maintain focus on overlapping practice transformation aims, including quality improvement, team formation, chronic care coordination, and patient engagement. Thus, minimal investments, initiative overlap, and an underlying focus on visit volume impede the ability to focus on reducing total spending, which is difficult when primary care practices drive small fractions of spending themselves and have incomplete control over where and when their patients utilize care.

Nonetheless, the literature on impact of payment reform on total spending remains mixed and may depend on organizational and patient characteristics (Veet et al., 2020). For example, some integrated delivery systems have improved outcomes, and low-income patients have improved clinical outcomes (van den Berk-Clark et al., 2018). Many payer-reported efforts have suggested savings (Jabbarpour et al., 2017), but most peer-reviewed published analyses have been more widely divergent or null in their findings (Jackson et al., 2013; Sinaiko et al., 2017). One study with a 6-year observation period and another that took place after up to 9 years of implementation both found significant savings (Maeng et al., 2016; Saynisch et al., 2021). A key area of overlapping conclusion is that potential savings are concentrated in patients with multiple comorbidities and chronic conditions, where regression to the mean is possible.

This imperative to demonstrate short-term health care cost savings serves as a key challenge to child health–focused primary care models, as high-cost pediatric patients make up a much smaller proportion of the population. For example, just 5 percent of children account for about 50 percent of Medicaid spending for children (Berry et al., 2014). Most often, health care savings realized by primary care transformation may result as children and adolescents age into healthier young adults, with healthier behaviors (e.g., lower smoking rates, higher immunization rates) and fewer chronic illnesses (less obesity, lower rates of depression). Savings may also be realized outside of health care, in education (greater graduation rates, less need for special education services) (Zimmerman and Woolf, 2014), the workforce, and the criminal justice system (Wen et al., 2014). These, of course, are not costs that are considered in time-limited evaluations of primary care transformation. Thus, a recent review of child-focused ACOs concluded that the area of child health requires specific payment models to account for these issues (Perrin et al., 2017).

Ten years of experience with CMMI hybrid reimbursement models has generated some key lessons for future primary care model development (Peikes et al., 2020):

- Though participating practices valued the care delivery innovations, they often struggled to find the time or resources necessary to fully implement desired changes, even with multi-payer models.
- Busy primary care clinicians need education about what they are required to implement and why. They also require simplified and harmonized reporting requirements across payers to reduce administrative burden on practices.
- Practices need some flexibility from payers to adapt payment models to their circumstances.
- Involving an extended care team other than those in primary care can enhance model impact.
- The redesign of care can take time to yield impact.

Layering care management fees and shared savings on a largely unchanged chassis of FFS does not drive robust and focused practice change to reduce expensive specialty and hospital-based use; practices largely continue to operate within the confines of FFS, visit-based mentality (Bitton et al., 2012). Alternative payment models need to have stronger incentives to counter FFS, and multi-payer participation with more substantial shifts away from FFS toward risk-based contracting can help achieve this (Burton et al., 2018; Martin et al., 2020). However, many practices may not be immediately able to take on complex risk. Payments need to be clearly defined, relatively simple, and transparent. Data and feedback on performance are necessary, but they must be salient and actionable, and training on using data effectively may be necessary for model participants.

Particularly in the wake of the COVID-19 pandemic, attention has focused on another advantage to partially capitated models: they ensure a steady and predictable cash flow in times of severe service disruption (Phillips et al., 2020). To the extent that the declines of pandemic-induced visit volumes remain, greater implementation of hybrid payment arrangements would forestall the closure of primary care practices or their absorption into larger, more expensive health systems with no corresponding improvement in service value.

Findings for Option 2

- FFS models discourage successful engagement of primary care practices in structure and process improvements.

- Hybrid payment models in support of advanced primary care mitigate FFS incentives for increased use and provide resources for team-based care and non-PFS services, though this produces modest to no reductions in spending and use in the short term.
- With adequate time, hybrid reimbursement models show improvements in care and reductions in use, particularly for people with multiple complex chronic conditions.
- The likelihood of practice improvement increases in markets where one payer has a large market share or when multiple payers align.

Option 3: Broad Risk-Sharing Models

The types of organizations delivering primary care vary greatly, as discussed throughout this report. In 2018, health systems employed nearly half of primary care clinicians, and this number continues to grow (Abelson, 2019), with potential acceleration from the COVID-19 pandemic. In health care systems, primary care clinicians are often employees and operate under contracts established by the system at large. In those instances, where health care organizations have greater capability and often experience with financial risk, they can assume accountability for overall use and spending. Referred to collectively as "risk sharing"—where risk is the probability of the assigned population using medical services—practices can assume risk accountability in their own contracts, form new entities to participate in risk-sharing models, or participate as part of a larger medical group or integrated delivery system.

Accountable Care Organizations

ACOs are groups of clinicians participating in capitated or shared-risk contracts paired with incentives for quality performance. CMS manages several ACO programs[7] that have implications for primary care payment, and many commercial payers have ACO programs as well (Peiris et al., 2016). In 2019, there were 1,588 existing public and private ACO contracts covering almost 44 million lives (Muhlestein et al., 2019). When an ACO succeeds in both delivering high-quality care and spending health care dollars more wisely, it will share the savings. Some ACO contracts also include shared risk if spending exceeds targets (Peck et al., 2019). Under an ACO

---

[7] CMS and CMMI manage multiple types of ACOs, including the Medicare Shared Savings Program, the ACO Investment Model, and the Advance Payment Model for qualifying Medicare Shared Savings Program ACOs; the Comprehensive ESRD Care Initiative for beneficiaries receiving dialysis services; the Next Generation ACO Model for ACOs experienced in managing care for populations of patients; the Pioneer ACO Model (no longer active); and the Vermont All-Payer ACO Model.

contract, payments to clinicians typically continue on an FFS basis, and the ACO assumes the performance risk and associated incentives. Primary care is a central component of ACOs, and organizations differ in the extent to which they emphasize, incorporate, pay for, and support it.

In general, research on the impact of ACOs shows modest savings in total spending alongside quality and patient satisfaction improvements. Research has demonstrated that ACOs with a higher share of PCMH practices (Jabbarpour et al., 2018) and a greater proportion of PCPs perform better on cost and quality outcomes (Albright et al., 2016; Ouayogodé et al., 2017). Similarly, physician-led ACOs, compared to hospital-integrated ACOs, produce greater savings (Bleser et al., 2018; McWilliams et al., 2018). Medicaid ACO arrangements now exist in 14 states, showing mixed results (CHCS, 2017; McConnell et al., 2017; NAACOS, 2020). The Alternative Quality Contract, BlueCross BlueShield's Medicaid ACO program in Massachusetts, has shown consistent improvement in quality and savings (Song et al., 2019), while the same commercial ACO program showed little effect in care quality or spending in children (Chien et al., 2014). However, Partners for Kids, a pediatric ACO in Ohio taking full risk for Medicaid enrollees, demonstrated a lower rate of cost growth without reduced quality measures or outcomes (Kelleher et al., 2015). Minnesota's Medicaid ACO also showed promising results in the pediatric population (Christensen and Payne, 2016). ACO programs also show some evidence of reducing disparities (McConnell et al., 2018; Song et al., 2017).

ACOs have different structures for distributing performance-based payments across participants that can affect compensation of PCPs (Siddiqui and Berkowitz, 2014). ACO-affiliated practices are more likely than unaffiliated practices to use performance improvement strategies, such as feedback of quality data to clinicians, yet performance measures contribute little to physician compensation (Peiris et al., 2016; Rosenthal et al., 2019).

Primary Care Contracting

In response to the piecemeal efforts and heterogeneous results of hybrid payment models, recent Medicare payment reform efforts focus less on streamlining primary care transformation and more on total cost-of-care reductions. In 2019, CMMI announced several new risk-sharing models that will begin in 2021. Primary Care First combines capitated and reduced FFS payments, with greater potential for shared savings and expansion to a larger number of geographic regions (CMS, 2020f). The payments include performance-based incentives that use regional and historical benchmarks for spending, quality, and hospital use (CMS, 2020g). The capitated payment was calibrated to constitute about 60 percent of primary care payments.

CMMI also announced it would enable direct contracting models, which are capitated or partially capitated models that are broad in scope and touch on primary care in several ways (CMS, 2020c). The program has two voluntary risk-based payment arrangements. The professional option offers organizations capitated, risk-adjusted monthly payment for a defined set of enhanced primary care services. The global option provides the highest risk-sharing arrangements in exchange for capitated, risk-adjusted monthly payments for all services provided by a direct contracting entity and its preferred providers.

Direct primary care models typically work by charging patients a monthly, quarterly, or annual fee to cover all or most services, including preventive care, basic illness treatment for acute and chronic conditions, clinical and laboratory services, consultative services, care coordination, and comprehensive care management (AAFP, 2020; Doherty et al., 2015). Many direct primary care practices also arrange access to other discounted services, such as prescription drugs, laboratory tests, and imaging (Busch et al., 2020).

Patients from all segments of the health insurance market—commercially insured, uninsured, and beneficiaries of Medicare, Medicare Advantage, and Medicaid—can be direct primary care members. Additionally, employers can offer a direct primary care option through their self-insured group health benefit plans, where they cover the fees. As a result of the relative newness of direct primary care, the literature assessing outcomes is small. In addition, studies are plagued by the difficulty of adjusting for the selection of healthy patients into these practices. One recent study found that after adjusting for differences in health status, a matched employer-based direct primary care cohort experienced a statistically significant reduction in total claim costs relative to the traditional cohort during the same period, meaning that enrollment in direct primary care was associated with reduced overall demand for health services. Direct primary care has similarities to concierge care, but key differentiators are direct primary care practices have lower membership fees and do not bill third parties on an FFS basis (Busch et al., 2020).

Finally, other primary care payment models have been proposed but not broadly tested, such as the Comprehensive Primary Care Payment Calculator (George et al., 2019), AAFP's Advanced Primary Care Model (AAFP, 2017b), an Innovative Model for Primary Care Office Payment (Antonucci, 2018), and the Comprehensive Care Physician Payment Model (Meltzer, 2018; Tingley, 2018).

Findings for Option 3

- With almost half of primary care clinicians employed in health systems, attention should be paid to primary care payment methods in those settings. Many ACOs continue to pay primary care internally based on FFS, even though the larger organization may participate in risk-sharing models.
- ACOs have demonstrated modest savings in total spending alongside quality and patient satisfaction improvements. ACOs that are predominately primary care, PCMH based, or physician led achieve better performance than other ACOs. Some evidence indicates that pediatric-focused ACO models are effective for pediatric populations.
- Medicare is developing models to engage primary care practices more directly in managing the cost and quality of their care. These broad risk-sharing models have yet to be implemented.

Option 4: Increase the Allocation of Spending to Primary Care

The poor performance of the United States in many areas of population health has in part been attributed to a lack of "primary care orientation" of the country's health system (Friedberg et al., 2010). Clear evidence suggests that systems oriented toward primary care in both policy and relative resource allocation show improved population outcomes and better efficiency over time (Bitton et al., 2017; Shi, 2012). One way to measure primary care orientation is simple: the portion of total health care expenses spent on primary care services. Although comparisons are difficult, it appears the United States spends a smaller (Koller and Khullar, 2017; PCC, 2018) to similar proportion (Berenson et al., 2020) of total expenses compared to other Organisation for Economic Co-operation and Development (OECD) countries, depending on the definition (OECD, 2018). In 2016, the year for which the most recent comparable data are available, the United States spent approximately 5.4 percent of total health expenditure on primary care, compared with an average among 22 OECD countries of 7.8 percent (OECD, 2019). Within the United States, higher state-level proportions of health care spending devoted to primary care are associated with fewer emergency department visits, total hospitalizations, and hospitalizations for ambulatory care–sensitive conditions (Jabbarpour et al., 2019). Given this, a fourth option for influencing the flow of funds to primary care teams focuses on a desired policy priority of increasing the share of health care spending devoted to primary care. To achieve this priority, policy makers would direct third-party payers to increase the proportion devoted to primary care and hold them accountable to achieving it.

This strategy was first developed in Rhode Island for commercial insurers as part of a set of Affordability Standards promulgated by the Office of the Health Insurance Commissioner (Koller et al., 2010). The original iteration of the Affordability Standards called on commercial insurers to raise their "primary care spend figure" by 1 percentage point per year for 5 consecutive years without adding to overall premiums. It also required the increased spending not be accomplished through FFS increases and authorized specific uses as qualifying, notably a statewide health information exchange. Oregon has now followed Rhode Island's lead, and at least six other states have passed laws for public measurement and sometimes set targets for insurers (Jabbarpour et al., 2019). For example, Delaware, at the end of 2020, released a report through its Department of Insurance developing affordability standards for health insurance premiums and setting targets for insurance carrier investment (Delaware DOI, 2020).

Achieving the goal of implementing high-quality primary care through a strategy of regulating the proportion of spend devoted to primary care offers several advantages. It increases available funds, a key constraint to implementing high-quality primary care, and though the portion to be reallocated is a relatively small amount of total health care expenses, it would have large marginal effects in the primary care sector. It also addresses the failure of private health plan negotiations or Medicare to recognize the collective social value of primary care. In addition, this approach is relatively simple to understand and focuses public prioritization of primary care and the social benefits it delivers (Bolnick et al., 2020).

However, operational and policy challenges to such a strategy remain:

- Defining the policy goal: Target additional resources toward all primary care or specifically the desired elements of it? Are all means of distribution of equal merit? For example, Rhode Island specifically directed that the increase not be in FFS rates.
- What constitutes an acceptable rate of spend? Current spend differs by payer type because of population characteristics—an older and sicker population, such as with Medicare, consumes a greater share of health care resources on acute care, while a younger, healthier child population consumes considerably smaller levels of resources, with a resulting much greater share to primary care (AHRQ, 2020; Rui and Okeyode, 2016).
- Administering the measure requires a standard, administrable definition of primary care, and oversight and enforcement mechanisms.
- Is the state willing and able to coordinate its policy levers? Rhode Island's work was for commercially insured populations only and did not extend to Medicaid or its public employees.

- The strategy is inherently redistributive, and while the amounts may be small, this strategy will generate public discussion and conflict over the relative value of different health care services.
- The multi-payer nature of U.S. health care financing dictates that any spending increase by one payer type will have only an incremental effect on overall spending on primary care services.

Since Rhode Island enacted its spending mandate, the share of commercial insurance spending going to primary care has risen from 5.7 percent in 2008 to 12.3 percent in 2018, with more than 55 percent of these payments now in non-FFS methods (OHIC, 2020). Unlike Rhode Island, Oregon's statute extends to health insurers in Medicare and Medicaid and requires health insurance carriers and the risk-bearing provider organizations in Medicaid to allocate at least 12 percent of their health care expenditures to primary care by 2023. As of 2018, insurers had met these requirements (OHA, 2019).

Researchers investigating the effects of Rhode Island's Affordability Standards have also found that since their implementation, commercial health insurance costs rose at a slower rate than in a matched comparison group (Baum et al., 2019). They attributed most of this effect to hospital price inflation caps rather than the primary care spend requirement but noted declines in outpatient use that are not statistically significant and could have resulted from more comprehensive primary care services. Oregon's primary care spend requirement has been coupled with the creation of a primary care transformation office in state government that establishes and implements statewide standards for patient-centered primary care homes (PCPCHs) and a statutorily established oversight commission. Evaluations of the PCPCH program have shown positive results on cost and quality (OHA, 2015).

Rhode Island's and Oregon's efforts show that it is possible to use government action to increase the portion of health care expenses going to primary care. Both initiatives have attempted to influence how this additional money is spent, without being overly prescriptive, and both have been underpinned by state law or regulation and public support, oversight, and accountability. Public oversight has enabled both states to build political support to continue with these policies despite the lack of objective evidence conclusively identifying their positive effects on spending and quality. This support is based on public recognition of the value of primary care, a compelling argument that an insufficient share of resources is dedicated to it, an acceptance that this imbalance will not be corrected without public action, and directionally favorable evidence (Koller and Khullar, 2017).

Implementing a primary care spend requirement remains vexing, however, primarily because the local leadership required to build political support and the overlapping state and federal authorities attenuate a requirement's effects. While oversight of commercial health insurance and Medicaid are the province of state officials, Medicare, Medicare Advantage, and self-insured arrangements remain the responsibility of federal authorities. Because health plans often administer self-insured arrangements and tend to operate with a common provider contract for both commercial and self-insured populations, there may be spillover effects to self-insured populations. Furthermore, with the notable exception of Rhode Island, commercial statutory standards for health insurers do not include system-wide affordability efforts, circumscribing regulators' authority to impose spending requirements without additional statute.

Although these remain fundamental barriers to any systemic approach to health care delivery system reform in the United States, existing state reforms have generated significant additional dollars flowing into primary care. To the extent that these are coordinated across multiple payment types, as is the case in Oregon, any resulting benefits in improved primary care capacity and performance are shared across all populations.

Findings for Option 4

- At a national level, primary care–oriented health care systems are associated with better population health and lower spending.
- The portion of total health care expenses going to primary care is a way to measure primary care orientation. By this measure, the United States is at or below the proportion in other developed countries.
- State-level policies to increase primary care spending rates have been politically sustainable, resulted in significant additional resources for primary care through non-FFS mechanisms, and supported statewide efforts to build primary care capacity. When coupled in Rhode Island with hospital price inflation caps to pay for increasing funds to primary care, there were attributable spending reductions.

PAYMENT AS A FACILITATOR OF HIGH-QUALITY PRIMARY CARE

In developing recommendations for payment policies to implement high-quality primary care—in addition to the evidence and experience on the effects of payment on cost, population health, and consumer experience—design considerations must be assessed, including the models' effect on the development and deployment of interprofessional teams, the delivery of integrated care across settings, the patient's relationship with the primary care team, and equity.

Primary Care Team–Patient Relationships

Throughout this report (most notably in Chapter 4), the committee has underscored the importance of the relationship between the primary care team and the patient. Ideally, this relationship is built on a foundation of trust and, relevant to payment specifically, a lack of conflict of interest (Emanuel and Dubler, 1995). The managed care era featured a concern over the erosion of clinician–patient relationships and patient trust (Gray, 1997; Mechanic, 1996; Mechanic and Schlesinger, 1996; Sulmasy, 1992), though few studies have measured the effect of payment models on clinician–patient relationships. One found that FFS patients had slightly higher levels of trust than those in salary, capitated, or managed care plans (Kao et al., 1998b). Most patients, however, did not know how their physician was paid, potentially indicating that payment model is not a salient issue for patients (Kao et al., 1998a). Patient trust and good interpersonal relationships with clinicians are major predictors of patient satisfaction and loyalty in primary care (Platonova et al., 2008), and many pay-for-performance programs include patient satisfaction measures. ACO and PCMH models have shown mixed effects on patient satisfaction, with some studies showing improvements (McWilliams et al., 2014b; Sarinopoulos et al., 2017) and others no association (Hong et al., 2018; Martsolf et al., 2012). Considering patient trust and satisfaction in any payment model design is of paramount importance, yet we have little evidence to guide payment based on research to date.

Finding

- Little consistent evidence suggests that payment models affect patient experience or clinician trust, but these considerations should be central to payment design.

Interprofessional Teams and Integrated Delivery of Care

Considerable evidence shows that high-quality primary care is best delivered by interprofessional teams in multiple settings (see Chapter 6). Chronic care, for example, requires routine telephonic or video access to nurse care managers, and the acutely ill need access to sophisticated diagnostic skills. Pregnant women often benefit from in-home education by community health workers, and children and families benefit from care within a medical home with team members focused on preventive care services and care coordination for children with medical and social complexity. FFS payment is not compatible with the committee's definition of high-quality primary care, in that it discourages person-centered, team-based care by requiring the identification of specific services delivered by contracted clinicians in permitted settings. Part of the appeal of capitated or bundled payment is the flexibility they offer for care in multiple settings from an integrated, interprofessional care team. This notion echoes that of the "New Primary Care Paradigm" (AAFP et al., 2020), a joint statement from seven PCP societies and boards that called for a shift from FFS payment to models that are compatible with care that is more person centered, team based, and integrated.

A specific example of this flexibility is the ability to integrate behavioral health care into primary care. Behavioral health care, when fully integrated, is effective in improving population health by addressing the underlying behavioral conditions that often manifest as somatic complaints (Basu et al., 2017; Reiss-Brennan et al., 2010, 2016). A meta-analysis of randomized controlled trials of integrated primary care–behavioral health models for children and adolescents demonstrated better outcomes for the integrated care model compared with usual care, with the strongest effects for collaborative care models in which PCPs, care managers, and mental health specialists took a team-based approach (Asarnow et al., 2015). FFS payment models, particularly when paired with subcontracts by insurers for the management of behavioral health benefits, can discourage this integration by imposing licensing and billing restrictions. In addition, research has shown that current payment models cannot sustain integrated behavioral health care (Reiss-Brennan et al., 2016).

Primary care practices organized in response to FFS payment maximize revenue-producing in-person visits but are not configured to provide the integrated team-based care necessary to address the comprehensive preventive and chronic care needs of people and families, which must include behavioral, social, and oral health. Most attempts to develop these capacities in practices have recognized that it is insufficient to merely begin to pay practices differently; it is also necessary to invest in sustainable transformation resources, such as technical assistance and reimbursing practices for revenues forfeited as a result of staff development time. Medicare's CPC+ payment model provides these additional resources through a combination of consultant payments and care management fees. Oregon has an office of primary care transformation funded through its Medicaid waiver. Some commercial insurance PCMH programs have provided similar transformation resources that are financed individually or jointly. Evidence has emerged that facilitating practice transformation improves and sustains the change process (Baskerville et al., 2012; Bitton, 2018; Harder et al., 2016). The ACA authorized a Primary Care Extension Program designed to support practice transformation facilitation. Though it was not funded, it became the basis for EvidenceNOW, a multi-state practice transformation trial funded by the Agency for Healthcare Research and Quality.

Findings

- FFS payment methods can discourage the integration of services in primary care.
- Payment support for external, supporting services, such as practice facilitation, is important for helping practices evolve but difficult to support with traditional FFS payments.

Equity

Equity is a critical element of high-quality primary care and financial barriers, along with structural and procedural characteristics, can enhance or limit equitable access to health care. However, the precise effects of payment models on access to care are elusive. Each payment method presents risks to equitable access that must be managed by the payer, often through contract terms and oversight.

Addressing SDOH, including housing, nutrition, and education, has been an important piece of improving equity in recent years. A recent National Academies report set forth specific recommendations for how health care organizations can integrate care that addresses SDOH (NASEM, 2019a). These activities, such as assisting in referrals to social services and aligning services with them, do have a cost, and practices must fund them through their revenues. Primary care–based models that have undertaken these activities, such as Vermont's Blueprint for Health, Rhode Island's Community Health Teams, and various Oregon coordinated care organizations, have relied on flexible payment arrangements, including capitation, that encourage team-based care.

A systematic review found reimbursement models have limited effects on socioeconomic and racial inequity in access, use, and quality of primary care. The review found capitation has a small beneficial impact on inequity in access to primary care and number of ambulatory care–sensitive admissions compared to FFS but performed worse on patient satisfaction (Tao et al., 2016). Another survey found only 16 percent of physician practices (including primary care practices) screened for SDOH. Among practices, federally qualified health centers, bundled payment participants, participants in primary care improvement models, and Medicaid ACOs had higher rates of screening for all needs (Fraze et al., 2019). By targeting health disparities as measures of performance, enabling fair comparisons among interprofessional teams based on their patient populations, and incorporating community input in payment design, payment models can promote equity (Crumley and McGinnis, 2019). See Chapter 5 for more on integrating social needs into primary care delivery.

Finding

- Enhanced primary care payments delivered through non-FFS mechanisms can improve the ability of primary care teams to coordinate social services and address inequitable access to services.

TECHNICAL CONSIDERATIONS

When thinking about options for payment reform, several technical aspects must be considered, including alignment of multiple payers, attribution of patients to health care organizations, and risk adjustment.

Multi-Payer Alignment

As noted earlier in this chapter, the committee is making recommendations based on the current reality in the United States of a fragmented hybrid public–private financing system. Two large public payers—Medicaid and Medicare—constitute close to 50 percent of health care payments and are often represented by many contracted MCOs (CMS, 2019c). The rest comes from the hundreds of insurers and third-party administrators who act as intermediaries for employers and other purchasers.

To accommodate this mix, a primary care office may have scores of insurance contracts, each potentially with different administrative rules, payment standards, and quality or cost measures. Setting aside the administrative expenses incurred by this system, the office operates in a sea of confusing financial incentives from insurers that not only have no incentive to coordinate payment terms but often see their payment methodologies as a source of competitive differentiation.

To influence a practice, any payment methodology that facilitates the implementation of high-quality primary care must be implemented consistently and at sufficiently broad scale. Some authors estimate the required penetration to be 60 percent of the practice's patients (CMS, 2011; Friedberg et al., 2015, 2018) to change its economic incentives (Anglin et al., 2017). This dictates that payers align payment practices, because apart from closed models, such as the Veterans Health Administration, no one payer, not even Medicare, reaches this figure.

Even if insurers in each geographic market accept the desirability of multi-payer alignment, they are forbidden from explicitly coordinating under federal antitrust laws (Takach et al., 2015). Several attempts to address this barrier have been undertaken. State officials may invoke a state action exemption, permissible under federal laws, and declare it in the state's interests for competing insurers to share certain information in a process actively overseen by state government, with a goal of aligning payment methodologies to primary care. Many states used this authority to secure multi-payer participation in PCMH models (AcademyHealth, 2010; Takach et al., 2015).

Under its CPC and CPC+ payment initiatives, CMMI has required multi-payer participation and alignment, rather than payment coordination. Payers make a commitment to payment models similar to CMMI's as a precondition to participation, with similarity adjudicated by CMMI based on a confidential review of the proposed model. The effects of the models' multi-payer design have not been assessed independent of the rest of the components, such as payment amounts and methodology, practice transformation resources, and practice feedback tools. Anecdotally, a multi-payer forum often facilitated by the CPC payment models to address areas of common concern and improvement, such as quality measurement alignment, practice transformation and feedback, and health information exchange, has been beneficial in markets for promoting both better payer/clinician relations and high-quality primary care.

Finally, the CMMI-funded Healthcare Payment Learning and Action Network has been an attempt to facilitate national multi-payer discussions focused on speeding the adoption of alternative payment models by public and private payers. Lacking authority, however, and subject to varying levels of interest and support in the succeeding administration, it remains a relatively weak lever for aligning payer activities.

In terms of fostering multi-payer alignment, the broad historical influence of Medicare's payment policies for physicians, hospitals, and ancillary providers on commercial and Medicaid payers is instructive. FFS physician payments predominate in the United States because of Medicare's policies and size—where it goes, other payers inevitably follow. CMMI's primary care payment models have defined the field of experimentation and yielded instructive experience. Other payers have also tested payment and delivery models and provided important technical support to practices, yet information about these models is less available in the public domain. The sooner Medicare can move from voluntary models to mandatory ones—agreeing on how to pay all primary care teams for Medicare beneficiaries—the more likely other payers are to fall in line. This alignment can then be facilitated by market-based efforts focused on other elements of primary care transformation, including measurement and feedback alignment.

Attribution

As discussed in Chapter 6, empanelment is an important component to high-quality primary care. It can be defined as a continuous, iterative set of processes that identify and assign populations to practices, care teams, or clinicians that have a responsibility to know their assigned population and proactively deliver coordinated primary care (Bearden et al., 2019). Under hybrid reimbursement or risk-sharing models, payers and clinicians need a clear definition of the people the risk-sharing entity is responsible for in order to measure cost and quality. Making sure any capitated payment goes to the correct practice when a patient retains full freedom of choice of clinician, as in traditional Medicare, Medicare Advantage, and commercial preferred provider organizations, and in many Medicaid programs, is necessary and challenging.

Payers use two processes to assign patients to clinicians: voluntary alignment and attribution. In voluntary alignment, patients document whom they consider to be their primary care clinician. Alternatively, they can be attributed to clinician organizations using care patterns in insurance claims data. Where possible, voluntary alignment is likely to be more compatible with the goals of high-quality primary care, by virtue of engaging people and their preferences, yet the process is administratively complex and rarely used (MedPAC, 2018a).

Claims-based attribution based on care patterns can be prospective, meaning that clinicians are given a list of whom they are responsible for in the beginning of the year, or retrospective, when they are notified at the end of the year. Most attribution rules assign patients based on the plurality of their outpatient visits, while some focus specifically on primary care services. The details are important; the specific services that qualify for attribution (only outpatient evaluation and management codes or a larger set of services), how the quantity of services is measured (e.g., number of visits or allowed charges), how clinicians are grouped into teams to determine plurality (by the system, practice, or individually), whether specialists or associates count toward attribution, and whether any preference is given to primary care clinicians each impact who is attributed and resulting outcomes.

Research has found substantial turnover in attribution year over year, yet most patients are attributable using retrospective methodology (e.g., 88 percent of Medicare beneficiaries are attributable based on evaluation and management visits) (Hsu et al., 2016; McWilliams et al., 2014a; Ouayogodé et al., 2018). One study found that although both prospective and retrospective attribution have benefits and drawbacks, retrospective attribution yielded greater overlap of attributed patients and those treated during the year and resulted in a higher proportion of care concentrated within an ACO (Lewis et al., 2013). Furthermore, certain patient populations are difficult to capture via attribution, including the healthy, who use few qualifying health care services, and those at the end of life (Ouayogodé et al., 2018).

Most of these research studies had no "gold standard" attribution to compare the alignment of various methodologies. An exception is a study of empaneled patients at The Mayo Clinic, where researchers compared five methods and found the proportion of patients correctly attributed to their paneled clinician was 22–45 percent, with ACO attribution capturing the most empaneled patients and marked variation in use and spending by method (McCoy et al., 2018). All stakeholders need to understand how differences in attribution method affect the way that health care is measured, evaluated, and reported (Higuera and Carlin, 2017; McCoy et al., 2016; Mehrotra et al., 2010; NQF, 2019).

Risk Adjustment

In any model where a portion of the payment is not FFS, or those services vary in intensity based on the illness and case complexity, risk adjustment is of paramount importance. Risk adjustment involves quantifying the patient's complexity based on observable data in order to adjust the payment. In the absence of strong risk adjustment for health status, clinicians might "cream-skim," or shun sicker, costlier patients who would take up more time and resources in favor of healthier ones for whom payment would be the same (Berenson et al., 2016).

Risk adjustment must address the time and effort clinicians provide for patients of different complexity. Risk adjustment for primary care capitation as a full replacement for PFS payment needs to be a much more accurate predictor of performance risk than in hybrid payment models that continue to include a substantial percentage of PFS payments; PFSs serve as a reasonably effective form of risk adjustment for most patients (because more complex patients typically generate more visits).

Some payment models adopt the standard hierarchical condition category (HCC) model of risk adjustment that was initially used for full risk Medicare Advantage plans (Pope et al., 2004). HCCs were designed to adjust payment via a dominant factor of predicting hospitalization spending. This tool makes sense if the primary care practice were held accountable for the total cost of care but may not be the best measure of the relative effort and practice-based resource expenditures for primary care teams managing patients with different complexities.

An alternative view is that primary care capitation should seek to adjust for "activity level," the care that primary care clinicians *should* provide, accounting for the variation between healthy and complex patients (Goroll et al., 2007). An assessment of one risk adjustment approach to support this payment model found that the predicted and apparent costs of providing comprehensive primary care vary more than 100-fold across patients. It also showed that sophisticated risk adjustment is required to adequately distinguish across such differences (Ash and Ellis, 2012).

Current methods of risk adjustment relying on diagnosis- and use-based algorithms to predict future use may not capture nonclinical contributors to patient complexity (Berry et al., 2015; Fuentes and Coker, 2018; Hong et al., 2015), which should include SDOH. Patients identified as complex by physicians had only modest overlap with those identified using claims data, because clinicians consider medical, behavioral, and socioeconomic complexity domains. Primary care clinicians' qualitative assessment of future hospitalization risk among patients in their panels was an important independent predictor of subsequent hospitalization (Hwang et al., 2017). A study of primary care practices participating in CPC found that adding clinical intuition to clinical algorithms was associated with higher enrollment in care management within primary care practices (Reddy et al., 2017). Other models have proposed simple risk assessment methods, such as relying on "How's Your Health" self-assessments of pain, emotional issues, medical complexity (polypharmacy), medication side effects, and health care confidence (Antonucci, 2018). Self-reported health measures may also provide a promising way to prospectively profile likely health care needs (Wherry et al., 2014). In the future, more electronic health record or self-reported measures could be added to risk adjustment, but the technology does not exist yet to do this comprehensively.

A payment formula that accounts for medical problems but ignores social risk can underpay for vulnerable populations, potentially exacerbating inequality (Ash et al., 2017; Schrager et al., 2016). Building on studies that found neighborhood deprivation was associated with worse health status, recent work has progressed in risk adjustment for social factors (Nobel et al., 2017). In 2016, Massachusetts began adjusting payments based on SDOH, adding predictors describing housing instability, behavioral health issues, disability, and neighborhood-level stressors (Ash, 2016; Ash and Mick, 2016). Medical spending in residents of the most stressed neighborhoods was more than 23 percent higher than that in the least stressed neighborhoods. Overall, the model including these social factors performed slightly better than the diagnosis-based model, explaining most spending variation and reducing underpayments for vulnerable populations (Ash et al., 2017). In addition to adjusting for the proportion of a practices' patients covered by Medicaid, Vermont uses an indicator variable for members with more than $500 in annual payments for "special Medicaid services" (day treatment, residential treatment, case management services, and special school services covered by the U.S. Department of Education) to adjust payments for social needs. This is in addition to adjustment for the proportion of a practice's patients covered by Medicaid insurance and an interaction term for Medicaid coverage and use of maternity services, given the high risk for poor outcomes (Finison et al., 2017).

Findings for Technical Considerations

- Multi-payer alignment across financial incentives, quality measurement, and data feedback is critical but challenging.
- The federal government plays an important role in convening and guiding multi-payer alignment.
- Antitrust law can be a barrier to multi-payer alignment, yet states can act to facilitate it.
- Reliable patient attribution at the practice level is fundamental to any non-FFS primary care payment methodology.
- Risk adjustment of any capitation payment is important for fair payment; the greater the share of payment made by capitation, the more important risk adjustment precision is. Diagnosis use-based algorithms are the most common. Mechanisms using social risk adjustment factors are being tested and have shown promise.

GOALS AND MEASURES OF SUCCESS FOR PRIMARY CARE PAYMENT

The measure of whether a payment system for primary care is effective requires an understanding of the goals of payment design. The delivery of high-quality primary care as defined by the committee should drive the design of a payment system to support it adequately and effectively. In the United States, unfortunately, the converse has been true for the last four decades: an idiosyncratic, not-fit-for-purpose payment system has driven the design of a volume- and visit-based delivery system unable to support the provision of continuous long-term relationships or a strong connection between primary care, the rest of the health care system, and relevant parts of public health. If adequately supported, primary care will offer societal benefits as well as individual ones. For this reason, the committee believes primary care should be a common good and that payment models should reflect this. Furthermore, as the COVID-19 pandemic has demonstrated, the current, piecemeal system built on a chassis of FFS is unable to withstand health or volume shocks, making primary care particularly vulnerable at moments when it is most needed to be consistently effective. The underlying FFS basis, with layers of value-based payment reform and complex and sometimes competing incentives to an already stretched workforce, often yields mixed results or unsustainable improvements.

Effective primary care will require higher levels of predictable payment that allow patients to build, maintain, and access long-term relationships with integrated care teams. As has been discussed in previous chapters, such relationships are formed in different clinician settings based on patient circumstances, and payment should be flexible to support all of them.

Getting to a level of adequate spending to support relationship-based care will take time and experimentation with a variety of hybrid models. As this chapter has shown, all payment designs have pros and cons. Multi-payer collaboration to create a mix of approaches that minimizes the drawbacks and effectively blends incentives matched to a particular community of patients and clinicians will likely work best, though this will need further empirical testing and validation. Furthermore, careful attribution and risk adjustment, including for social factors, will be key to ensure that primary care practices are paid sufficiently and equitably to take care of a clearly defined population for which they will be appropriately and fairly held accountable and to precipitate unintended consequences that could result in expanding, not diminishing, disparities in care.

The organization of primary care in the United States is quite diverse, and primary care payment models must match the capacity and capabilities of different organizations. Payers should continue to maintain a portfolio of primary care payment methods to accommodate different organizational structures, geographic cultural variations, and community realities, yet the hybrid reimbursement models reviewed here should constitute alternative base payment models, with an option remaining for the assumption of more financial risk. Primary care models oriented to comprehensive care for a broad population have different financial needs and risk tolerance than those focused on narrow segmentation for high-cost, high-need patients or a pediatric population, in which costs savings are a more long-term horizon and often attributed to sectors outside of health care. The committee believes it is important to maintain the diversity of primary care practice settings that currently exist but that a base-level, multi-payer hybrid reimbursement model, with reimbursement levels adequate to support an integrated, team-based care, should be the default rather than FFS.

Measuring the ultimate success of increasing both the levels and trends in primary care spending, while changing the type, is necessarily multimodal. At the practice level, it should encourage accountability and high performance for standards set forth in Chapter 8. Workforce measures, such as attrition, burnout, practice closure, and recruitment into the field, tell a deeply discouraging story (Steinwald et al., 2018), especially in underserved or historically marginalized communities. The ability and interest of primary care practices, especially independent ones, to continue to serve their communities despite often overwhelming pandemic and financial shocks is another measure of the success, or failure, of near-term payment reform.

Primary care alone should not be saddled with the burden of reducing the excessive costs of health care in the United States. Clear evidence (Song and Gondi, 2019) is emerging that primary care transformation and payment reform does not reduce total costs of care in the short or medium term, despite many stakeholders' best wishes. Over the long term, clear national and global evidence suggests that primary care–oriented systems with more robust primary care payment are more efficient than specialty-oriented and FFS payment models, but it can take decades to achieve these results (WHO, 2018). While in the medium term, strengthening primary care can achieve cost savings by reducing ambulatory care–sensitive emergency room visits and hospitalizations (Maeng et al., 2016; OECD, 2020; Saynisch et al., 2021), system-wide changes that reorient the health care workforce and practice patterns to primary care can take much longer (Friedberg et al., 2010). Thus, primary care payment reform should serve to start to rebalance the specialist–generalist ratios and spending in the United States but not have to assume that it can "pay for itself" in the short term.

Fundamentally, primary care payment reform should be thought of as an *investment* in future health asset capacity and equity production, instead of a simplistic return on investment for near-term savings. If cost savings are paramount, other means are more effective at reducing costs. What should motivate interested stakeholders more are the measures of population health, equitable outcomes, changing mortality and chronic disease prevalence trends, and overall increased health and well-being for individuals and families (OECD, 2020; WHO, 2018) that primary care can produce with larger, more predictable, payment (Basu et al., 2018).

Findings for Goals and Measures of Success

- Long-term payment reform plus redistribution toward primary care can deliver a reorientation of the entire health system toward more equitable and efficient goals.
- Primary care payment reform can be seen as an investment in future health system capacities and orientation, as opposed to a short-term driver of cost savings.
- Prospective, population-based payment can serve as a source of predictable revenue during times of crisis and service disruption.

FINDINGS AND CONCLUSIONS

Evidence shows that the dominant FFS payment mechanism, in combination with the process CMS uses to set relative prices for primary care and other services in the PFS, continues to devalue and shortchange primary care relative to its population health benefit, resulting in the large and widening gaps between primary care and specialty care compensation. In fact, using the portion of total health care expenses going to primary care as a measure of primary care orientation, the United States is at or below the proportion in other developed countries. This widening compensation gap is associated with reductions in medical trainees' likelihood of choosing primary care careers and with hospitals' graduate medical education training priorities. However, if CMS is provided with adequate leadership and resources to establish its own data collection and valuation tools, rather than relying on the RUC recommendations that reflect the dominance of specialty care in RUC membership, it has the authority to address the weaknesses of the current system and generate payment levels aligned with high-quality primary care.

Such action, however, would not negate the inherent shortcomings of FFS payment models. Evidence supports the finding that FFS models discourage successful engagement of primary care practices in structure and process improvements and the integration of other services into primary care, while hybrid payment models can mitigate FFS incentives for increased use and provide resources for integrated, team-based care and non-FFS services consistent with the committee's definition of high-quality primary care. In that respect, hybrid payment models should be seen as a mechanism to support high-quality care rather than a means of reducing spending and use in the short term. That said, in the long run, hybrid reimbursement models have potential to improve care and reduce use, particularly when they are aligned across payers and for people with multiple complex chronic conditions.

With almost half of primary care clinicians employed in health systems, attention should be paid to primary care payment methods in those settings. Many ACOs, which have demonstrated modest savings in total spending alongside quality and patient satisfaction improvements, continue to pay primary care internally based on FFS, even though the larger organization itself may participate in risk-sharing models. ACOs that are predominately primary care, PCMH based, or physician led achieve better performance (better population health and lower spending) than other ACOs. Some evidence indicates that pediatric-focused ACO models are effective.

State-level policies to increase primary care spending rates, which have been politically sustainable, resulted in significant additional resources for primary care through non-FFS mechanisms and supported statewide efforts to build primary care capacity. When coupled in Rhode Island with hospital price inflation caps to pay for increasing funds to primary care, there were attributable spending reductions. In addition, state-level action can address antitrust-associated barriers that can encourage multi-payer alignment across financial incentives, quality measurement, and data feedback, which can increase the likelihood of practice improvement in markets that lack one dominant payer. The federal government can also play an important role in convening and guiding multi-payer alignment.

In summary, primary care payment reform is an investment in future health system capacities and orientation. Long-term payment reforms plus redistribution toward primary care can reorient the entire health system, resulting in improved population health and greater health equity. While such reform may reduce health care expenditures in the long run, short-term cost savings should not be the priority policy outcome.

REFERENCES

AAFP (American Academy of Family Physicians). 2017a. *AAFP member survey provides valuable perspective.* https://www.aafp.org/news/blogs/inthetrenches/entry/20170801ITT_Survey.html (accessed September 4, 2020).

AAFP. 2017b. *Advanced primary care: A foundational alternative payment model (APC-APM) for delivering patient-centered, longitudinal, and coordinated care; a proposal to the Physician-Focused Payment Model Technical Advisory Committee.* Leawood, KS: American Academy of Family Physicians.

AAFP. 2020. *Direct primary care.* https://www.aafp.org/family-physician/practice-and-career/delivery-payment-models/direct-primary-care.html (accessed November 23, 2020).

AAFP, AAP (American Academy of Pediatrics), ABFM (American Board of Family Medicine), ABIM (American Board of Internal Medicine), ABP (American Board of Pediatrics), ACP (American College of Physicians), and SGIM (Society of General Internal Medicine). 2020. *A new primary care paradigm.* https://www.newprimarycareparadigm.org (accessed December 23, 2020).

AAP (American Academy of Pediatrics). 2019. *Pediatricians' practice and personal characteristics: U.S. only, 2018–2019.* https://www.aap.org/en-us/professional-resources/Research/pediatrician-surveys/Pages/Personal-and-Practice-Characteristics-of-Pediatricians-US-only.aspx (accessed December 18, 2020).

AAPA (American Academy of Physician Assistants). 2020. *Top 10 paying specialties in the PA profession.* https://www.aapa.org/news-central/2020/12/top-10-paying-specialties-in-the-pa-profession (accessed December 17, 2020).

Abelson, R. 2019. High medical bills are at center of hospital group's trial. *The New York Times,* October 3. https://www.nytimes.com/2019/10/03/health/sutter-hospitals-medical-bills.html (accessed December 18, 2020).

AcademyHealth. 2010. *Navigating antitrust concerns in multi-payer initiatives.* Washington, DC: AcademyHealth.

AHRQ (Agency for Healthcare Research and Quality). 2020. *Mean events per person by age groups, United States, 1996–2018.* https://www.meps.ahrq.gov/mepstrends/hc_use (accessed October 19, 2020).

Albright, B. B., V. A. Lewis, J. S. Ross, and C. H. Colla. 2016. Preventive care quality of Medicare accountable care organizations: Associations of organizational characteristics with performance. *Medical Care* 54(3):326–335.

Altman, S. H. 2012. The lessons of Medicare's prospective payment system show that the bundled payment program faces challenges. *Health Affairs* 31(9):1923–1930.

AMA (American Medical Association). 2016. *Composition of the RVS update committee (RUC).* https://www.ama-assn.org/about/rvs-update-committee-ruc/composition-rvs-update-committee-ruc (accessed September 8, 2020).

Anglin, G., H. A. Tu, K. Liao, L. Sessums, and E. F. Taylor. 2017. Strengthening multipayer collaboration: Lessons from the Comprehensive Primary Care Initiative. *Milbank Quarterly* 95(3):602–633.

Antonucci, J. 2018. *An innovative model for primary care office payment.* https://aspe.hhs.gov/system/files/pdf/255906/ProposalAntonucci.pdf (accessed February 1, 2021).

Asarnow, J. R., M. Rozenman, J. Wiblin, and L. Zeltzer. 2015. Integrated medical-behavioral care compared with usual primary care for child and adolescent behavioral health: A meta-analysis. *JAMA Pediatrics* 169(10):929–937.

Ash, A. 2016. *Masshealth risk adjustment model social determinants of health.* Boston, MA: Executive Office of Health & Human Services.

Ash, A. S., and R. P. Ellis. 2012. Risk-adjusted payment and performance assessment for primary care. *Medical Care* 50(8):643–653.

Ash, A., and E. Mick. 2016. *UMass risk adjustment project for Masshealth payment and care delivery reform: Describing the 2017 payment mode.* Worcester, MA: UMass Medical School Center for Health Policy and Research.

Ash, A. S., E. O. Mick, R. P. Ellis, C. I. Kiefe, J. J. Allison, and M. A. Clark. 2017. Social determinants of health in managed care payment formulas. *JAMA Internal Medicine* 177(10):1424–1430.

Baskerville, N. B., C. Liddy, and W. Hogg. 2012. Systematic review and meta-analysis of practice facilitation within primary care settings. *Annals of Family Medicine* 10(1):63–74.

Basu, S., B. E. Landon, J. W. Williams, Jr., A. Bitton, Z. Song, and R. S. Phillips. 2017. Behavioral health integration into primary care: A microsimulation of financial implications for practices. *Journal of General Internal Medicine* 32(12):1330–1341.

Basu, S., R. S. Phillips, A. Bitton, Z. Song, and B. E. Landon. 2018. Finance and time use implications of team documentation for primary care: A microsimulation. *Annals of Family Medicine* 16(4):308–313.

Basu, S., S. A. Berkowitz, R. L. Phillips, A. Bitton, B. E. Landon, and R. S. Phillips. 2019. Association of primary care physician supply with population mortality in the United States, 2005–2015. *JAMA Internal Medicine* 179(4):506–514.

Basu, S., R. S. Phillips, R. Phillips, L. E. Peterson, and B. E. Landon. 2020. Primary care practice finances in the United States amid the COVID-19 pandemic. *Health Affairs* 10.1377/hlthaff.2020.00794.

Baum, A., Z. Song, B. E. Landon, R. S. Phillips, A. Bitton, and S. Basu. 2019. Health care spending slowed after Rhode Island applied affordability standards to commercial insurers. *Health Affairs* 38(2):237–245.

Bearden, T., H. Ratcliffe, J. Sugarman, A. Bitton, L. Anaman, G. Buckle, M. Cham, D. Chong Woei Quan, F. Ismail, B. Jargalsaikhan, W. Lim, N. Mohammad, I. Morrison, B. Norov, J. Oh, G. Riimaadai, S. Sararaks, and L. Hirschhorn. 2019. Empanelment: A foundational component of primary health care. *Gates Open Research* 3(1654).

Berenson, R. A. 1989. Physician payment reform: Congress's turn. *Annals of Internal Medicine* 111(5):351–353.

Berenson, R. A., and J. D. Goodson. 2016. Finding value in unexpected places—fixing the Medicare physician fee schedule. *New England Journal of Medicine* 374(14):1306–1309.

Berenson, R. A., D. K. Upadhyay, S. F. Delbanco, and R. Murray. 2016. *Payment methods: How they work.* Washington, DC: Urban Institute.

Berenson, R. A., A. Shartzer, and R. C. Murray. 2020. *Strengthening primary care delivery through payment reform.* Paper commissioned by the Committee on Implementing High-Quality Primary Care. https://www.nap.edu/catalog/25983 (accessed May 4, 2021).

Berry, J. G., M. Hall, J. Neff, D. Goodman, E. Cohen, R. Agrawal, D. Kuo, and C. Feudtner. 2014. Children with medical complexity and Medicaid: Spending and cost savings. *Health Affairs* 33(12):2199–2206.

Berry, J. G., M. Hall, E. Cohen, M. O'Neill, and C. Feudtner. 2015. Ways to identify children with medical complexity and the importance of why. *Journal of Pediatrics* 167(2):229–237.

Bianco, D., C. Demars, L. Miller, and E. Sites. 2020. *The impact of federal value-based primary care programs on participating Oregon practices: A snapshot.* New York: Milbank Memorial Fund.

Bitton, A. 2018. Finding a parsimonious path for primary care practice transformation. *Annals of Family Medicine* 16(Suppl 1):S16–S19.

Bitton, A., C. Martin, and B. E. Landon. 2010. A nationwide survey of patient centered medical home demonstration projects. *Journal of General Internal Medicine* 25(6):584–592.

Bitton, A., G. R. Schwartz, E. E. Stewart, D. E. Henderson, C. A. Keohane, D. W. Bates, and G. D. Schiff. 2012. Off the hamster wheel? Qualitative evaluation of a payment-linked patient-centered medical home (PCMH) pilot. *Milbank Quarterly* 90(3):484–515.

Bitton, A., H. L. Ratcliffe, J. H. Veillard, D. H. Kress, S. Barkley, M. Kimball, F. Secci, E. Wong, L. Basu, C. Taylor, J. Bayona, H. Wang, G. Lagomarsino, and L. R. Hirschhorn. 2017. Primary health care as a foundation for strengthening health systems in low- and middle-income countries. *Journal of General Internal Medicine* 32(5):566–571.

Bleser, W. K., R. S. Saunders, D. Muhlestein, S. Q. Morrison, H. H. Pham, and M. McClellan. 2018. ACO quality over time: The MSSP experience and opportunities for system-wide improvement. *American Journal of Accountable Care* 6(1):e1–e15.

Bodenheimer, T. 2006. Primary care—will it survive? *New England Journal of Medicine* 355(9):861–864.

Bodenheimer, T. 2008. Coordinating care—a perilous journey through the health care system. *New England Journal of Medicine* 358(10):1064–1071.

Bolnick, H. J., A. L. Bui, A. Bulchis, C. Chen, A. Chapin, L. Lomsadze, A. H. Mokdad, F. Millard, and J. L. Dieleman. 2020. Health-care spending attributable to modifiable risk factors in the USA: An economic attribution analysis. *The Lancet Public Health* 5(10):e525–e535.

BPC (Bipartisan Policy Center). 2020. *Advancing comprehensive primary care in Medicaid.* Washington, DC: Bipartisan Policy Center.

Brown, C. C., and J. M. Tilford. 2020. *Value-based primary care: Insights from a commercial insurer in Arkansas.* New York: Milbank Memorial Fund.

Burton, R., R. Berenson, and S. Zuckerman. 2017. *Medicare's evolving approach to paying for primary care.* Washington, DC: Urban Institute.

Burton, R. A., N. M. Lallemand, R. A. Peters, and S. Zuckerman. 2018. Characteristics of patient-centered medical home initiatives that generated savings for Medicare: A qualitative multi-case analysis. *Journal of General Internal Medicine* 33(7):1028–1034.

Busch, F., D. Grzeskowiak, and E. Huth. 2020. *Direct primary care: Evaluating a new model of delivery and financing.* Schaumburg, IL: Society of Actuaries.

Calsyn, M., and M. Twomey. 2018. *Rethinking the RUC: Reforming how Medicare pays for doctors' services.* https://www.americanprogress.org/issues/healthcare/reports/2018/07/13/453159/rethinking-the-ruc (accessed December 7, 2020).

Carlo, A. D., L. Drake, A. D. H. Ratzliff, D. Chang, and J. Unützer. 2020. Sustaining the collaborative care model (COCM): Billing newly available COCM CPT codes in an academic primary care system. *Psychiatric Services* 71(9):972–974.

CHCS (Center for Health Care Strategies). 2017. *Medicaid ACO programs: Promising results from leading-edge states.* Trenton, NJ: Center for Health Care Strategies.

Chien, A. T., Z. Song, M. E. Chernew, B. E. Landon, B. J. McNeil, D. G. Safran, and M. A. Schuster. 2014. Two-year impact of the alternative quality contract on pediatric health care quality and spending. *Pediatrics* 133(1):96–104.

Christensen, E. W., and N. R. Payne. 2016. Effect of attribution length on the use and cost of health care for a pediatric Medicaid accountable care organization. *JAMA Pediatrics* 170(2):148–154.

Clemens, J., and J. D. Gottlieb. 2014. Do physicians' financial incentives affect medical treatment and patient health? *American Economic Review* 104(4):1320–1349.

Clemens, J., J. D. Gottlieb, and T. L. Molnár. 2015. *The anatomy of physician payment: Contracting subject to complexity.* Cambridge, MA: National Bureau of Economic Research.

CMS (Centers for Medicare & Medicaid Services). 2011. *Solicitation for the comprehensive primary care initiative.* Baltimore, MD: Centers for Medicare & Medicaid Services.

CMS. 2019a. *HHS news: HHS to delivery value-based transformation in primary care.* https://www.cms.gov/newsroom/press-releases/hhs-news-hhs-deliver-value-based-transformation-primary-care (accessed November 30, 2020).

CMS. 2019b. *National health expenditures 2019 highlights.* Baltimore, MD: Centers for Medicare & Medicaid Services.

CMS. 2019c. *National health expenditure data (by source of funds).* https://www.cms.gov/Research-Statistics-Data-and-Systems/Statistics-Trends-and-Reports/NationalHealth ExpendData/NationalHealthAccountsHistorical (accessed July 22, 2020).

CMS. 2020a. *Comprehensive primary care initiative.* https://innovation.cms.gov/innovation-models/comprehensive-primary-care-initiative (accessed July 20, 2020).

CMS. 2020b. *Comprehensive primary care plus.* https://innovation.cms.gov/innovation-models/comprehensive-primary-care-plus (accessed September 3, 2020).

CMS. 2020c. *Direct contracting model options.* https://innovation.cms.gov/innovation-models/direct-contracting-model-options (accessed September 3, 2020).

CMS. 2020d. Final rule and interim final rule: Medicare program; CY 2021 payment policies under the physician fee schedule and other changes to Part B payment policies; etc. As published on December 28, 2020. *Federal Register* 85(248). https://www.govinfo.gov/content/pkg/FR-2020-12-28/pdf/2020-26815.pdf (accessed March 11, 2021).

CMS. 2020e. Final rule: Medicaid program; Medicaid and Children's Health Insurance Program (CHIP) managed care. As published on November 13, 2020. *Federal Register* 85(220):72802–72807. https://www.govinfo.gov/content/pkg/FR-2020-11-13/pdf/2020-24758.pdf (accessed February 26, 2021).

CMS. 2020f. *Primary Care First model options.* https://innovation.cms.gov/innovation-models/primary-care-first-model-options (accessed September 3, 2020).

CMS. 2020g. *Primary Care First: Payment webinar.* Baltimore, MD: Centers for Medicare & Medicaid Services.

COGME (Council on Graduate Medical Education). 2010. *Advancing primary care.* Rockville, MD: Council on Graduate Medical Education.

Colla, C. H., T. Ajayi, and A. Bitton. 2020. Potential adverse financial implications of the merit-based incentive payment system for independent and safety net practices. *JAMA* 324(10):948–950.

Commonwealth Fund Task Force on Payment and Delivery System Reform. 2020. *Health care delivery system reform: Six policy imperatives.* Washington, DC: The Commonwealth Fund.

Coulam, R. F., and G. L. Gaumer. 1991. Medicare's prospective payment system: A critical appraisal. *Health Care Financing Review* (Annual Supplement):45–77.

Cromwell, J., and J. B. Mitchell. 1986. Physician-induced demand for surgery. *Journal of Health Economics* 5(4):293–313.

Crumley, D., and T. McGinnis. 2019. *Advancing health equity in Medicaid: Emerging value-based payment innovations.* https://www.chcs.org/advancing-health-equity-in-medicaid-emerging-value-based-payment-innovations (accessed July 20, 2020).

Cunningham, P., and J. May. 2006. Medicaid patients increasingly concentrated among physicians. *Tracking Report* (16):1–5.

Davis, K., M. Abrams, and K. Stremikis. 2011. How the Affordable Care Act will strengthen the nation's primary care foundation. *Journal of General Internal Medicine* 26(10):1201–1203.

Decker, S. L. 2012. In 2011 nearly one-third of physicians said they would not accept new Medicaid patients, but rising fees may help. *Health Affairs* 31(8):1673–1679.

Delaware DOI (Department of Insurance). 2020. *Delaware health care affordability standards: An integrated approach to improve access, quality and value.* Dover, DE: Delaware Department of Insurance.

Dewar, S., J. Bynum, and J. A. Batsis. 2020. Uptake of obesity intensive behavioral treatment codes in Medicare beneficiaries, 2012–2015. *Journal of General Internal Medicine* 35(1):368–370.

Doherty, R., N. S. Damle, J. A. Blehm, C. M. Reimer, M. Auron, E. Barrett, J. W. Fincher, A. L. Fuisz, C. S. Hunter, M. D. Leahy, M. D. Mignoli, R. McLean, A. L. Clark, M. Newman, J. O'Neill, Jr., C. M. Soppet, F. Syed, and M. P. Tschanz. 2015. Assessing the patient care implications of "concierge" and other direct patient contracting practices: A policy position paper from the American College of Physicians. *Annals of Internal Medicine* 163(12):949–952.

Dowd, B. E., and M. J. Laugesen. 2020. Fee-for-service payment is not the (main) problem. *Health Services Research* 55(4):491–495.

Doximity. 2019. *2019 physician compensation report: Third annual study.* San Francisco, CA: Doximity.

Dulsky Watkins, L. 2019. *Comprehensive primary care in Ohio and Kentucky—positive findings.* https://www.milbank.org/2019/01/comprehensive-primary-care-in-ohio-and-kentucky-positive-findings (accessed July 20, 2020).

Dwyer-Lindgren, L., A. Bertozzi-Villa, R. W. Stubbs, C. Morozoff, J. P. Mackenbach, F. J. van Lenthe, A. H. Mokdad, and C. J. L. Murray. 2017. Inequalities in life expectancy among U.S. counties, 1980 to 2014: Temporal trends and key drivers. *JAMA Internal Medicine* 177(7):1003–1011.

Edwards, S. T., A. Bitton, J. Hong, and B. E. Landon. 2014. Patient-centered medical home initiatives expanded in 2009–13: Providers, patients, and payment incentives increased. *Health Affairs* 33(10):1823–1831.

Ellis, R. P., and T. G. McGuire. 1990. Optimal payment systems for health services. *Journal of Health Economics* 9(4):375–396.

Emanuel, E. J., and N. N. Dubler. 1995. Preserving the physician–patient relationship in the era of managed care. *JAMA* 273(4):323–329.

Finison, K., M. Mohlman, C. Jones, M. Pinette, D. Jorgenson, A. Kinner, T. Tremblay, and D. Gottlieb. 2017. Risk-adjustment methods for all-payer comparative performance reporting in Vermont. *BMC Health Services Research* 17(1):58.

Fraze, T. K., A. L. Brewster, V. A. Lewis, L. B. Beidler, G. F. Murray, and C. H. Colla. 2019. Prevalence of screening for food insecurity, housing instability, utility needs, transportation needs, and interpersonal violence by us physician practices and hospitals. *JAMA Network Open* 2(9):e1911514.

Friedberg, M. W., P. S. Hussey, and E. C. Schneider. 2010. Primary care: A critical review of the evidence on quality and costs of health care. *Health Affairs* 29(5):766–772.

Friedberg, M. W., P. G. Chen, C. White, O. Jung, L. Raaen, S. Hirshman, E. Hoch, C. Stevens, P. B. Ginsburg, L. P. Casalino, M. Tutty, C. Vargo, and L. Lipinski. 2015. *Effects of health care payment models on physician practice in the United States.* Santa Monica, CA: RAND Corporation.

Friedberg, M. W., P. G. Chen, M. M. Simmons, T. Sherry, P. Mendel, L. Raaen, J. Ryan, P. Orr, C. Vargo, L. Carlasare, C. Botts, and K. Blake. 2018. *Effects of health care payment models on physician practice in the United States: Follow-up study.* Santa Monica, CA: RAND Corporation.

Fuentes, M., and T. R. Coker. 2018. Social complexity as a special health care need in the medical home model. *Pediatrics* 142(6).

Fujisawa, R., and G. Lafortune. 2008. The remuneration of general practitioners and specialists in 14 OECD countries. *OECD Health Working Papers* No. 14.

Galewitz, P. 2018. *Medicare advantage plans shift their financial risk to doctors.* https://www.modernhealthcare.com/article/20181008/NEWS/181009920/medicare-advantage-plans-shift-their-financial-risk-to-doctors (accessed October 17, 2020).

GAO (U.S. Government Accountability Office). 2012. *Higher use of advanced imaging services by providers who self-refer costing Medicare millions.* Washington, DC: U.S. Government Accountability Office.

GAO. 2015. *Medicare physician payment rates: Better data and greater transparency could improve accuracy.* Washington, DC: U.S. Government Accountability Office.

George, A., N. Sachdev, J. Hoff, S. Borg, T. Weida, M. O'Connor, and K. N. Davis. 2019. Development, value, and implications of a comprehensive primary care payment calculator for family medicine report from Family Medicine for America's Health Payment Tactic Team. *Family Medicine* 51(2):185–192.

Goroll, A. H., R. A. Berenson, S. C. Schoenbaum, and L. B. Gardner. 2007. Fundamental reform of payment for adult primary care: Comprehensive payment for comprehensive care. *Journal of General Internal Medicine* 22(3):410–415.

Gray, B. H. 1997. Trust and trustworthy care in the managed care era. *Health Affairs* 16(1):34–49.

Gruber, J., J. Kim, and D. Mayzlin. 1998. Physician fees and procedure intensity: The case of cesarean delivery. *NBER Working Paper Series* (Working Paper 6744).

Hadley, J. 2003. Sicker and poorer—the consequences of being uninsured: A review of the research on the relationship between health insurance, medical care use, health, work, and income. *Medical Care Research and Review* 60(Supplement to June 2003):3S–75S; discussion 76S–112S.

Harder, V. S., W. E. Long, S. E. Varni, J. Samuelson, and J. S. Shaw. 2016. Pediatric-informed facilitation of patient-centered medical home transformation. *Clinical Pediatrics* 56(6):564–570.

HCPLAN (Health Care Payment Learning & Action Network). 2019. *Measuring progress: Adoption of alternative payment models in commercial, Medicaid, Medicare Advantage, and traditional Medicare programs.* McLean, VA: The MITRE Corporation.

Hellinger, F. J. 1996. The impact of financial incentives on physician behavior in managed care plans: A review of the evidence. *Medical Care Research and Review* 53(3):294–314.

Higuera, L., and C. Carlin. 2017. A comparison of retrospective attribution rules. *American Journal of Managed Care* 23(6):e180–e185.

Hinton, E., R. Rudowitz, M. Diaz, and N. Singer. 2019. *10 things to know about Medicaid managed care.* San Francisco, CA: Kaiser Family Foundation.

Holgash, K., and M. Heberlein. 2019. Physician acceptance of new Medicaid patients: What matters and what doesn't. *Health Affairs Blog.* https://www.healthaffairs.org/do/10.1377/hblog20190401.678690/full (accessed December 18, 2020).

Hong, C. S., S. J. Atlas, J. M. Ashburner, Y. Chang, W. He, T. G. Ferris, and R. W. Grant. 2015. Evaluating a model to predict primary care physician-defined complexity in a large academic primary care practice-based research network. *Journal of General Internal Medicine* 30(12):1741–1747.

Hong, Y. R., K. Sonawane, S. Larson, A. G. Mainous, and N. M. Marlow. 2018. Impact of provider participation in ACO programs on preventive care services, patient experiences, and health care expenditures in U.S. adults aged 18–64. *Medical Care* 56(8):711–718.

Hsiao, W. C., D. L. Dunn, and D. K. Verrilli. 1993. Assessing the implementation of physician-payment reform. *New England Journal of Medicine* 328(13):928–933.

Hsu, J., M. Price, J. Spirt, C. Vogeli, R. Brand, M. E. Chernew, S. K. Chaguturu, N. Mohta, E. Weil, and T. Ferris. 2016. Patient population loss at a large Pioneer accountable care organization and implications for refining the program. *Health Affairs* 35(3):422–430.

Hwang, A., J. Ashburner, C. Hong, W. He, and S. Atlas. 2017. Can primary care physicians accurately predict the likelihood of hospitalization in their patients? *American Journal of Managed Care* 23:e127–e128.

IOM (Institute of Medicine). 2004. *Insuring America's health: Principles and recommendations*. Washington, DC: The National Academies Press.

IOM. 2009. *America's uninsured crisis: Consequences for health and health care*. Washington, DC: The National Academies Press.

Jabbarpour, Y., E. DeMarchis, A. Bazemore, and P. Grundy. 2017. *The impact of primary care practice transformation on cost, quality, and utilization*. Washington, DC: Patient-Centered Primary Care Collaborative, Robert Graham Center.

Jabbarpour, Y., M. Coffman, A. Habib, Y. Chung, W. Liaw, S. B. Gold, H. Jackson, A. Bazemore, and W. D. Marder. 2018. *Advanced primary care: A key contributor to successful ACOs*. Washington, DC: Patient-Centered Primary Care Collaborative.

Jabbarpour, Y., A. Greiner, A. Jetty, M. Coffman, C. Jose, S. Petterson, K. Pivaral, R. Phillips, A. Bazemore, and A. Neumann Kane. 2019. *Investing in primary care: A state-level analysis*. Washington, DC: Patient-Centered Primary Care Collaborative.

Jackson, G. L., B. J. Powers, R. Chatterjee, J. P. Bettger, A. R. Kemper, V. Hasselblad, R. J. Dolor, R. J. Irvine, B. L. Heidenfelder, A. S. Kendrick, R. Gray, and J. W. Williams. 2013. The patient centered medical home. A systematic review. *Annals of Internal Medicine* 158(3):169–178.

Jacobson, M., C. C. Earle, M. Price, and J. P. Newhouse. 2010. How Medicare's payment cuts for cancer chemotherapy drugs changed patterns of treatment. *Health Affairs* 29(7):1391–1399.

Kao, A. C., D. C. Green, N. A. Davis, J. P. Koplan, and P. D. Cleary. 1998a. Patients' trust in their physicians: Effects of choice, continuity, and payment method. *Journal of General Internal Medicine* 13(10):681–686.

Kao, A. C., D. C. Green, A. M. Zaslavsky, J. P. Koplan, and P. D. Cleary. 1998b. The relationship between method of physician payment and patient trust. *JAMA* 280(19):1708–1714.

Katz, S., and G. Melmed. 2016. How relative value units undervalue the cognitive physician visit: A focus on inflammatory bowel disease. *Gastroenterology & Hepatology* 12(4):240–244.

Kelleher, K. J., J. Cooper, K. Deans, P. Carr, R. J. Brilli, S. Allen, and W. Gardner. 2015. Cost saving and quality of care in a pediatric accountable care organization. *Pediatrics* 135(3):e582–e589.

Kern, L. M., A. Edwards, and R. Kaushal. 2016. The patient-centered medical home and associations with health care quality and utilization: A 5-year cohort study. *Annals of Internal Medicine* 164(6):395–405.

Kern, L. M., M. Rajan, H. A. Pincus, L. P. Cassalino, and S. S. Stuard. 2020. Health care fragmentation in Medicaid managed care vs. fee for service. *Population Health Management* 23(1):53–58.

KFF (Kaiser Family Foundation). 2019. *An overview of Medicare*. San Francisco, CA: Kaiser Family Foundation.

KFF. 2020. *Total Medicaid MCO enrollment: 2018*. https://www.kff.org/other/state-indicator/total-medicaid-mco-enrollment (accessed November 5, 2020).

Koller, C. F., and D. Khullar. 2017. Primary care spending rate—a lever for encouraging investment in primary care. *New England Journal of Medicine* 377(18):1709–1711.

Koller, C. F., T. A. Brennan, and M. H. Bailit. 2010. Rhode Island's novel experiment to rebuild primary care from the insurance side. *Health Affairs* 29(5):941–947.

Kralewski, J., E. Rich, R. Feldman, B. Dowd, T. Bernhardt, C. Johnson, and W. Gold. 2000. The effects of medical group practice and physician payment methods on costs of care. *Health Services Research* 35:591–613.

LaBonte, C. T., P. Payne, W. Rollow, M. W. Smith, A. Nissar, P. Holtz, and L. L. Sessums. 2019. Performance on electronic clinical quality measures in the Comprehensive Primary Care Initiative. *American Journal of Medical Quality* 34(2):119–126.

Laugesen, M. J. 2016. *Fixing medical prices: How physicians are paid*. Cambridge, MA: Harvard University Press.

Laugesen, M. J., R. Wada, and E. M. Chen. 2012. In setting doctors' medicare fees, CMS almost always accepts the relative value update panel's advice on work values. *Health Affairs* 31(5):965–972.

Lebrun-Harris, L. A., L. Shi, J. Zhu, M. T. Burke, A. Sripipatana, and Q. Ngo-Metzger. 2013. Effects of patient-centered medical home attributes on patients' perceptions of quality in federally supported health centers. *Annals of Family Medicine* 11(6):508–516.

Lewis, V. A., A. B. McClurg, J. Smith, E. S. Fisher, and J. P. Bynum. 2013. Attributing patients to accountable care organizations: Performance year approach aligns stakeholders' interests. *Health Affairs* 32(3):587–595.

Lopez, E., T. Neuman, and L. Levitt. 2020. *How much more than Medicare do private insurers pay? A review of the literature*. https://www.kff.org/medicare/issue-brief/how-much-more-than-medicare-do-private-insurers-pay-a-review-of-the-literature (accessed November 5, 2020).

Macinko, J., B. Starfield, and L. Shi. 2007. Quantifying the health benefits of primary care physician supply in the United States. *International Journal of Health Services* 37(1):111–126.

MACPAC (Medicaid and CHIP Payment and Access Commission). 2011. Section C: Managed care plans. In *Report to the Congress: The evolution of managed care in Medicaid*. Washington, DC: Medicaid and CHIP Payment and Access Commission. Pp. 41–54.

MACPAC. 2013. Medicaid primary care physician payment increase. In *Report to the Congress on Medicaid and CHIP*. Washington, DC: Medicaid and CHIP Payment and Access Commission. Pp. 47–60.

MACPAC. 2020. *Provider payment and delivery systems*. https://www.macpac.gov/medicaid-101/provider-payment-and-delivery-systems (accessed October 17, 2020).

Maeng, D. D., J. P. Sciandra, and J. F. Tomcavage. 2016. The impact of a regional patient-centered medical home initiative on cost of care among commercially insured population in the U.S. *Risk Management and Healthcare Policy* 9:67–74.

Martin, S., R. L. Phillips, Jr., S. Petterson, Z. Levin, and A. W. Bazemore. 2020. Primary care spending in the United States, 2002–2016. *JAMA Internal Medicine* 180(7):1019–1020.

Martsolf, G. R., J. A. Alexander, Y. Shi, L. P. Casalino, D. R. Rittenhouse, D. P. Scanlon, and S. M. Shortell. 2012. The patient-centered medical home and patient experience. *Health Services Research* 47(6):2273–2295.

McCall, N., J. Cromwell, and P. Braun. 2006. Validation of physician survey estimates of surgical time using operating room logs. *Medical Care Research and Review* 63(6):764–777.

McCarty, N. 2013. Complexity, capacity, and capture. In *Preventing regulatory capture: Special interest influence and how to limit it*, edited by D. Carpenter and D. A. Moss. Cambridge, UK: Cambridge University Press. Pp. 99–123.

McConnell, K. J., S. Renfro, B. K. S. Chan, T. H. A. Meath, A. Mendelson, D. Cohen, J. Waxmonsky, D. McCarty, N. Wallace, and R. C. Lindrooth. 2017. Early performance in Medicaid accountable care organizations: A comparison of Oregon and Colorado. *JAMA Internal Medicine* 177(4):538–545.

McConnell, K. J., C. J. Charlesworth, T. H. A. Meath, R. M. George, and H. Kim. 2018. Oregon's emphasis on equity shows signs of early success for black and American Indian Medicaid enrollees. *Health Affairs* 37(3):386–393.

McCoy, R. G., S. M. Tulledge-Scheitel, J. M. Naessens, A. E. Glasgow, R. J. Stroebel, S. J. Crane, K. S. Bunkers, and N. D. Shah. 2016. The method for performance measurement matters: Diabetes care quality as measured by administrative claims and institutional registry. *Health Services Research* 51(6):2206–2220.

McCoy, R. G., K. S. Bunkers, P. Ramar, S. K. Meier, L. L. Benetti, R. E. Nesse, and J. M. Naessens. 2018. Patient attribution: Why the method matters. *American Journal of Managed Care* 24(12):596–603.

McWilliams, J. M., M. E. Chernew, J. B. Dalton, and B. E. Landon. 2014a. Outpatient care patterns and organizational accountability in Medicare. *JAMA Internal Medicine* 174(6):938–945.

McWilliams, J. M., B. E. Landon, M. E. Chernew, and A. M. Zaslavsky. 2014b. Changes in patients' experiences in Medicare accountable care organizations. *New England Journal of Medicine* 371(18):1715–1724.

McWilliams, J. M., L. A. Hatfield, B. E. Landon, P. Hamed, and M. E. Chernew. 2018. Medicare spending after 3 years of the Medicare shared savings program. *New England Journal of Medicine* 379(12):1139–1149.

Mechanic, D. 1996. Changing medical organization and the erosion of trust. *Milbank Quarterly* 74(2):171–189.

Mechanic, D., and M. Schlesinger. 1996. The impact of managed care on patients' trust in medical care and their physicians. *JAMA* 275(21):1693–1697.

MedPAC (Medicare Payment Advisory Commission). 2006. *Report to the Congress: Medicare payment policy.* Washington, DC: Medicare Payment Advisory Commission.

MedPAC. 2015. *Report to the Congress: Medicare payment policy.* Washington, DC: Medicare Payment Advisory Commission.

MedPAC. 2018a. *Comment letter to CMS re: File code CMS-1701-P.* http://www.medpac. gov/docs/default-source/comment-letters/10152018_aco_2018_medpac_comment_v2_ sec283312adfa9c665e80adff00009edf9c.pdf (accessed February 1, 2021).

MedPAC. 2018b. *Report to the Congress: Medicare and the health care delivery system.* Washington, DC: Medicare Payment Advisory Commmission.

MedPAC. 2019. *Report to the Congress: Medicare and the health care delivery system.* Washington, DC: Medicare Payment Advisory Commission.

MedPAC. 2020a. *A data book: Health care spending and the Medicare program.* Washington, DC: Medicare Payment Advisory Commission.

MedPAC. 2020b. *Report to the Congress: Fact sheet (updated).* Washington, DC: Medicare Payment Advisory Commission.

Mehrotra, A., J. L. Adams, J. W. Thomas, and E. A. McGlynn. 2010. The effect of different attribution rules on individual physician cost profiles. *Annals of Internal Medicine* 152(10):649–654.

Meltzer, D. O. 2018. *The Comprehensive Care Physician Payment Model (CCP-PM).* Chicago, IL: The University of Chicago.

Merrell, K., C. Schur, and T. Oberlander. 2014. *Analysis of physician time use patterns under the Medicare fee schedule.* Washington, DC: Social & Scientific Systems, Urban Institute.

Muhlestein, D., W. K. Bleser, R. S. Saunders, R. Richards, E. Singletary, and M. B. Mcclellan. 2019. Spread of ACOs and value-based payment models in 2019: Gauging the impact of pathways to success. *Health Affairs Blog.* https://www.healthaffairs.org/do/10.1377/ hblog20191020.962600/full (accessed December 18, 2020).

Mulcahy, A. W., T. Gracner, and K. Finegold. 2018. Associations between the Patient Protection and Affordable Care Act Medicaid primary care payment increase and physician participation in Medicaid. *JAMA Internal Medicine* 178(8):1042–1048.

Mulcahy, A. W., K. Merrell, and A. Mehrotra. 2020. Payment for services rendered—updating Medicare's valuation of procedures. *New England Journal of Medicine* 382(4):303–306.

NAACOS (National Association of ACOs). 2020. *State ACO activities.* https://www.naacos. com/medicaid-acos (accessed October 17, 2020).

NASEM (National Academies of Sciences, Engineering, and Medicine). 2019a. *Integrating social care into the delivery of health care: Moving upstream to improve the nation's health.* Washington, DC: The National Academies Press.

NASEM. 2019b. *Vibrant and healthy kids: Aligning science, practice, and policy to advance health equity.* Washington, DC: The National Academies Press.

Navathe, A. S., E. J. Emanuel, A. Bond, K. Linn, K. Caldarella, A. Troxel, J. Zhu, L. Yang, S. E. Matloubieh, E. Drye, S. Bernheim, E. O. Lee, M. Mugiishi, K. T. Endo, J. Yoshimoto, I. Yuen, S. Okamura, M. Stollar, J. Tom, M. Gold, and K. G. Volpp. 2019. Association between the implementation of a population-based primary care payment system and achievement on quality measures in Hawaii. *JAMA* 322(1):57–68.

Nicholson, S., and N. S. Souleles. 2001. *Physician income expectations and specialty choice.* Cambridge, MA: National Bureau of Economic Research.

Nobel, L., W. M. Jesdale, J. Tjia, M. E. Waring, D. C. Parish, A. S. Ash, C. I. Kiefe, and J. J. Allison. 2017. Neighborhood socioeconomic status predicts health after hospitalization for acute coronary syndromes: Findings from TRACE-CORE (transitions, risks, and actions in coronary events-center for outcomes research and education). *Medical Care* 55(12):1008–1016.

NQF (National Quality Forum). 2019. *Attribution: Principles and approaches.* Washington, DC: National Quality Forum.

Nurse.org. 2020. *15 highest paying nursing jobs in 2021.* https://nurse.org/articles/15-highest-paying-nursing-careers (accessed December 17, 2020).

OECD (Organisation for Economic Co-operation and Development). 2018. *Spending on primary care: First estimates.* Paris, France: Organisation for Economic Co-operation and Development.

OECD. 2019. *Deriving preliminary estimates of primary care spending under the SHA 2011 framework.* Paris, France: Organisation for Economic Co-operation and Development.

OECD. 2020. *Realising the potential of primary health care.* Paris, France: Organisation for Economic Co-operation and Development.

OHA (Oregon Health Authority). 2015. *The Oregon Health Authority patient-centered primary care home program: 2014–2015 annual report.* Salem, OR: Oregon Health Authority.

OHA. 2019. *Primary care spending in Oregon: A report to the Oregon legislature.* Salem, OR: Oregon Health Authority.

OHIC (Office of the Health Insurance Commissioner). 2020. *Primary care spending data update.* Cranston, RI: Office of the Health Insurance Commissioner.

Ouayogodé, M. H., C. H. Colla, and V. A. Lewis. 2017. Determinants of success in shared savings programs: An analysis of ACO and market characteristics. *Healthcare* 5(1–2):53–61.

Ouayogodé, M. H., E. Meara, C. H. Chang, S. R. Raymond, J. P. W. Bynum, V. A. Lewis, and C. H. Colla. 2018. Forgotten patients: ACO attribution omits those with low service use and the dying. *American Journal of Managed Care* 24(7):e207–e215.

PAI (Physicians Advocacy Institute). 2020. *2020 Merit-Based Incentive Payment System (MIPS) overview.* Raleigh, NC: Physicians Advocacy Institute.

Park, S., J. F. Figueroa, P. Fishman, and N. B. Coe. 2020. Primary care utilization and expenditures in traditional Medicare and Medicare Advantage, 2007–2016. *Journal of General Internal Medicine* 35(8):2480–2481.

PCC (Primary Care Collaborative). 2018. *Fact sheet: Spending for primary care.* Washington, DC: Primary Care Collaborative.

Peck, K. A., B. Usadi, A. J. Mainor, E. S. Fisher, and C. H. Colla. 2019. ACO contracts with downside financial risk growing, but still in the minority. *Health Affairs* 38(7):1201–1206.

Peikes, D., G. Anglin, S. Dale, E. F. Taylor, A. O'Malley, A. Ghosh, K. Swankoski, J. Crosson, R. Keith, A. Mutti, S. Hoag, P. Singh, H. Tu, T. Grannemann, M. Finucane, A. Zutshi, L. Vollmer, and R. Brown. 2018. *Evaluation of the Comprehensive Primary Care Initiative: Fourth annual report.* Princeton, NJ: Mathematica Policy Research.

Peikes, D., E. F. Taylor, A. S. O'Malley, and E. C. Rich. 2020. The changing landscape of primary care: Effects of the ACA and other efforts over the past decade. *Health Affairs* 39(3):421–428.

Peiris, D., M. C. Phipps-Taylor, C. A. Stachowski, L. S. Kao, S. M. Shortell, V. A. Lewis, M. B. Rosenthal, and C. H. Colla. 2016. ACOs holding commercial contracts are larger and more efficient than noncommercial ACOs. *Health Affairs* 35(10):1849–1856.

Perrin, J. M., E. Zimmerman, A. Hertz, T. Johnson, T. Merrill, and D. Smith. 2017. Pediatric accountable care organizations: Insight from early adopters. *Pediatrics* 139(2):e20161840.

Perrin, J. M., G. M. Kenney, and S. Rosenbaum. 2020. Medicaid and child health equity. *New England Journal of Medicine* 383(27):2595–2598.

Phillips, R. L., Jr., and A. W. Bazemore. 2010. Primary care and why it matters for U.S. health system reform. *Health Affairs* 29(5):806–810.

Phillips, R. L., Jr., M. Dodoo, S. Petterson, I. Xierali, A. Bazemore, B. Teevan, K. Bennett, C. Legagneur, J. Rudd, and J. Phillips. 2009. *Specialty and geographic distribution of the physician workforce: What influences medical student and resident choices?* Washington, DC: Robert Graham Center.

Phillips, R. L., Jr., A. Bazemore, and A. Baum. 2020. The COVID-19 tsunami: The tide goes out before it comes in. *Health Affairs Blog.* https://www.healthaffairs.org/do/10.1377/hblog20200415.293535/full (accessed December 18, 2020).

Platonova, E. A., K. N. Kennedy, and R. M. Shewchuk. 2008. Understanding patient satisfaction, trust, and loyalty to primary care physicians. *Medical Care Research and Review* 65(6):696–712.

Polsky, D., M. Richards, S. Basseyn, D. Wissoker, G. M. Kenney, S. Zuckerman, and K. V. Rhodes. 2015. Appointment availability after increases in Medicaid payments for primary care. *New England Journal of Medicine* 372(6):537–545.

Pope, G. C., J. Kautter, R. P. Ellis, A. S. Ash, J. Z. Ayanian, L. I. Lezzoni, M. J. Ingber, J. M. Levy, and J. Robst. 2004. Risk adjustment of Medicare capitation payments using the CMS-HCC model. *Health Care Financing Review* 25(4):119–141.

Quinn, K. 2015. The 8 basic payment methods in health care. *Annals of Internal Medicine* 163(4):300–306.

Rama, A. 2017. *Payment and delivery in 2016: The prevalence of medical homes, accountable care organizations, and payment methods reported by physicians.* Chicago, IL: American Medical Association.

Reddy, A., L. Sessums, R. Gupta, J. Jin, T. Day, B. Finke, and A. Bitton. 2017. Risk stratification methods and provision of care management services in Comprehensive Primary Care Initiative practices. *Annals of Family Medicine* 15(5):451–454.

Reddy, A., L. M. Marcotte, L. Zhou, S. D. Fihn, and J. M. Liao. 2020. Use of chronic care management among primary care clinicians. *Annals of Family Medicine* 18(5):455–457.

Reid, R., C. Damberg, and M. W. Friedberg. 2019. Primary care spending in the fee-for-service Medicare population. *JAMA Internal Medicine* 179(7):977–980.

Reiff, J., N. Brennan, and J. Fuglesten Biniek. 2019. Primary care spending in the commercially insured population. *JAMA* 322(22):2244–2245.

Reiss-Brennan, B., P. C. Briot, L. A. Savitz, W. Cannon, and R. Staheli. 2010. Cost and quality impact of Intermountain's mental health integration program. *Journal of Healthcare Management* 55(2):97–113; discussion 113–114.

Reiss-Brennan, B., K. D. Brunisholz, C. Dredge, P. Briot, K. Grazier, A. Wilcox, L. Savitz, and B. James. 2016. Association of integrated team-based care with health care quality, utilization, and cost. *JAMA* 316(8):826–834.

Rice, T. H. 1983. The impact of changing Medicare reimbursement rates on physician-induced demand. *Medical Care* 21(8):803–815.

Robinson, J. C. 2001. Theory and practice in the design of physician payment incentives. *Milbank Quarterly* 79(2):iii, 149–177.

Rosenbaum, S. 2009. *Medicaid payment rate lawsuits: Evolving court views mean uncertain future for Medi-Cal.* Sacramento, CA: California Health Care Foundation.

Rosenbaum, S. 2020. Children and Medicaid: Will the courts be there when they need them? *Academic Pediatrics* 20(2):157–159.

Rosenthal, M., S. Shortell, N. D. Shah, D. Peiris, V. A. Lewis, J. A. Barrera, B. Usadi, and C. H. Colla. 2019. Physician practices in accountable care organizations are more likely to collect and use physician performance information, yet base only a small proportion of compensation on performance data. *Health Services Research* 54(6):1214–1222.

Rui, P., and T. Okeyode. 2016. *National Ambulatory Medical Care Survey: 2016 national summary tables*. Atlanta, GA: Centers for Disease Control and Prevention.

Salzberg, C. A., A. Bitton, S. R. Lipsitz, C. Franz, S. Shaykevich, L. P. Newmark, J. Kwatra, and D. W. Bates. 2017. The impact of alternative payment in chronically ill and older patients in the patient-centered medical home. *Medical Care* 55(5):483–492.

Sarinopoulos, I., D. L. Bechel-Marriott, J. M. Malouin, S. Zhai, J. C. Forney, and C. L. Tanner. 2017. Patient experience with the patient-centered medical home in Michigan's statewide multi-payer demonstration: A cross-sectional study. *Journal of General Internal Medicine* 32(11):1202–1209.

Saynisch, P. A., G. David, B. Ukert, A. Agiro, S. H. Scholle, and T. Oberlander. 2021. Model homes: Evaluating approaches to patient-centered medical home implementation. *Medical Care* 59(3):206–212.

Schlenker, R. E., M. C. Powell, and G. K. Goodrich. 2005. Initial home health outcomes under prospective payment. *Health Services Research* 40(1):177–193.

Schrager, S. M., K. C. Arthur, J. Nelson, A. R. Edwards, J. M. Murphy, R. Mangione-Smith, and A. Y. Chen. 2016. Development and validation of a method to identify children with social complexity risk factors. *Pediatrics* 138(3).

Schroeder, S. A., and W. Frist. 2013. Phasing out fee-for-service payment. *New England Journal of Medicine* 368(21):2029–2032.

Shapiro, S. 2008. Does the amount of participation matter? Public comments, agency responses and the time to finalize a regulation. *Policy Sciences* 41(1):33–49.

Shi, L. 2012. The impact of primary care: A focused review. *Scientifica* 2012:432892.

Siddiqui, M., and S. A. Berkowitz. 2014. Shared savings models for ACOs—incentivizing primary care physicians. *Journal of General Internal Medicine* 29(6):832–834.

Sinaiko, A. D., M. B. Landrum, D. J. Meyers, S. Alidina, D. D. Maeng, M. W. Friedberg, L. M. Kern, A. M. Edwards, S. P. Flieger, P. R. Houck, P. Peele, R. J. Reid, K. McGraves-Lloyd, K. Finison, and M. B. Rosenthal. 2017. Synthesis of research on patient-centered medical homes brings systematic differences into relief. *Health Affairs* 36(3):500–508.

Song, Z., and S. Gondi. 2019. Will increasing primary care spending alone save money? *JAMA* 322(14):1349–1350.

Song, Z., S. Rose, M. E. Chernew, and D. G. Safran. 2017. Lower- versus higher-income populations in the Alternative Quality Contract: Improved quality and similar spending. *Health Affairs* 36(1):74–82.

Song, Z., Y. Ji, D. G. Safran, and M. E. Chernew. 2019. Health care spending, utilization, and quality 8 years into global payment. *New England Journal of Medicine* 381(3):252–263.

Steinwald, B., P. Ginsburg, C. Brandt, S. Lee, and K. Patel. 2018. *Medicare graduate medical education funding is not addressing the primary care shortage: We need a radically different approach*. Washington, DC: The Brookings Institution.

Sulmasy, D. P. 1992. Physicians, cost control, and ethics. *Annals of Internal Medicine* 116(11):920–926.

Takach, M., C. Townley, R. Yalowich, and S. Kinsler. 2015. Making multipayer reform work: What can be learned from medical home initiatives. *Health Affairs* 34(4):662–672.

Tao, W., J. Agerholm, and B. Burstrom. 2016. The impact of reimbursement systems on equity in access and quality of primary care: A systematic literature review. *BMC Health Services Research* 16(1):542.

The Larry A. Green Center and PCC (Primary Care Collaborative). 2020. *Quick COVID-19 primary care survey: Clinician series 9 fielded May 8–11, 2020.* https://www.green-center. org/covid-survey (accessed September 15, 2020).

The Lewin Group. 2015. *Health practitioner bonuses and their impact on the availability and utilization of primary care services.* Falls Church, VA: The Lewin Group.

Tingley, K. 2018. Trying to put a value on the doctor-patient relationship. *The New York Times Magazine.* https://www.nytimes.com/interactive/2018/05/16/magazine/health-is-sue-reinvention-of-primary-care-delivery.html (accessed December 18, 2020).

Trish, E., P. Ginsburg, L. Gascue, and G. Joyce. 2017. Physician reimbursement in Medicare Advantage compared with traditional Medicare and commercial health insurance. *JAMA Internal Medicine* 177(9):1287–1295.

van den Berk-Clark, C., E. Doucette, F. Rottnek, W. Manard, M. A. Prada, R. Hughes, T. Lawrence, and F. D. Schneider. 2018. Do patient-centered medical homes improve health behaviors, outcomes, and experiences of low-income patients? A systematic review and meta-analysis. *Health Services Research* 53(3):1777–1798.

Veet, C. A., T. R. Radomski, C. D'Avella, I. Hernandez, C. Wessel, E. C. S. Swart, W. H. Shrank, and N. Parekh. 2020. Impact of healthcare delivery system type on clinical, utilization, and cost outcomes of patient-centered medical homes: A systematic review. *Journal of General Internal Medicine* 35(4):1276–1284.

Weida, N. A., R. L. Phillips, Jr., and A. W. Bazemore. 2010. Does graduate medical education also follow green? *Archives of Internal Medicine* 170(4):389–390.

Wen, H., J. M. Hockenberry, and J. R. Cummings. 2014. The effect of substance use disorder treatment use on crime: Evidence from public insurance expansions and health insurance parity mandates. *NBER Working Paper Series* (Working Paper No. 20537).

Wherry, L. R., M. E. Burns, and L. J. Leininger. 2014. Using self-reported health measures to predict high-need cases among Medicaid-eligible adults. *Health Services Research* 49(2):2147–2172.

WHO (World Health Organization). 2018. *Building the economic case for primary health care: A scoping review.* Geneva, Switzerland: World Health Organization.

Wynn, B. O., L. F. Burgette, A. W. Mulcahy, E. N. Okeke, I. Brantley, N. Iyer, T. Ruder, and A. Mehrotra. 2015. *Development of a model for the validation of work relative value units for the Medicare physician fee schedule.* Santa Monica, CA: RAND Corporation.

Zabar, S., A. Wallach, and A. Kalet. 2019. The future of primary care in the United States depends on payment reform. *JAMA Internal Medicine* 179(4):515–516.

Zimmerman, E., and S. H. Woolf. 2014. *Understanding the relationship between education and health.* Discussion Paper, Institute of Medicine, Washington, DC. https://nam.edu/perspectives-2014-understanding-the-relationship-between-education-and-health (accessed April 12, 2021).

Zuckerman, S., and D. Goin. 2012. *How much will Medicaid physician fees for primary care rise in 2013? Evidence from a 2012 survey of Medicaid physician fees.* Washington, DC: Kaiser Family Foundation.

Zuckerman, S., K. Merrell, R. A. Berenson, N. Cafarella Lallemand, and J. Sunshine. 2015. *Realign physician payment incentives in Medicare to achieve payment equity among specialties, expand the supply of primary care physicians, and improve the value of care for beneficiaries.* Washington, DC: Urban Institute, Social & Scientific Systems Inc.

Zuckerman, S., K. Merrell, R. Berenson, S. Mitchel, D. Upadhyay, and R. Lewis. 2016. *Collecting empirical physician time data: Piloting an approach for validating work relative value units.* Washington, DC: Urban Institute.

Zuckerman, S., L. Skopec, and M. Epstein. 2017. *Medicaid physician fees after the ACA primary care fee bump: 19 states continue the Affordable Care Act's temporary policy change.* Washington, DC: Urban Institute.

Zuvekas, S. H., and J. W. Cohen. 2016. Fee-for-service, while much maligned, remains the dominant payment method for physician visits. *Health Affairs* 35(3):411–414.

10

Enhancing Research
in Primary Care

Primary care is the only function within the health care system responsible for all people in the population. It is the platform where more than one-third of all health care visits are made (Johansen et al., 2016), and, for many, the only place they seek care. Nonetheless, with few exceptions, primary care largely depends on evidence derived from research on subspecialty care, hospital settings, or single-disease cohorts (Petterson et al., 2014). Primary care practice–based research networks (Hickner and Green, 2015; Phillips et al., 2007b) have famously turned our understanding of disease and treatment on its head regarding brown recluse bites (Mold and Thompson, 2004), depression, upper respiratory infections, heart failure, unstable angina, and radiologic examinations of headaches, among many other topics (Westfall et al., 2007), by studying the epidemiology of symptoms, conditions, and treatments in the settings where illness often first presents (Westfall et al., 2007). Research has also demonstrated that how primary care clinical data are collected and organized can enable translating electronic clinical data into probability engines for clinical decision making and research into how symptoms become disease and how disease treatment affects outcomes (Eberl et al., 2008; Soler et al., 2008).

The neglect of basic primary care research (PCR), and lack of research that draws on primary care–specific databases, such as clinical registries, not only adversely affects primary care outcomes but also leads to the lack of a population-based understanding of illness and disease along the health care spectrum. Better PCR support could lead to answers to questions that are critically important for improving population health. For example, adequate support could propel pioneering work regarding how best to incorporate data on the social determinants of health (SDOH) into clinical decision making. Such studies could also help health care systems and society at large better address patients' important social needs as a means of improving health outcomes (Cottrell et al., 2018; DeVoe et al., 2016; Gold et al., 2017).

Many leading experts in biomedical and scientific inquiry predict that future scientific breakthroughs and advancements will require transdisciplinary collaboration (Méndez, 2015; NRC, 2015). PCR teams are naturally transdisciplinary and span the boundaries of the biological, physical, and social sciences. Primary care and health care have "wicked" problems that have not been addressed with traditional methods and siloed researchers (Camillus, 2008); tackling them will require alliance building and collaboration with a range of expertise in both qualitative and quantitative research designs. Moreover, once discoveries are made in a few settings, important questions about how to most effectively disseminate, implement, and scale evidence-based interventions will be key, demonstrating the critical role of implementation scientists on PCR teams.

Returning to the fundamental question of why PCR is needed, Richard Hobbs of the Nuffield Department of Primary Care Health Sciences at Oxford University summarized it well:

> Given that most patient contacts originate and end in primary care in most developed health systems, the necessity to research more within primary care is obvious. The full spectrum of disease is represented, the long trajectory of disease is discoverable, and the patient subjects are representative of the total population and demonstrate the full range of behaviours … care in the community should be based on evidence from community populations, whether for diagnostic test performance and thresholds or for therapeutic interventions. (Hobbs, 2019, p. 424)

Taking this one step further, care in the community should be based on evidence from community populations that is gathered in partnership with community-based research teams that understand the context and players and bring both a primary care and an equity lens to their work.

THE 1996 INSTITUTE OF MEDICINE REPORT

The report *Primary Care: America's Health in a New Era* (IOM, 1996) declared that the science base for primary care is modest and the infrastructure underlying the knowledge base is skeletal at best. It added that current clinical research may have little to offer to primary care clinicians, lessons from well-done PCR are not available to inform the larger picture of health care organization and delivery, and the paucity of PCR and development leaves primary care insufficiently prepared to confront the challenges and opportunities inherent in the committee's definition of primary care. The current committee believes that these three findings remain unchanged.

These findings led to four recommendations in the 1996 Institute of Medicine (IOM) report that the current committee still finds relevant:

Recommendation 8.1 Federal Support for Primary Care Research called for a declaration of a lead PCR agency and adequate research infrastructure funding.

Recommendation 8.2 National Database and Primary Care Data Set called for a new national health care needs database beyond existing national health surveys.

Recommendation 8.3 Research in Practice-Based Primary Care Research Networks called for providing "adequate and stable financial support to practice-based primary care research networks" (p. 12).

Recommendation 8.4 Data Standards called for new data standards for primary care clinical data collection akin to the International Classification for Primary Care, particularly for capturing episodes of care.

The first recommendation remains relevant because there is still no federal agency charged with developing and advancing a robust program of PCR and funded to support that mission. (See later in this chapter for more on Recommendation 8.1.) For 8.2, the 1996 report's findings about relying on important but insufficient national health surveys to assess the health of the general public, their care-seeking behaviors, their care use, and the quality of the care they receive still hold true. In fact, the difficulties with response rates and sampling challenges have only grown since 1996. Re-evaluating these surveys and considering alternative ways to sample population and primary care data remain a priority.

Practice-based research networks (PBRNs) (Recommendation 8.3) are increasingly important for frontline health and health equity research, and yet they continue to struggle to find infrastructure and sustain funding (Gaglioti et al., 2016; Goldstein et al., 2018; Hall-Lipsy et al., 2018; Westfall et al., 2019).

Finally, for Recommendation 8.4, the electronic health record (EHR) evolved to optimize payment for delivering health care, but it has not fulfilled its potential to support research and improve health care or population health. Criticism of EHRs is abundant, but their lack of functionality to capture and organize data in a way that could inform primary care is notably problematic (Krist et al., 2014, 2015; Phillips et al., 2015). Currently, researchers rely on the National Ambulatory Medical Care Survey (NAMCS) from the National Center for Health Statistics, which samples some 3,000 physicians, to capture what is happening in outpatient care. In 2016, the criteria were sufficiently outdated that nearly half the initial sample needed to be excluded. As a result, 1 week in the lives of 209 primary care physicians (263 if obstetrics and gynecology is included) has been used to determine most of what is known about more than 400 million visits (Rui and Okeyode, 2016). In an era when nearly 90 percent of office-based primary care physicians use EHRs (ONC, 2019) and an increasing number of EHRs collect patient-reported outcomes, the nation has opportunities to assimilate large regional and national databases, standardize and normalize these data, and use this information to enhance the understanding of population health and health disparities and the relationship of primary care to both. Tapping EHR and claims data fully for research would meet the 1996 IOM report's data recommendation partway, but doing so fully also requires having better data sources on people who do not seek care. NAMCS remains incomplete for capturing the contribution of other primary care team members, and EHR and/or claims data could be assembled to better characterize their contributions and care effects.

THE STATUS OF RESEARCH SUPPORT IN PRIMARY CARE

As noted in the previous section, the 1996 IOM report recommended that the U.S. Department of Health and Human Services (HHS) should "identify a lead agency for primary care research and ... the Congress of the United States [should] appropriate funds for this agency in an amount adequate to both build the infrastructure required to conduct primary care research and fund high-priority research projects" (p. 11). Today, the Agency for Healthcare Research and Quality (AHRQ) is the only federal agency with a mandate for PCR, but its National Center for Excellence in Primary Care has consistently had no specific research funding and a nebulous structure, at best, limiting its ability to meaningfully contribute to the field (CAFM, 2019). In 2018, the National Academies held a workshop on the Future of Health Services Research (NASEM, 2018b). As in the 1996 report, primary care was presented as highly overlapping with health services research (HSR), as both share struggles for support, though with some distinctly different needs. This workshop also discussed strategies to develop quality measures and embedding research skills in care delivery, along with models of engaging care-seekers and communities throughout the research process. Central to the discussion was the lack of federal investment in studying the process of health care delivery and factors that influence effective delivery and positive outcomes. This workshop also highlighted that current support for HSR focuses mainly on hospital settings, with a minority of resources going to primary care.

Between 2002 and 2014, family medicine, the specialty that provides more than one-quarter of all outpatient visits across the health care system, consistently received around 0.2 percent of total research funding dollars and 0.3 percent of all awards by the National Institutes of Health (NIH) (Cameron et al., 2016). A related qualitative study found that NIH officials valued the clinical relationships in family medicine but saw no research home for it at NIH (Lucan et al., 2009). A later study of the Patient-Centered Outcome Research Institute (PCORI) found that primary care fared better there but that less than one-third of the studies it supported involved or were relevant to primary care (Mazur et al., 2016).

This long-standing lack of funding for PCR led to a provision in H.R. 1625, the Consolidated Appropriations Act of 2018,[1] which directed and authorized AHRQ to contract with an independent entity for a study on HSR and PCR supported by federal agencies.

> The goal of the study was to provide an independent assessment of the current breadth, scope, and impact of HSR and PCR supported by HHS' 11 operating divisions and the Department of Veterans Affairs (VA) since fiscal year 2012. In support of this goal, the study was to identify research gaps and propose recommendations to AHRQ for maximizing the outcomes, value, and impact of HSR and PCR investments during the next five to 20 years. (Mendel et al., 2020a, p. 1)

The study, completed by the RAND Corporation in 2020, found that between 2012 and 2018, federal agencies had funded 1,090 primary care projects and another 8,845 that could be classified as HSR and/or PCR. Of the studies that were purely about PCR, NIH funded 750, and the VA was second at 150; however, across all research agencies, PCR represented only 1 percent of all funded projects (Mendel et al., 2020a).

RAND noted that AHRQ's distinct focus on health care systems, synthesis of evidence, and dissemination of innovations across settings and populations is unique among government agencies, most of which (including NIH) tend to focus on more specific topics, such as diseases, populations, or settings. The RAND study offered recommendations for HSR and PCR (Mendel et al., 2020a) (see Box 10-1).

The RAND report also noted that PCR has emerged as a distinct field in its own right, addressing a central component of the health care system. Study participants mentioned challenges to coordination of HSR and PCR portfolios, including the breadth and volume of research activities across the federal HSR and PCR enterprise, differing research time frames among agencies, and the lack of targeted funding for a lead agency to coordinate PCR in particular.

The committee agrees that a separate interagency prioritization process for PCR would ensure that the country's vital needs for primary care

---

[1] Consolidated Appropriations Act of 2018, Public Law 115-141 (March 23, 2018).

BOX 10-1
Recommendations from the Health Services
and Primary Care Research Study

Crosscutting recommendations for federally funded health services re-search and primary care research include suggestions for improving the relevance and timeliness of research, dissemination of actionable and find-able results, and interagency prioritization and coordination of research

- Create funding mechanisms that support more rapid, engaged research approaches.
- Expand funding for mixed qualitative and quantitative methods suited to generating evidence on implementation of change in complex health systems.
- Create funding mechanisms that support innovative high-risk, high-re-ward research.
- Train and assist researchers in effectively communicating results in formats readily usable by health care delivery stakeholders.
- Fund research to identify the most effective channels to communicate research results for different audiences and users.
- Require researchers to consider implementation issues early in study design and explicitly apply theories of change.
- Expand funding for the synthesis of evidence across research projects.
- Initiate a strategic planning process across federal agencies to prioritize HSR investments.
- Establish a review process and data systems to proactively identify potential overlaps across agency research portfolios.
- Maintain the Agency for Healthcare Research and Quality as an inde-pendent agency within HHS to serve as the funded hub of federal HSR to ensure its unique and central role.

Primary care research–specific recommendations include the following

- Initiate a strategic planning process across federal agencies specifically to prioritize PCR investments.
- Establish a review process to proactively identify potential overlaps across agency research portfolios, focused on maximizing limited federal funding available for PCR.
- Provide targeted funding for a hub for federal PCR to adequately support research on core functions of primary care and coordinate PCR across federal agencies.

SOURCE: Adapted from Mendel et al., 2020a.

knowledge and evidence base are attended to, incorporating the stakeholders needed to inform prioritization and spanning the full breadth of the primary care basic research questions. Federal PCR efforts are not yet aligned but could be by coordinating both PCR across federal agency research portfolios and the funding to achieve it (Mendel et al., 2020b). As discussed in Chapter 8, this committee notes that one role of a Secretary's Council, supported by an advisory committee formed under the Federal Advisory Committee Authority, could be to coordinate PCR activities. One of the tasks of the Council and the advisory committee would be to assess the adequacy of PCR support across HHS agencies and to direct interagency efforts to support PCR and research infrastructure (see Chapter 12 for the committee's recommendation related to this).

The current structure and priority setting of institutes within NIH and programs within AHRQ often overlook the need for knowledge about integrating, personalizing, and prioritizing whole-person care (Thomas et al., 2018). These essential primary care functions require a science base able to support the work of primary care as a force for integration in a fragmented health care system (Cebul et al., 2008; Hughes et al., 1977; Stange, 2009b). In addition, there is a prevalent but unfounded notion that primary care is simple (Martin and Sturmberg, 2009; Muche-Borowski et al., 2017), and can be supported merely by adding up knowledge gained from outside settings and disease- or organ-specific research studies (Creighton, 2013). These factors have led to a diminished appreciation for the generalist function in health care (Alston et al., 2019; Gerard et al., 2008; Mazzone et al., 2015; Tuggy et al., 2015) and left it insufficiently supported by a relevant knowledge base (IOM, 1996; Stange et al., 2001). The lack of support for the mechanisms by which primary care functions has resulted in a devaluing of relationship-centered whole-person care (Beach and Inui, 2006; Rudebeck, 2019) and an increasing commodification (Heath, 2006; Lown, 2007; NASEM, 2018a) and depersonalization of the health care enterprise (Rotenstein et al., 2018; Shippee et al., 2018).

Disease-specific knowledge can be very useful in informing many aspects of primary care. However, most clinical trials exclude people with the comorbid conditions (Fortin et al., 2006), social and medical complexity (Peek et al., 2009; Ronis et al., 2019), and undifferentiated illness (Epstein et al., 2006; Heath, 1995) that are the norm in primary care. Evidence-based guidelines ignore the complexity of primary care (Casalino, 1999), and the unintended consequences of focusing quality improvement only on narrowly defined evidence are profound (Galvin, 2006; Lipsitz, 2012; McDonald and Roland, 2009; Sutton et al., 2009). No current funding home exists to support research on the integrating, personalizing, and prioritizing functions that provide much of the added value of primary care in functional health care systems.

Where the RAND report judged that the risks associated with moving AHRQ into NIH outweigh the potential advantages, a both/and strategy may be warranted as their individual foci are distinct. The 2007 series of IOM reports on emergency medicine (IOM, 2007a,b,c) are credited on the NIH website (NIH, 2019) for the formation of the Office of Emergency Care Research, which has the important task of working across NIH institutes to identify, coordinate, and support research relevant to emergency medicine. The formation of an Office of Primary Care Research at NIH operating with similar goals and functions could be tremendously helpful to making PCR a more robust part of the NIH portfolio. This would not obviate the need for the National Center for Excellence in PCR at AHRQ; it could still fill this important role, but only if Congress and HHS dedicate resources to it. This would allow AHRQ to continue as a focused funder of PCR but build an internal advocacy and coordination unit within NIH to frame categorical (e.g., disease-specific) PCR relevant to particular Institutes and propose crosscutting primary care/generalist research questions.

There are precedents for new investment in big challenges that create distributed innovation networks and that the committee believes could serve as models for future NIH commitments to support PCR. For example, the National Cancer Act of 1971[2] created 71 National Cancer Institute (NCI)-designated Cancer Centers, 58 of which have research as a focus (NCI, 2019). In 2006, NIH launched the Clinical and Translational Science Awards (CTSA) program with the goals or increasing the quality of clinical and translational research through scientific breakthroughs and enhancing collaborations among institutions, disciplines, and researchers (Frechtling et al., 2012). In 2011, NIH swept these into a new NIH center, the National Center for Advancing Translational Sciences, building a network of more than 50 institutional hubs.

NEEDED RESEARCH IN PRIMARY CARE

The preceding chapters of this report have identified specific PCR needs. All of these foci of functionality suffer from a lack of research infrastructure and sustained support within primary care. This section focuses on these fundamental needs and the inflexibility of national research infrastructure, including funding agencies, to address them.

Primary Care Basic Research

PCR methods, laboratories, and theories exist but are largely unsupported. PCR has been a pioneer in the integration of quantitative and

---

[2] National Cancer Act of 1971, Public Law 218 (December 23, 1971).

qualitative methods (Crabtree and Miller, 1999; Stange and Zyzanski, 1989; Stange et al., 1994) and in participatory methods (Borkan, 2004; Creswell and Hirose, 2019; Macaulay and Nutting, 2006; Westfall et al., 2009) that bring together the numbers and narratives and the diverse perspectives needed to understand how care can be integrated for whole people, families, and communities (Aungst et al., 2019; Homa et al., 2015; Macaulay et al., 1999; Stange et al., 2017).

Primary care also has a robust theoretical basis (Brown et al., 1986; Checkland, 2007; Donner-Banzhoff, 2018; Greenhalgh, 2007; McWhinney, 1972, 1977; Miller et al., 2010; Starfield, 1992, 1996, 1998, 2001) but has suffered from having to force a fit between interest in relationship-centered, family-centered, whole-person care and disease- and organ-based, reductionist worldviews and methods in order to be funded. Relevant theories grounded in the wisdom of practice (Green and Lutz, 1990; Stange, 2009a) and in complexity science (Grant et al., 2011; Greenhalgh and Papoutsi, 2018; Litaker et al., 2006; Peek et al., 2009) are worthy of testing but typically seen as out of scope by categorical funders (Stange et al., 2001). The growing recognition of the inadequacy of the science base (Fortin et al., 2005) to understand and support care for the large number of Americans living with multiple chronic conditions (Parekh et al., 2011; Tinetti et al., 2019; Ward and Schiller, 2013) shows the need for research on this vital use case for primary care.

Primary Care Basic Science Research Questions

Many PCR questions can be pursued through categorical funding mechanisms, such as those available through NIH and the HSR tracks at AHRQ. Research questions that use primary care in service of a narrowly focused disease or medical condition question tend to be advantaged over those needed to build primary care delivery knowledge (Slawson et al., 2001), advantaged in the review processes that value a narrow focus, and advantaged by the tacit assumption that rigor must be equated with rigid adherence to prespecified protocols over identifying processes and outcomes that emerge from participatory and complex system processes (deGruy et al., 2015; Peek et al., 2014). The current research funding environment has prevented addressing meaningful questions critical to the advancement of primary care. No meaningful area of medicine or science can survive and thrive without sufficient support for discovery and innovation.

Here are a few examples of research questions that go unasked in the current limited funding and peer-review environment:

- What are the mechanisms by which primary care works to advance the health of people and populations, while controlling health care costs and increasing equity and system-level quality of care?

- How do we explain the paradox of primary care—that despite the apparently poorer quality of care for disease-specific measures, health care systems based on primary care have greater population health, equity, and quality of care, at lower cost?
- What are the outcomes of investing in health care as a relationship rather than as a series of transactions?
- How can care be integrated for people living with multiple chronic conditions?
- How do continuity, comprehensiveness, and coordination of care work together to affect person and system outcomes?
- How do primary care clinicians approach prioritizing care, particularly for those who have multiple conditions with potentially competing evidence-based guidelines?
- How are trust and trustworthiness developed over time in relationships between care-seekers, families, and communities and their primary care clinicians? What are the trade-offs and outcomes?
- How do we measure what matters in/from care of the whole person, not just their individual diseases?
- How does primary care prioritize care based on a whole-person focus, and how does that affect person and system outcomes?
- How can we network the primary care platform to share best evidence and best practices for prioritizing and managing care during a public health crisis or pandemic?
- What kind of variability in primary care is useful? How do we distinguish between variability that involves personalizing care and variability that represents missing opportunities for evidence-based care that affects outcomes?
- What are the new information management and science roles required in a high-performing primary care setting?
- How can primary care serve as a force for integration in a fragmented health care system and society?
- How do we prioritize individual patient-directed goals with guideline recommendations and quality metrics?
- What does it mean to provide care in the context of family and community? How do different approaches affect outcomes?
- How should training of primary care clinicians change in order to stress the benefits of a whole-person approach to care, rather than approaching the care of people as a sum of what we learn in pieces, studying their organs and systems?
- By what mechanisms does primary care affect health care and health equity?
- How can care be optimized for people presenting with early, undifferentiated illness?

- How does primary care best provide care for the many people whose illnesses don't fit into current disease categories?
- Are intermediate clinical outcomes the best approach for assessing quality and value in primary care?
- How can primary care of whole people be best supported—at the level of the community, practice, local health care system, and state and national policy?
- How do we make it easier for clinicians to consistently deliver the right care at the right time?

In thinking about the need for the types of studies listed above, it is clear that the questions cannot be answered by one discipline alone. The complexity of primary care requires a transdisciplinary approach that brings together scientists from medicine and other health professions but also public health, psychology, sociology, economics, social justice, and equity, to name a few.

Epidemiologic Research

Basic research about the prevalence and presentation of symptoms and illness is largely driven by sample surveys when it no longer need be. The basic understanding of the content and complexity of primary care is woefully lacking. For example, SDOH inform whether someone stays healthy, seeks care, carries out treatment or prevention strategies, and needs acute care and receives it in a timely manner. Epidemiological methods to capture the complex layers of factors that influence health and illness trajectories are unfortunately lagging behind the recognition of their importance. Understanding how SDOH, or drivers, affect health and testing upstream interventions to protect at-risk people has a natural fit in primary care. Moving toward interventions needs information on prevalence and effects that remains largely unexplored in primary care.

Clinical Research

Studies of diagnostic and therapeutic strategies should be relevant to primary care, incorporate the individual's perspective with respect to acceptability and feasibility, and incorporate, rather than exclude, multimorbidity (De Maeseneer et al., 2003). The Primary Care and Interventions Unit of the United Kingdom's National Health Service occasionally asks primary care physicians about gaps in research that would help them care for people (Lecky et al., 2020). The United States has no such systematic inquiry. Given that many of the guidelines and therapeutic options for specific diseases are created based on studies of populations without multiple conditions, studies are critically needed for patients in primary care who typically have more than one condition to understand the real-world risks and benefits of care pathways.

Practice-Based Research Networks

A 2007 *JAMA* article, "Practice-Based Research—'Blue Highways' on the NIH Roadmap," effectively made the case for the need for connections between the "interstates" of academic science and ambulatory practices (Westfall et al., 2007, p. 404):

> A potential solution to these problems is the expansion of practice-based research, which is grounded in, informed by, and intended to improve practice. Practice-based research occurs in the office, where most patients receive most of their care most of the time and may be the essential link between bench discoveries, bedside efficacy, and everyday clinical effectiveness. Practice-based research and practice-based research networks (PBRNs) may help because they can (1) identify the problems that arise in daily practice that create the gap between recommended care and actual care; (2) demonstrate whether treatments with proven efficacy are truly effective and sustainable when provided in the real-world setting of ambulatory care; and (3) provide the "laboratory" for testing system improvements in primary care to maximize the number of patients who benefit from medical discovery.

The authors offered a model (see Figure 10-1) that has led to greater engagement with NIH by using their language and imagery, but the impact has been limited. A few related NIH programs have been launched to formalize laboratories for implementation science, including NCI's Implementation Science Centers in Cancer Control, but these are not limited to primary care, and many have been established in academic health center systems.

> The current NIH Roadmap for Medical Research includes two major research laboratories (bench and bedside) and two translational steps (T1 and T2). Historically, moving new medical discoveries into clinical practice (T2) has been haphazard, occurring largely through continuing medical education programs, pharmaceutical detailing, and guideline development. Proposed expansion of the NIH Roadmap (blue) includes an additional research laboratory (practice-based research) and translational step (T3) to improve incorporation of research discoveries into day-to-day clinical care. The research roadmap is a continuum, with overlap between sites of research and translational steps. The figure [10-1] includes examples of the types of research common in each research laboratory and translational

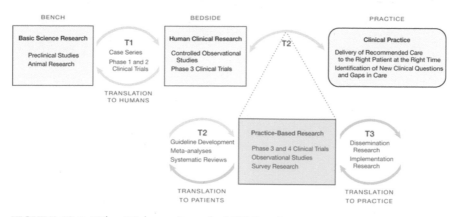

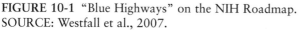

FIGURE 10-1 "Blue Highways" on the NIH Roadmap.
SOURCE: Westfall et al., 2007.

step. This map is not exhaustive; other important types of research that might be included are community-based participatory research, public health research, and health policy analysis. (Westfall et al., 2007, p. 405)

PBRNs are vital participatory community laboratories for "reuniting practice and research around the problems most of the people have most of the time" (Nutting and Green, 1994, p. 335). PBRNs overcome the problem of translating research into practice (Brownson et al., 2012; Cohen et al., 2008; Davis and Taylor-Vaisey, 1997) by making the research questions, settings, and populations served immediately relevant to the real problems faced by patients and primary care practices (DeVoe and Sears, 2013; Westfall et al., 2011). These reasons suggest the nation should establish and maintain an infrastructure to support PBRNs and use them to conduct research to generate the real-world evidence that primary care clinicians need to practice effectively.

AHRQ provided early support for PBRNs (AHRQ, 2012), as did the CTSA program in its early years (Fagnan et al., 2010), but AHRQ support for PBRNs has dwindled, and the CTSA program currently sees clinical practice networks primarily as vehicles for enrolling participants in clinical trials (Riley-Behringer et al., 2017). Despite its importance to the health and health care of the nation, no ongoing primary care cohort or data source exists outside of high-level health service use data. NIH's investments in CTSA flow through the National Center for Advancing Translational Sciences, dedicated solely to this distributed research mechanism. This model could work nicely for PCR centers or PBRNs.

Secondary Data

As noted above, EHRs lack functionality to capture and organize data in a way that could inform primary care. In addition, data are currently privatized and monetized by EHR and digital health vendors. Primary care practices and even primary care researchers struggle to access existing clinical data, and they have to ask vendors for them. This unacceptable situation is stifling PCR. Clinicians and patients should be able to access and share their data with primary care researchers. These data hold great promise with adequate investment and an organized PCR infrastructure to harness them.

Health information exchanges hold a large volume of ambulatory data, and a few clinical registries do too, but these were rarely systematically used for research before the COVID-19 pandemic, and even most of these studies are based on hospital data (Lavery et al., 2020). AHRQ supports secondary research on the Medical Expenditure Panel Survey, and the National Library of Medicine has recently made notice of supporting EHR data research, but there has not been systematic support of basic studies of data collected in primary care that would harness data from more than 450 million visits per year. The capacity to apply sophisticated analyses, including machine learning, to these data could replace reliance on national surveys for understanding patterns of symptoms, illness, and treatment and offer far greater reliability.

Even so, researchers struggle with the utility of the data because of the way they are captured and classified. Clinical classification codes used worldwide have become increasingly specific because they are critical to health care business transactions, but this drastically reduces their utility for understanding patterns of care and outcomes in primary care. As noted earlier, the International Classification for Primary Care captures reason for visit and episodes of conditions, key elements for studying how symptoms relate to disease, which medications are effective or dangerous, which tests are useful, and likely outcomes for patients (Okkes et al., 2002b). This classification is in use in more than 30 countries (Basílio et al., 2016; Okkes et al., 2002a; PH3C, 2011; USYD, 2020; van Boven et al., 2017), but it has no foothold in the United States despite being in the Unified Medical Language System of the National Library of Medicine (NLM, 2020), recognized by the World Health Organization, integrated into the Systematized Nomenclature of Medicine, and able to produce *International Classification of Diseases* codes in the course of care.

A shared primary care data model would facilitate the accurate capture of clinical processes and enable accurate assessment for individuals, families, and communities within the larger health care enterprise (Green and Klinkman, 2015). The United States currently relies on an outdated Framingham Study, clinical trials in other settings, or meta-analysis to create decision support tools. With the right methods and research, existing primary care data could radically improve the ability to use probabilistic, predictive models at point of care, manage panels of patients, and inform population health work (Phillips et al., 2007a).

Research Capacity

It is difficult to find primary care researchers who have not pivoted to disease-specific research to fit the NIH or PCORI models or HSR to fit AHRQ's paradigm (Robinson and Westfall, 2011). Successful PCR departments exist around the country, and many share common characteristics that could be replicated with support (Liaw et al., 2019). Fellowship funding supports successful research training centers, often with Institutional Career Development Awards or T32 National Research Service Award mechanisms (NIH, 2020b). National Research Service Award Fellowships are also important but do not support faculty salaries (NIH, 2020a). Stimulating Access to Research in Residency Transition Scholar awards are also being implemented in some primary care residency programs. The mechanisms are in place, but without a particular preference for primary care and the limited hubs for PCR, the pipeline for primary care researchers will remain small and lacking in significant and sustained investment.

Other countries have successfully organized research around primary care, and the United States often relies on their research. Leading examples include the Netherlands Institute for Health Services Research, which grew out of general practice but has migrated increasingly toward HSR and a broader, European focus. Nevertheless, it has produced some of the most important research about the strength of primary care across developed countries and relationship to outcomes (NIVEL, 2020). The United Kingdom has a specific focus on PCR within the National Institute for Health Research, which funded 562 primary care studies through its Clinical Research Network in 2018 and 2019; these represented 9.2 percent of the 6,106 studies conducted by the network (NIHR, 2020). Similarly, the Canadian Institutes of Health Research has initiatives focused on community-based primary health care and primary and integrated health care innovations (CIHR, 2020).

FINDINGS AND CONCLUSIONS

Given the data showing that primary care accounts for one-third of all health care visits and the paucity of published PCR, a substantial need is clear for primary care–oriented research that could identify the practices that improve the delivery of high-quality primary care. With few exceptions, the committee has determined that primary care largely depends on evidence derived from research done in subspecialty care, hospital settings, or among single-disease cohorts, even though primary care PBRNs have famously yielded important insights regarding many health conditions and treatments. While disease-specific knowledge can be useful in informing many aspects of primary care, most clinical trials exclude people with the comorbid conditions, social and medical complexity, and undifferentiated illness that are the norm in primary care. Evidence-based guidelines ignore the complexity of primary care, and the unintended consequences of focusing quality improvement only on narrowly defined evidence are profound.

The neglect of basic PCR, and lack of research that draws on primary care–specific databases, such as clinical registries, not only adversely affects primary care outcomes but also leads to the lack of a population-based understanding of illness and disease along the health care spectrum. However, better support of PCR could lead to answers to questions that are critically important for improving population health, such as how to incorporate data on SDOH into clinical decision making.

This situation is not new, as it was noted in the 1996 IOM report. Nonetheless, 25 years later, current clinical research has little to offer to primary care clinicians. Moreover, lessons from well-done PCR are not available to inform the larger picture of health care organization and delivery. As a result, the paucity of PCR and development leaves primary care insufficiently prepared to confront the challenges and opportunities inherent in this committee's definition.

An important reason for the neglect PCR suffers is that no federal agency is charged with developing and advancing a robust PCR program and funded to support that mission. In fact, PBRNs continue to struggle to find infrastructure and sustained funding, even though they are increasingly important for frontline health and health equity research. While AHRQ has a federal mandate to conduct PCR, its National Center for Excellence in Primary Care has consistently had no specific research funding and is under constant budgetary threat, limiting its ability to meaningfully contribute to the field. Family medicine, the primary care specialty that accounts for more than 25 percent of all outpatient visits, has consistently received some 0.2 percent of total research and 0.3 percent of all NIH awards. A dedicated office of PCR at NIH could ensure that PCR becomes a more robust part of the NIH portfolio.

In summary, while primary care is the most widely used service in health care, research that could improve its delivery is in need of a significant boost in emphasis and funding. The lack of an agency or office within the federal government whose primary mission is to emphasize, coordinate, and fund research on primary care is a critical impediment to generating the type of knowledge that would benefit both those who provide care in the primary setting and all Americans who receive most of their care in that same setting.

REFERENCES

AHRQ (Agency for Healthcare Research and Quality). 2012. *Primary care practice-based research networks: An AHRQ initiative.* https://www.ahrq.gov/research/findings/factsheets/primary/pbrn/index.html (accessed December 23, 2020).

Alston, M., J. Cawse-Lucas, L. S. Hughes, T. Wheeler, and A. Kost. 2019. The persistence of specialty disrespect: Student perspectives. *PRiMER* 3:1.

Aungst, H., M. Baker, C. Bouyer, B. Catalano, M. Cintron, N. B. Cohen, P. A. Gannon, J. Gilliam, H. Gullett, K. Hassmiller-Lich, S. C. Horner, R. N. Karmali, Ó. B. Kristjánsdóttir, R. Martukovich, J. Mirkovic, J. E. Misak, S. M. Moore, N. Ponyicky, A. Reichsman, M. C. Ruhe, C. Ruland, D. S. Schaadt, K. C. Stange, U. Stenberg, S. A. Sweeney, A. van der Meulen, R. F. Weinberger, J. Williams, and J. Yokie. 2019. *Identifying personal strengths to help patients manage chronic illness.* Washington, DC: Patient-Centered Outcomes Research Institute (PCORI).

Basílio, N., C. Ramos, S. Figueira, and D. Pinto. 2016. Worldwide usage of international classification of primary care use. *Revista Brasileira de Medicina de Família e Comunidade* 11:1.

Beach, M. C., and T. Inui. 2006. Relationship-centered care. A constructive reframing. *Journal of General Internal Medicine* 21(Suppl 1):S3–S8.

Borkan, J. M. 2004. Mixed methods studies: A foundation for primary care research. *Annals of Family Medicine* 2(1):4–6.

Brown, J., M. Stewart, E. McCracken, I. R. McWhinney, and J. Levenstein. 1986. The patient-centered clinical method. 2. Definition and application. *Family Practice* 3(2):75–79.

Brownson, R. C., G. A. Colditz, and E. K. Proctor, eds. 2012. *Dissemination and implementation research in health: Translating science to practice.* New York: Oxford University Press.

CAFM (Council of Academic Family Medicine). 2019. *Fund AHRQ's primary care research center.* Washington, DC: Council of Academic Family Medicine.

Cameron, B. J., A. W. Bazemore, and C. P. Morley. 2016. Lost in translation: NIH funding for family medicine research remains limited. *Journal of the American Board of Family Practice* 29(5):528–530.

Camillus, J. C. 2008. *Strategy as a wicked problem.* https://hbr.org/2008/05/strategy-as-a-wicked-problem (accessed November 18, 2020).

Casalino, L. P. 1999. The unintended consequences of measuring quality on the quality of medical care. *New England Journal of Medicine* 341(15):1147–1150.

Cebul, R. D., J. B. Rebitzer, L. J. Taylor, and M. E. Votruba. 2008. Organizational fragmentation and care quality in the U.S. healthcare system. *Journal of Economic Perspectives* 22(4):93–113.

Checkland, K. 2007. Understanding general practice: A conceptual framework developed from case studies in the UK NHS. *British Journal of General Practice* 57(534):56–63.

CIHR (Canadian Institutes of Health Research). 2020. *About us.* https://cihr-irsc.gc.ca/e/37792.html (accessed November 11, 2020).

Cohen, D. J., B. F. Crabtree, R. S. Etz, B. A. Balasubramanian, K. Donahue, L. C. Leviton, E. C. Clark, N. F. Isaacson, K. C. Stange, and L. W. Green. 2008. Fidelity versus flexibility: Translating evidence-based research into practice. *American Journal of Preventive Medicine* 35:S381–S389.

Cottrell, E. K., R. Gold, S. Likumahuwa, H. Angier, N. Huguet, D. J. Cohen, K. D. Clark, L. M. Gottlieb, and J. E. DeVoe. 2018. Using health information technology to bring social determinants of health into primary care: A conceptual framework to guide research. *Journal of Health Care for the Poor and Underserved* 29(3):949–963.

Crabtree, B. F., and W. L. Miller, eds. 1999. *Doing qualitative research.* 2nd ed. Thousand Oaks, CA: Sage Publications.

Creighton, S. 2013. "Why waste a medical education on primary care?" *Op-Med.* https://opmed.doximity.com/articles/why-waste-a-medical-education-on-primary-care-edc497 ed-fc19-4ddf-be32-a86533975a21 (accessed December 22, 2020).

Creswell, J. W., and M. Hirose. 2019. Mixed methods and survey research in family medicine and community health. *Family Medicine and Community Health* 7(2):e000086.

Davis, D. A., and A. Taylor-Vaisey. 1997. Translating guidelines into practice. A systematic review of theoretic concepts, practical experience and research evidence in the adoption of clinical practice guidelines. *Canadian Medical Association Journal* 157(4):408–416.

De Maeseneer, J. M., M. L. van Driel, L. A. Green, and C. van Weel. 2003. The need for research in primary care. *The Lancet* 362(9392):1314–1319.

deGruy, F. V., B. Ewigman, J. E. DeVoe, L. Hughes, P. James, F. D. Schneider, J. Hickner, K. Stange, T. Van Fossen, A. J. Kuzel, and R. Mullen. 2015. A plan for useful and timely family medicine and primary care research. *Family Medicine* 47(8):636–642.

DeVoe, J. E., and A. Sears. 2013. The Ochin Community Information Network: Bringing together community health centers, information technology, and data to support a patient-centered medical village. *Journal of the American Board of Family Practice* 26(3):271–278.

DeVoe, J. E., A. W. Bazemore, E. K. Cottrell, S. Likumahuwa-Ackman, J. Grandmont, N. Spach, and R. Gold. 2016. Perspectives in primary care: A conceptual framework and path for integrating social determinants of health into primary care practice. *Annals of Family Medicine* 14(2):104–108.

Donner-Banzhoff, N. 2018. Solving the diagnostic challenge: A patient-centered approach. *Annals of Family Medicine* 16(4):353–358.

Eberl, M. M., R. L. Phillips, Jr., H. Lamberts, I. Okkes, and M. C. Mahoney. 2008. Characterizing breast symptoms in family practice. *Annals of Family Medicine* 6(6):528–533.

Epstein, R. M., C. G. Shields, S. C. Meldrum, K. Fiscella, J. Carroll, P. A. Carney, and P. R. Duberstein. 2006. Physicians' responses to patients' medically unexplained symptoms. *Psychosomatic Medicine* 68(2):269–276.

Fagnan, L. J., M. Davis, R. A. Deyo, J. J. Werner, and K. C. Stange. 2010. Linking practice-based research networks and clinical and translational science awards: New opportunities for community engagement by academic health centers. *Academic Medicine* 85(3):476–483.

Fortin, M., L. Lapointe, C. Hudon, and A. Vanasse. 2005. Multimorbidity is common to family practice: Is it commonly researched? *Canadian Family Physician* 51:244–245.

Fortin, M., J. Dionne, G. Pinho, J. Gignac, J. Almirall, and L. Lapointe. 2006. Randomized controlled trials: Do they have external validity for patients with multiple comorbidities? *Annals of Family Medicine* 4(2):104–108.

Frechtling, J., K. Raue, J. Michie, A. Miyaoka, and M. Spiegelman. 2012. *The CTSA national evaluation final report.* Rockville, MD: Westat.

Gaglioti, A. H., J. J. Werner, G. Rust, L. J. Fagnan, and A. V. Neale. 2016. Practice-based research networks (PBRNs) bridging the gaps between communities, funders, and policymakers. *Journal of the American Board of Family Medicine* 29(5):630–635.

Galvin, R. 2006. Pay-for-performance: Too much of a good thing? A conversation with Martin Roland. Interview by Robert Galvin. *Health Affairs* 25(5):w412–w419.

Gerard, K., C. Salisbury, D. Street, C. Pope, and H. Baxter. 2008. Is fast access to general practice all that should matter? A discrete choice experiment of patients' preferences. *Journal of Health Services Research and Policy* 13(2):3–10.

Gold, R., E. Cottrell, A. Bunce, M. Middendorf, C. Hollombe, S. Cowburn, P. Mahr, and G. Melgar. 2017. Developing electronic health record (EHR) strategies related to health center patients' social determinants of health. *Journal of the American Board of Family Practice* 30(4):428–447.

Goldstein, K. M., D. Vogt, A. Hamilton, S. M. Frayne, J. Gierisch, J. Blakeney, A. Sadler, B. M. Bean-Mayberry, D. Carney, B. DiLeone, A. B. Fox, R. Klap, E. Yee, Y. Romodan, H. Strehlow, J. Yosef, and E. M. Yano. 2018. Practice-based research networks add value to evidence-based quality improvement. *Healthcare* 6(2):128–134.

Grant, R. W., J. M. Ashburner, C. C. Hong, Y. Chang, M. J. Barry, and S. J. Atlas. 2011. Defining patient complexity from the primary care physician's perspective. *Annals of Internal Medicine* 155(12):797–804.

Green, L. A., and M. Klinkman. 2015. Perspectives in primary care: The foundational urgent importance of a shared primary care data model. *Annals of Family Medicine* 13(4):303–311.

Green, L. A., and L. J. Lutz. 1990. Notions about networks: Primary care practices in pursuit of improved primary care. In *Primary care research: An agenda for the 90s*, edited by J. Mayfield and M. L. Grady. Washington, DC: Agency for Health Care Policy and Research. Pp. 125–132.

Greenhalgh, T. 2007. *Primary health care: Theory and practice.* Malden, MA: Blackwell/BMJ Books.

Greenhalgh, T., and C. Papoutsi. 2018. Studying complexity in health services research: Desperately seeking an overdue paradigm shift. *BMC Medicine* 16(1):1–6.

Hall-Lipsy, E., L. Barraza, and C. Robertson. 2018. Practice-based research networks and the mandate for real-world evidence. *American Journal of Law & Medicine* 44(2-3):219–236.

Heath, I. 1995. *The mystery of general practice.* London, UK: Nuffield Provincial Hospitals Trust.

Heath, I. 2006. Patients are not commodities. *BMJ* 332(7545):846–847.

Hickner, J., and L. A. Green. 2015. Practice-based research networks (PBRNs) in the United States: Growing and still going after all these years. *Journal of the American Board of Family Practice* 28(5):541–545.

Hobbs, R. 2019. Is primary care research important and relevant to GPs? *British Journal of General Practice* 69(686):424–425.

Homa, L., J. Rose, P. S. Hovmand, S. T. Cherng, R. L. Riolo, A. Kraus, A. Biswas, K. Burgess, H. Aungst, K. C. Stange, K. Brown, M. Brooks-Terry, E. Dec, B. Jackson, J. Gilliam, G. E. Kikano, A. Reichman, D. Schaadt, J. Hilfer, C. Ticknor, C. V. Tyler, A. Van der Meulen, H. Ways, R. F. Weinberger, and C. Williams. 2015. A participatory model of the paradox of primary care. *Annals of Family Medicine* 13(5):456–465.

Hughes, J. R., R. Grayson, and F. C. Stiles. 1977. Fragmentation of care and the medical home. *Pediatrics* 60(4):559.

IOM (Institute of Medicine). 1996. *Primary care: America's health in a new era.* Washington, DC: National Academy Press.

IOM. 2007a. *Emergency care for children: Growing pains.* Washington, DC: The National Academies Press.

IOM. 2007b. *Emergency medical services: At the crossroads.* Washington, DC: The National Academies Press.

IOM. 2007c. *Hospital-based emergency care: At the breaking point.* Washington, DC: The National Academies Press.

Johansen, M. E., S. M. Kircher, and T. R. Huerta. 2016. Reexamining the ecology of medical care. *New England Journal of Medicine* 374(5):495–496.

Krist, A. H., J. W. Beasley, J. C. Crosson, D. C. Kibbe, M. S. Klinkman, C. U. Lehmann, C. H. Fox, J. M. Mitchell, J. W. Mold, W. D. Pace, K. A. Peterson, R. L. Phillips, R. Post, J. Puro, M. Raddock, R. Simkus, and S. E. Waldren. 2014. Electronic health record functionality needed to better support primary care. *Journal of the American Medical Informatics Association* 21(5):764–771.

Krist, A. H., L. A. Green, R. L. Phillips, J. W. Beasley, J. E. DeVoe, M. S. Klinkman, J. Hughes, J. Puro, C. H. Fox, T. Burdick, and the NAPCRG Health Information Technology Working Group. 2015. Health information technology needs help from primary care researchers. *Journal of the American Board of Family Medicine* 28(3):306–310.

Lavery, A. M., L. E. Preston, J. Y. Ko, J. R. Chevinsky, C. L. DeSisto, A. F. Pennington, L. Kompaniyets, S. D. Datta, E. S. Click, T. Golden, A. B. Goodman, W. R. Mac Kenzie, T. K. Boehmer, and A. V. Gundlapalli. 2020. Characteristics of hospitalized COVID-19 patients discharged and experiencing same-hospital readmission—United States, March–August 2020. *Morbidity and Mortality Weekly Report* 69(45).

Lecky, D. M., S. Granier, R. Allison, N. Q. Verlander, S. M. Collin, and C. A. M. McNulty. 2020. Infectious disease and primary care research—what English general practitioners say they need. *Antibiotics (Basel)* 9(5).

Liaw, W., A. Eden, M. Coffman, M. Nagaraj, and A. Bazemore. 2019. Factors associated with successful research departments: A qualitative analysis of family medicine research bright spots. *Family Medicine* 51(2):87–102.

Lipsitz, L. A. 2012. Understanding health care as a complex system: The foundation for unintended consequences. *JAMA* 308(3):243–244.

Litaker, D., A. Tomolo, V. Liberatore, K. C. Stange, and D. C. Aron. 2006. Using complexity theory to build interventions that improve health care delivery in primary care. *Journal of General Internal Medicine* 21(Suppl 2):S30–S34.

Lown, B. 2007. The commodification of health care. *PNHP Newsletter* (Spring):40–44.

Lucan, S. C., F. K. Barg, A. W. Bazemore, and R. L. Phillips, Jr. 2009. Family medicine, the NIH, and the medical-research roadmap: Perspectives from inside the NIH. *Family Medicine* 41(3):188–196.

Macaulay, A. C., and P. A. Nutting. 2006. Moving the frontiers forward: Incorporating community-based participatory research into practice-based research networks. *Annals of Family Medicine* 4(1):4–7.

Macaulay, A. C., L. E. Commanda, W. L. Freeman, N. Gibson, M. L. McCabe, C. M. Robbins, and P. L. Twohig. 1999. Participatory research maximises community and lay involvement. North American primary care research group. *BMJ* 319(7212):774–778.

Martin, C., and J. Sturmberg. 2009. Complex adaptive chronic care. *Journal of Evaluation in Clinical Practice* 15(3):571–577.

Mazur, S., A. Bazemore, and D. Merenstein. 2016. Characteristics of early recipients of Patient-Centered Outcomes Research Institute funding. *Academic Medicine* 91(4):491–496.

Mazzone, M., N. Bhuyan, G. M. Dickson, J. W. Jarvis, L. Maxwell, W. F. Miser, K. Mitchell, S. Schultz, T. Shaffer, and M. Tuggy. 2015. A prescription to advocate for graduate medical education reform. *Annals of Family Medicine* 13(2):184–185.

McDonald, R., and M. Roland. 2009. Pay for performance in primary care in England and California: Comparison of unintended consequences. *Annals of Family Medicine* 7(2):121–127.

McWhinney, I. R. 1972. Beyond diagnosis: An approach to the integration of behavioral science and clinical medicine. *New England Journal of Medicine* 287(8):384–387.

McWhinney, I. R. 1977. The naturalist tradition in general practice. *Journal of Family Practice* 5(3):375–378.

Mendel, P., C. A. Gidengil, A. Tomoaia-Cotisel, S. Mann, A. J. Rose, K. J. Leuschner, N. S. Qureshi, V. Kareddy, J. L. Sousa, and D. Kim. 2020a. *Health services and primary care research study: Comprehensive report.* Santa Monica, CA: RAND Corporation.

Mendel, P., C. A. Gidengil, A. Tomoaia-Cotisel, S. Mann, A. J. Rose, K. J. Leuschner, N. S. Qureshi, V. Kareddy, J. L. Sousa, and D. Kim. 2020b. *Investing in the future of health care: A strategic assessment of federally funded health services research and primary care research.* Santa Monica, CA: RAND Corporation.

Méndez, F. 2015. Transdiscipline and research in health: Science, society and decision making. *Colombia Médica* 46(3):128–134.

Miller, W. L., B. F. Crabtree, P. A. Nutting, K. C. Stange, and C. R. Jaén. 2010. Primary care practice development: A relationship-centered approach. *Annals of Family Medicine* 8(Suppl 1):S68–S79, S92.

Mold, J. W., and D. M. Thompson. 2004. Management of brown recluse spider bites in primary care. *Journal of the American Board of Family Practice* 17(5):347–352.

Muche-Borowski, C., D. Lühmann, I. Schäfer, R. Mundt, H. O. Wagner, M. Scherer, and the Guideline Group of the German College of General Practice and Family Medicine (DEGAM). 2017. Development of a meta-algorithm for guiding primary care encounters for patients with multimorbidity using evidence-based and case-based guideline development methodology. *BMJ Open* 7(6):e015478.

NASEM (National Academies of Sciences, Engineering, and Medicine). 2018a. *Crossing the global quality chasm: Improving health care worldwide.* Washington, DC: The National Academies Press.

NASEM. 2018b. *The future of health services research: Advancing health systems research and practice in the United States.* Washington, DC: The National Academies Press.

NCI (National Cancer Institute). 2019. *NCI-designated cancer centers.* https://www.cancer.gov/research/infrastructure/cancer-centers (accessed December 14, 2020).

NIH (National Institutes of Health). 2019. *OECR history.* https://www.ninds.nih.gov/Current-Research/Trans-Agency-Activities/Office-Emergency-Care-Research/OECR-History (accessed November 3, 2020).

NIH. 2020a. *NIH National Research Service Award (NRSA) fellowships.* https://www.nlm.nih.gov/ep/NRSAFellowshipGrants.html (accessed November 11, 2020).

NIH. 2020b. *Ruth L. Kirschstein Institutional National Research Service Award.* https://researchtraining.nih.gov/programs/training-grants/T32 (accessed November 11, 2020).

NIHR (National Institute for Health Research). 2020. *Primary care.* https://www.nihr.ac.uk/explore-nihr/specialties/primary-care.htm (accessed November 11, 2020).

NIVEL (Netherlands Institute for Health Services Research). 2020. *QUALICOPC.* https://www.nivel.nl/en/international-projects/qualicopc (accessed November 11, 2020).

NLM (National Library of Medicine). 2020. *ICPC (International Classification of Primary Care)—synopsis.* https://www.nlm.nih.gov/research/umls/sourcereleasedocs/current/ICPC/index.html (accessed June 2, 2020).

NRC (National Research Council). 2015. *Enhancing the effectiveness of team science.* Washington, DC: The National Academies Press.

Nutting, P. A., and L. A. Green. 1994. Practice-based research networks: Reuniting practice and research around the problems most of the people have most of the time. *Journal of Family Practice* 38(4):335–336.

Okkes, I. M., S. K. Oskam, and H. Lamberts. 2002a. The probability of specific diagnoses for patients presenting with common symptoms to Dutch family physicians. *Journal of Family Practice* 51(1):31–36.

Okkes, I. M., G. O. Polderman, G. E. Fryer, T. Yamada, M. Bujak, S. K. Oskam, L. A. Green, and H. Lamberts. 2002b. The role of family practice in different health care systems: A comparison of reasons for encounter, diagnoses, and interventions in primary care populations in the Netherlands, Japan, Poland, and the United States. *Journal of Family Practice* 51(1):72–73.

ONC (Office of the National Coordinator for Health Information Technology). 2019. *Office-based physician electronic health record adoption.* dashboard.healthit.gov/quickstats/pages/physician-ehr-adoption-trends.php (accessed December 8, 2020).

Parekh, A. K., R. A. Goodman, C. Gordon, and H. K. Koh. 2011. Managing multiple chronic conditions: A strategic framework for improving health outcomes and quality of life. *Public Health Reports* 126(4):460–471.

Peek, C. J., M. A. Baird, and E. Coleman. 2009. Primary care for patient complexity, not only disease. *Families, Systems, & Health* 27(4):287–302.

Peek, C. J., R. E. Glasgow, K. C. Stange, L. M. Klesges, E. P. Purcell, and R. S. Kessler. 2014. The 5 R's: An emerging bold standard for conducting relevant research in a changing world. *Annals of Family Medicine* 12(5):447–455.

Petterson, S., B. F. Miller, J. C. Payne-Murphy, and R. L. Phillips Jr. 2014. Mental health treatment in the primary care setting: Patterns and pathways. *Families, Systems, & Health* 32(2):157–166.

PH3C (Primary Health Care Classification Consortium). 2011. *Members.* http://www.ph3c.org/4daction/w3_CatVisu/?wCatFonc=membres&chMembreNom=&chMembrePrenom=&chMembreAnnee=&chMembreActif=&aff=liste&wNbEnrPage=20&wNumPage=1&wCritTri=3 (accessed June 2, 2020).

Phillips, R. L., Jr., M. Klinkman, and L. A. Green. 2007a. *Conference report: Harmonizing primary care clinical classification and data standards.* Washington, DC: Robert Graham Center and Agency for Healthcare Research and Quality.

Phillips, R. L., Jr., J. Mold, and K. Peterson. 2007b. Research-based research networks. In *The learning healthcare system: Workshop summary,* edited by L. Olsen, D. Aisner, and J. M. McGinnis. Washington, DC: The National Academies Press.

Phillips, R. L., Jr., A. W. Bazemore, J. E. DeVoe, T. J. Weida, A. H. Krist, M. F. Dulin, and F. E. Biagioli. 2015. A family medicine health technology strategy for achieving the triple aim for US health care. *Family Medicine* 47(8):628–635.

Riley-Behringer, M., M. M. Davis, J. J. Werner, L. J. Fagnan, and K. C. Stange. 2017. The evolving collaborative relationship between practice-based research networks (PBRNs) and clinical and translational science awardees (CTSAs). *Journal of Clinical and Translational Science* 1(5):301–309.

Robinson, K., and J. Westfall. 2011. NAPCRG puts the increase of primary care research funding at the top of the priority list. *Annals of Family Medicine* 9(5):468–469.

Ronis, S. D., R. Grossberg, R. Allen, A. Hertz, and L. C. Kleinman. 2019. Estimated non-reimbursed costs for care coordination for children with medical complexity. *Pediatrics* 143(1).

Rotenstein, L. S., M. Torre, M. A. Ramos, R. C. Rosales, C. Guille, S. Sen, and D. A. Mata. 2018. Prevalence of burnout among physicians: A systematic review. *JAMA* 320(11):1131–1150.

Rudebeck, C. E. 2019. Relationship based care—how general practice developed and why it is undermined within contemporary healthcare systems. *Scandinavian Journal of Primary Health Care* 37(3):335–344.

Rui, P., and T. Okeyode. 2016. *National Ambulatory Medical Care Survey: 2016 national summary tables.* Atlanta, GA: Centers for Disease Control and Prevention.

Shippee, N. D., T. P. Shippee, P. D. Mobley, K. M. Fernstrom, and H. R. Britt. 2018. Effect of a whole-person model of care on patient experience in patients with complex chronic illness in late life. *American Journal of Hospice & Palliative Care* 35(1):104–109.

Slawson, D. C., A. F. Shaughnessy, and H. Barry. 2001. Which should come first: Rigor or relevance? *Journal of Family Practice* 50(3):209–210.

Soler, J. K., I. Okkes, M. Wood, and H. Lamberts. 2008. The coming of age of ICPC: Celebrating the 21st birthday of the international classification of primary care. *Family Practice* 25(4):312–317.

Stange, K. C. 2009a. The generalist approach. *Annals of Family Medicine* 7(3):198–203.

Stange, K. C. 2009b. The problem of fragmentation and the need for integrative solutions. *Annals of Family Medicine* 7(2):100–103.

Stange, K. C., and S. J. Zyzanski. 1989. Integrating qualitative and quantitative research methods. *Family Medicine* 21(6):448–451.

Stange, K. C., W. L. Miller, B. F. Crabtree, P. J. O'Connor, and S. J. Zyzanski. 1994. Multimethod research: Approaches for integrating qualitative and quantitative methods. *Journal of General Internal Medicine* 9(5):278–282.

Stange, K. C., W. L. Miller, and I. McWhinney. 2001. Developing the knowledge base of family practice. *Family Medicine* 33(4):286–297.

Stange, K. C., S. T. Cherng, R. L. Riolo, L. Homa, J. Rose, P. S. Hovmand, and A. Kraus. 2017. No longer looking just under the lamp post: Modeling the complexity of primary health care. In *Growing inequality: Bridging complex systems, population health, and health disparities*, edited by G. A. Kaplan, A. V. Diez Roux, C. P. Simon, and S. Galea. Washington, DC: Westphalia Press. Pp. 81–107.

Starfield, B. 1992. *Primary care: Concept, evaluation, and policy.* New York: Oxford University Press.

Starfield, B. 1996. A framework for primary care research. *Journal of Family Practice* 42(2):181–185.

Starfield, B. 1998. *Primary care: Balancing health needs, services, and technology.* Revised edition. New York: Oxford University Press.

Starfield, B. 2001. New paradigms for quality in primary care. *British Journal of General Practice* 51(465):303–309.

Sutton, M., R. Elder, B. Guthrie, and G. Watt. 2009. Record rewards: The effects of targeted quality incentives on the recording of risk factors by primary care providers. *Health Economics* 19(1):1–13.

Thomas, H., G. Mitchell, J. Rich, and M. Best. 2018. Definition of whole person care in general practice in the English language literature: A systematic review. *BMJ Open* 8(12):e023758.

Tinetti, M. E., A. R. Green, J. Ouellet, M. W. Rich, and C. Boyd. 2019. Caring for patients with multiple chronic conditions. *Annals of Internal Medicine* 170(3):199–202.

Tuggy, M., N. Bhuyan, G. M. Dickson, J. W. Jarvis, L. Maxwell, M. Mazzone, W. F. Miser, K. Mitchell, S. Schultz, and T. Shaffer. 2015. Training implications of family medicine for America's health: A preview. *Annals of Family Medicine* 13(1):91–92.

USYD (University of Sydney). 2020. *Bettering the evaluation and care of health (BEACH).* https://www.sydney.edu.au/medicine-health/our-research/research-centres/bettering-the-evaluation-and-care-of-health.html (accessed June 2, 2020).

van Boven, K., A. A. Uijen, N. van de Wiel, S. K. Oskam, H. J. Schers, and W. J. J. Assendelft. 2017. The diagnostic value of the patient's reason for encounter for diagnosing cancer in primary care. *Journal of the American Board of Family Medicine* 30(6):806–812.

Ward, B. W., and J. S. Schiller. 2013. Prevalence of multiple chronic conditions among us adults: Estimates from the National Health Interview Survey, 2010. *Preventing Chronic Disease* 10:E65.

Westfall, J. M., J. Mold, and L. Fagnan. 2007. Practice-based research—"blue highways" on the NIH roadmap. *JAMA* 297(4):403–406.

Westfall, J. M., L. J. Fagnan, M. Handley, J. Salsberg, P. McGinnis, L. K. Zittleman, and A. C. Macaulay. 2009. Practice-based research is community engagement. *Journal of the American Board of Family Practice* 22(4):423–427.

Westfall, J. M., L. Zittleman, E. W. Staton, B. Parnes, P. C. Smith, L. J. Niebauer, D. H. Fernald, J. Quintela, R. F. Van Vorst, L. M. Dickinson, and W. D. Pace. 2011. Card studies for observational research in practice. *Annals of Family Medicine* 9(1):63–68.

Westfall, J. M., R. Roper, A. Gaglioti, and D. E. Nease, Jr. 2019. Practice-based research networks: Strategic opportunities to advance implementation research for health equity. *Ethnicity & Disease* 29(Suppl 1):113–118.

11

The Committee's Approach to
an Implementation Strategy

The committee focused its work explicitly on the *implementation* of high-quality primary care. This charge was a response to the lack of implementation of many of the recommendations from the report *Primary Care: America's Health in a New Era* (IOM, 1996). The committee interpreted its task of developing an implementation plan as one that requires its recommendations to be explicit—recommendations must not only have an actor and action but include specific guidance as to how the actors should carry out the actions to effect change (see Chapter 12 for the committee's recommendations and implementation plan).

The specific actions the committee recommends to strengthen primary care are organized around a fundamental premise of high-quality care as a common good, an environmental assessment, a comprehensive analysis of the evidence for what constitutes high-quality primary care and its facilitators, lessons from implementation science and public policy studies, and a resulting three-part implementation strategy. As articulated in Chapter 2, the committee believes that high-quality primary care deserves status as a common good that merits public stewardship because of its unique capacity among health care services to improve population health and reduce health care inequities. Ongoing stressors in the U.S. health care system have continually weakened primary care and make attention to high-quality primary care delivery interventions a high public policy priority.

An implementation strategy must account for the environmental context in which it calls for implementing core objectives. The U.S. health care system is diverse and complex. Representing almost one-fifth of the U.S. economy (CMS, 2019), the health care system comprises multiple sources of payments from public and private payers, numerous mechanisms and means for delivering health care, and often conflicting governmental oversight at the federal, state, and local levels (NASEM, 2019). The committee does not aspire to eliminate this complexity but rather to adopt a complexity-informed implementation strategy that considers the multiple influences and forces that must be factored into any primary care change process (Braithwaite et al., 2018). While universal health insurance or a single payer system would go a long way to reduce much of this complexity and give primary care the common good status the committee believes it deserves, the committee developed its implementation plan to work within the realities of the current U.S. insurance marketplace. Thus, rather than calling for radical transformations throughout the health care system, the committee's implementation plan is made up of incremental changes that in combination would lead to a dramatic change to primary care in the United States.

In addition to defining high-quality primary care, the committee's scope requires it to articulate the key proven facilitators necessary for implementing its plan. As first set forth in Chapter 2, the analysis of research and evidence regarding integrated care, digital health care, clinical accountability, payment models, interprofessional care teams, and research constitutes the heart of the committee's report and resulting recommendations that target ways to effectively scale and implement successful innovations.

The committee's implementation strategy informs its recommendations and must account for the work described above. The aim of implementation science is to accelerate the systematic uptake of evidence into real-world practice (Fisher et al., 2016). The committee drew three fundamental lessons from science and practice to inform its recommendations:

- The need for a conceptual understanding that recognizes the adaptive and dynamic developmental processes through which recommendations are translated and implementation occurs (Braithwaite et al., 2018; Nilsen, 2015).
- The need for a feedback structure for accountability for the use, alignment, and effectiveness of recommended actions (Greenhalgh and Papoutsi, 2019; Holtrop et al., 2018).
- The need for policies that reinforce and promote actions that support recommended actions and are congruent with system goals (Stetler et al., 2008).

Public policy analysis also makes it clear that strong, evidence-based policy recommendations are necessary but not sufficient for successful implementation. A strategy that accounts for public perceptions and political opportunities is necessary as well.

Based on these considerations, the committee's implementation strategy includes three interrelated components: an implementation framework, an accountability framework, and a public policy–making framework.

AN IMPLEMENTATION FRAMEWORK

The committee draws from work by previous National Academies committees. In *Crossing the Quality Chasm: A New Health System for the 21st Century* (IOM, 2001), the recommendations targeted four levels of change in the health care system (see Table 11-1): individual, group or team, organization, and larger system or environment (Ferlie and Shortell, 2001). The 2019 National Academies report *Taking Action Against Clinician Burnout: A Systems Approach to Professional Well-Being* combined the individual and team levels but maintained its emphasis on system levels that

TABLE 11-1 Four Levels of Change for Improving Quality

Levels	Examples
Individual	Education Academic detailing Data feedback Benchmarking Guideline, protocol, pathway implementation Leadership development
Group/team	Team development Task redesign Clinical audits Breakthrough collaboratives Guideline, protocol, pathway implementation
Organization	Quality assurance Continuous quality improvement/total quality management Organization development Organization culture Organization learning Knowledge management/transfer
Larger system/environment	National bodies (NICE, CHI, AHRQ) Evidence-based practice centers Accrediting/licensing agencies (NCQA, Joint Commission) Public disclosure ("report cards," etc.) Payment policies Legal system

NOTE: AHRQ = Agency for Healthcare Research and Quality; CHI = Commission for Health Improvement; NCQA = National Committee for Quality Assurance; NICE = National Institute for Health and Care Excellence.
SOURCE: Ferlie and Shortell, 2001.

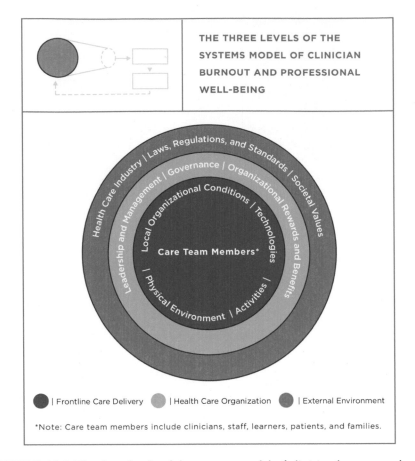

FIGURE 11-1 The three levels of the systems model of clinician burnout and professional well-being.
SOURCE: NASEM, 2019.

varied in their scope of focus (Ferlie and Shortell, 2001; NASEM, 2019) (see Figure 11-1). At the level of frontline care delivery, patients, families, and care teams interact at the point of care or virtually via technology. At the health care organization level, leadership and governance creates and maintains the processes and structures in which the frontline care delivery level operates. The external environment includes societal values, the greater health care industry, government, and the policies and standards that establish the parameters that the health care organizations and frontline care delivery levels must operate within.

This committee adopts a modified version of these three levels of an interrelated, complex system in which the committee distinguishes between

TABLE 11-2 The Committee's Implementation Framework

System Level	Public			Private	
	Example Actor	Example Actions	Example Actor	Example Actions	
Macro	Federal/state legislative branch	Policies; laws; funding	Coalitions; associations	Policy advocacy; public accountability; professional standards	
Meso	Federal, state, local executive branch; federal payers; public delivery systems; educators	Regulations; contracting; payment; administrative practices; training	Private delivery organizations; private payers; corporations; institutions; educators	Management policies and practices; training	
Micro	Individuals and interprofessional teams delivering care in public and government health systems; individuals and families seeking care	Self-education; quality assessment and improvement; behavior practice	Individuals and interprofessional teams delivering care; individuals and families seeking care	Self-education; quality assessment and improvement; behavior practice	

the public and private sectors within each of its three levels (see Table 11-2). Doing so accounts for the different actors and actions in the public and private sectors, each with different roles in the committee's implementation plan. In the committee's framework, the macro level includes federal and state governments and legislators, regulators, and coalitions and professional associations. The meso level includes the executive branches of federal, state, and local government; public and private payers; health care organizations; and community-based social services, health care corporations, and other health-affiliated institutions. The micro level includes interprofessional primary care teams that may operate in public- or private-sector organizations, patients, and their families. The implementation science lens focuses on the interconnections, interactions, and necessary bidirectional dialogue between and among actors at all three levels to effectively adopt core recommendations (Côté-Boileau et al., 2019; Fisher et al., 2016).

The implementation framework exists in the context of prevailing cultural and social values. With this context and framework in mind, the task of the committee became reviewing the evidence for actions that promote scalable high-quality primary care—as presented in the bulk of the preceding chapters—and then proposing a portfolio of evidence-based recommendations for the public and private sectors at all three system levels. Implementation is a process that occurs dynamically over time, so the framework should include not just the need for recommendations to engage actors across different system levels in the public and private sectors but also consideration for how recommendations will be adopted, monitored, and improved over time.

The committee has identified three distinct but interrelated and continuous phases for the implementation of any recommendation:

- During a **planning period,** recommendations are formally considered and elaborated upon with purposeful design. Designated actors identify and develop the steps and resource capacity required to implement the recommendation, and leadership sets the vision, mission, and "social message" these recommendations explicitly propagate.
- During an **adoption period,** recommendations are implemented in a carefully managed and circumscribed accountable environment. Based on predicted and actual experience and evaluation, the steps are adjusted and resources identified in the planning period.
- During a **scaling period,** recommendations and key, effective, facilitating elements replicated during the adoption period are implemented in more and progressively broader settings to reach the population as a whole.

Detailing the specifics of each implementation phase for each recommendation is beyond the committee's scope. However, implicit in each recommendation in Chapter 12 is the responsibility for the named actor to plan for building implementation capacity for all three phases.

AN ACCOUNTABILITY FRAMEWORK

For successful implementation, it is not enough have named actors and specific actions. A framework of accountability and feedback is required for those actors to communicate and cooperate (Berwick and Shine, 2020) regarding effective local adaption of recommended actions, assess implementation progress over time (Holtrop et al., 2018), and adapt practices as conditions change. Leaders are accountable for creating a learning, participatory culture that facilitates adoption through transparent evaluation methods. They promulgate open dialogue between delivery and policy through evaluating the intended impact and effectiveness of their implementation plan by assembling objective measures of performance; a process for collecting, using, and accelerating timely learnings from those measures; and an enforcement and reward system based on performance and social impact. Scaling effective primary care innovations, such as those described in this report, beyond a local context to ensure a common good for the U.S. population depends on leaders building implementation capacity to support, sustain, and improve the core recommendations.

Within a single organization, such an accountability framework is relatively easy to develop: it is implemented through an organizational structure and using tools of change management accountability, such as measurement, communications, and performance reviews and incentives for quality. Outcomes are monitored constantly and fed back to frontline clinicians to promote continuous learning and improvement (Forrest et al., 2014; Greene et al., 2012). Across a health care system spanning almost one-fifth of the U.S. economy, an accountability framework is somewhat more difficult, requiring assessment and feedback at multiple system levels. While the 1996 report recommended establishing an accountability structure (in the form of a public–private consortium), the recommendation did not specify which entities should participate or lead the proposed endeavor, and it was never created. As discussed in Chapter 1, this lack of accountability structure was a critical reason many of that report's recommendations went unimplemented.

However, systemic accountability can be facilitated by organizing constituents—those most affected by the success or failure of an implementation plan—for collective action related to implementation actions. Harnessing the local sensemaking capacities and actors' voices at all three levels promotes the systematic spread and accountable scale of successful innovations. This is often most readily accomplished by joint private and public assessment of iterative progress on the impact of implementation actions and communication of findings. The committee's implementation plan in Chapter 12 recommends ways to accomplish this.

A PUBLIC POLICY–MAKING FRAMEWORK

With primary care's status as a common good, a significant portion of implementation actions will be the responsibility of the public sector. But primary care is not the only common good—there are many claims upon limited resources and conflicting notions of what constitutes the public welfare. Actors in the public sector act through the public policy–making process that adjudicates these competing values and priorities.

The committee's implementation strategy draws from the frequently cited policy-making concept of the "policy window" (Kingdon, 1995), which proposes that regardless of the merits of a public policy proposal—in this case, a series of actions that advance high-quality primary care—three separate public policy streams (political imperative, effective policy, and a perceived problem) must align to create a window of opportunity for implementation (see Figure 11-2). Achieving this to produce the window of opportunity is only partially serendipitous, for actors that promote policy actions, known as "policy entrepreneurs," can create it (Guldbrandsson and Fossum, 2009; Kingdon, 1995). The committee's implementation plan does indeed rest in part on the success of policy entrepreneurs committed to high-quality primary care, but it does recommend strategies for such actors.

Effective policy identification is typically the domain of reports from the National Academies, and the committee has endeavored to develop the basis for those regarding high-quality primary care in previous chapters. But the charge to the committee of "implementation" requires it to consider the domains of public perception and political imperative. These domains

The Kingdon Model

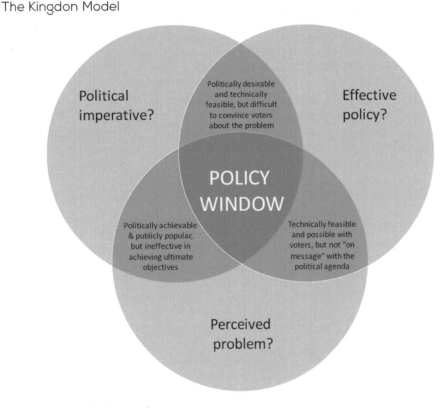

FIGURE 11-2 Windows of opportunity.
SOURCES: NZIER, 2018, based on Kingdon, 1995.

are, by their nature, often specific to a moment in time. While research adds to policy evidence, commonly perceived problems and political opportunities at the time of this report may fundamentally change in the future.

Given the need to consider all aspects of the policy window, the committee considered the commonly perceived problems its recommendations could address. There are lessons to be drawn from states that have been leading on primary care policy, such as Vermont, with its Blueprint for Health (Bielaszka-DuVernay, 2011; Jones et al., 2016), Rhode Island (Koller et al., 2010), and Oregon (Howard et al., 2015; OHA, 2019), with their mandated primary care spend levels. In each case, policy leaders pointed to an unbalanced health care delivery system with a specialty and institutional orientation in comparison to the best-performing national and international systems, successfully making the case for public policy prioritization of primary care for long-term benefits in terms of lower health care costs and better population health, similar to what is seen in other countries.

These lessons may be applicable for federal policies. National polling shows that while Americans are generally satisfied with the quality of their personal care, a significant portion have concerns about affordability and access (Newport, 2019). Few believe the U.S. health care system to be in crisis, but a majority believes it has "major problems" and worries about the affordability and availability of health care in the future.

Implementing high-quality primary care can be a way to address public concerns about the ongoing stability of the U.S. health care system. It is an evidence-based investment in strengthening primary care now, for later benefit. It avoids protracted conflicts over comprehensive health reform and threats of perceived loss of access or choice. Leaders can point to declining U.S. life expectancy despite outsized health care expenditures to crystallize those concerns and the evidence regarding primary care's significant positive benefits as a way to address them. For those policies that require expenditures, the relatively small proportion of health care expenses devoted to primary care then becomes an opportunity. A small absolute increase in primary care spending for the policies identified in this report, redistributed from the large expenses across the rest of the system, can have a high proportional effect on primary care. This redistribution argument will encounter resistance from the remainder of the system but is essential for leaders to address public concerns that health care is already too expensive.

The committee recognizes that the implementation of its plan may require new authorizations or changes to current federal or state law. While the committee's plan addresses the policy changes it believes are needed to achieve its vision of high-quality primary care in the United States, it was beyond the scope of its task to identify the specific legal changes that may be required for implementation.

The COVID-19 Pandemic as a Catalyst for Change

The COVID-19 pandemic has revealed much about what is broken in primary care and population health management. The imperative of addressing the lapses will be a useful and important mandate, in which private- and public-sector primary care champions could advance elements of the committee's implementation plan. Leaders can use the collective experience of the pandemic to demonstrate how it weakened primary care in the United States at precisely the point when it was most needed: to partner with public health; decompress crowded emergency rooms; monitor populations most vulnerable to infection; conduct testing; treat less acute cases and contact trace; administer vaccines; treat long-term sequelae; and prepare for the social and emotional fallout of a distressed and isolated population.

Instead, according to a weekly national survey, within 3 weeks of the March 13, 2020, declaration of a national emergency, half of primary care practices reported a severe effect. Some 90 percent were limiting chronic and acute care visits, and the large majority were switching to predominantly telehealth visits, despite a mostly deficient technology infrastructure beyond basic telephone services (The Larry A. Green Center and PCC, 2020a). Saddled with a fee-for-service reimbursement system at a time when in-person visits were actively discouraged, just 1 month into the pandemic, nearly half of primary care practices were unsure if they had enough cash to remain open, 47 percent had laid off or furloughed staff, and 85 percent reported dramatic decreases in visit volume and corresponding income. Three-fifths of practices noted that the majority of their work was not reimbursable, even as they responded to COVID-19's effects on patients' physical, psychological, and financial well-being (The Larry A. Green Center and PCC, 2020b).

Soon, one can anticipate sweeping federal policies in the aftermath of the pandemic, much as Congress acted in the wake of the September 11, 2001, terrorist attacks, the flooding of New Orleans by Hurricane Katrina, and the economic collapse of 2008. The realms of action might include public health investments and pandemic preparation, health care system strengthening and pandemic resiliency, and economic recovery. This recovery and rebuilding effort can constitute the political imperative required to advance the committee's policy recommendations, given skillful and committed champions in positions of influence who can communicate the missed potential of primary care to assist in the pandemic and capitalize on public concerns about the future sustainability of our health care system.

A strategy is a well-considered plan, not an assurance of results. While the evidence of the value of primary care for population health and its weakened state in the United States is incontrovertible, evidence-based recommendations alone are insufficient to effect change and promote high-quality primary care. An implementation framework, a model for accountability, and a public policy–making framework provide a guide to select recommendations and increase the likelihood of their adoption, the rate of their implementation, and the speed with which the resulting benefits will accrue to the nation over time.

REFERENCES

Berwick, D. M., and K. Shine. 2020. Enhancing private sector health system preparedness for 21st-century health threats: Foundational principles from a National Academies initiative. *JAMA* 323(12):1133–1134.

Bielaszka-DuVernay, C. 2011. Vermont's blueprint for medical homes, community health teams, and better health at lower cost. *Health Affairs* 30(3):383–386.

Braithwaite, J., K. Churruca, J. C. Long, L. A. Ellis, and J. Herkes. 2018. When complexity science meets implementation science: A theoretical and empirical analysis of systems change. *BMC Medicine* 16(1):63.

CMS (Centers for Medicare & Medicaid Services). 2019. *National health expenditure data.* https://www.cms.gov/Research-Statistics-Data-and-Systems/Statistics-Trends-and-Reports/NationalHealthExpendData/NationalHealthAccountsHistorical (accessed July 22, 2020).

Côté-Boileau, E., J.-L. Denis, B. Callery, and M. Sabean. 2019. The unpredictable journeys of spreading, sustaining and scaling healthcare innovations: A scoping review. *Health Research Policy and Systems* 17(1):84.

Ferlie, E. B., and S. M. Shortell. 2001. Improving the quality of health care in the United Kingdom and the United States: A framework for change. *Milbank Quarterly* 79(2):281–315.

Fisher, E. S., S. M. Shortell, and L. A. Savitz. 2016. Implementation science: A potential catalyst for delivery system reform. *JAMA* 315(4):339–340.

Forrest, C. B., P. Margolis, M. Seid, and R. B. Colletti. 2014. PEDSnet: How a prototype pediatric learning health system is being expanded into a national network. *Health Affairs* 33(7):1171–1177.

Greene, S. M., R. J. Reid, and E. B. Larson. 2012. Implementing the learning health system: From concept to action. *Annals of Internal Medicine* 157(3):207–210.

Greenhalgh, T., and C. Papoutsi. 2019. Spreading and scaling up innovation and improvement. *BMJ* 365:l2068.

Guldbrandsson, K., and B. Fossum. 2009. An exploration of the theoretical concepts policy windows and policy entrepreneurs at the Swedish public health arena. *Health Promotion International* 24(4):434–444.

Holtrop, J. S., B. A. Rabin, and R. E. Glasgow. 2018. Dissemination and implementation science in primary care research and practice: Contributions and opportunities. *Journal of the American Board of Family Practice* 31(3):466–478.

Howard, S. W., S. L. Bernell, J. Yoon, J. Luck, and C. M. Ranit. 2015. Oregon's experiment in health care delivery and payment reform: Coordinated care organizations replacing managed care. *Journal of Health Politics, Policy & Law* 40(1):245–255.

IOM (Institute of Medicine). 1996. *Primary care: America's health in a new era.* Washington, DC: National Academy Press.

IOM. 2001. *Crossing the quality chasm: A new health system for the 21st century.* Washington, DC: National Academy Press.

Jones, C., K. Finison, K. McGraves-Lloyd, T. Tremblay, M. K. Mohlman, B. Tanzman, M. Hazard, S. Maier, and J. Samuelson. 2016. Vermont's community-oriented all-payer medical home model reduces expenditures and utilization while delivering high-quality care. *Population Health Management* 19(3):196–205.

Kingdon, J. 1995. *Agendas, alternatives, and public policies.* New York: Longman.

Koller, C. F., T. A. Brennan, and M. H. Bailit. 2010. Rhode Island's novel experiment to re-build primary care from the insurance side. *Health Affairs* 29(5):941–947.

NASEM (National Academies of Sciences, Engineering, and Medicine). 2019. *Taking action against clinician burnout: A systems approach to professional well-being.* Washington, DC: The National Academies Press.

Newport, F. 2019. *Americans' mixed views of healthcare and healthcare reform.* https://news.gallup.com/opinion/polling-matters/257711/americans-mixed-views-healthcare-healthcare-reform.aspx (accessed November 20, 2020).

Nilsen, P. 2015. Making sense of implementation theories, models and frameworks. *Implementation Science* 10(1):53.

NZIER (New Zealant Institute of Economic Research). 2018. *Population ageing: Do we understand and accept the challenge?* Wellington, NZ: Chartered Accountants Australia and New Zealand.

OHA (Oregon Health Authority). 2019. *Primary care spending in Oregon: A report to the Oregon legislature.* Salem, OR: Oregon Health Authority.

Stetler, C. B., L. McQueen, J. Demakis, and B. S. Mittman. 2008. An organizational framework and strategic implementation for system-level change to enhance research-based practice: QUERI series. *Implementation Science* 3(1):30.

The Larry A. Green Center and PCC (Primary Care Collaborative). 2020a. *Quick COVID-19 primary care survey: Clinician series 3 fielded March 27–30, 2020.* https://www.green-center.org/covid-survey (accessed September 15, 2020).

The Larry A. Green Center and PCC. 2020b. *Quick COVID-19 primary care survey: Clinician series 7 fielded April 24–27, 2020.* https://www.green-center.org/covid-survey (accessed September 15, 2020).

12

A Plan for Implementing High-Quality Primary Care

Primary care is the heart of a high-functioning health care system. Properly done, it serves the majority of most people's health care needs the majority of times, with continuous, coordinated, comprehensive, and convenient care. It also serves as a vital navigator to assist people and their families in obtaining external services care.

Primary care is the only component of health care where an increased supply is associated with better population health and more equitable outcomes. Neither hospitals nor specialty care can make this claim. For this reason, the committee considers primary care to be a common good, making the strength and quality of U.S. primary care services a public concern.

Yet there are many characteristics of today's U.S. health care system that are weakening primary care. Provider payment policy for publicly financed care, such as Medicare and Medicaid, and market-based negotiations for privately financed care reward those parts of the system with political and economic power, while the primary care sector has neither. One result is that primary care teams deliver 55 percent of ambulatory care services but only receive about 5 percent of total health care spending—a figure that continues to decline (Martin et al., 2020; PCPCC, 2018; Reiff et al., 2019). Visits to primary care clinicians are declining, and the workforce pipeline is shrinking, with physicians and other clinicians opting to specialize in more lucrative health care fields.

This weakening of primary care comes at a time when the country needs it more than ever.

- The number of individuals in the United States with chronic health conditions is increasing, and U.S. life expectancy is steadily declining. Primary care is associated with improved management of chronic health issues and longer life expectancy.
- COVID-19 has revealed the vulnerabilities of the U.S. health care system and stressed many parts to the breaking point. High-quality primary care can reduce demands on other parts of the health system, allowing for more efficient deployment of scarce resources. Yet, primary care practices, paid predominantly by the visit and denied COVID-19 federal relief funds, have struggled to keep their doors open.
- The United States is experiencing a period of racial unrest and growing economic inequity. High-quality primary care, widely distributed, can reduce health care disparities.

This report aims to address the shortcomings of the current health care systems that have devalued primary care by offering a vision for high-quality primary care and a set of evidence-based recommendations that will strengthen the heart of the health care system at a time of great need. The committee declared its vision for high-quality primary care in the United States with the definition it stated in Chapter 2:

High-quality primary care is the provision of whole-person, integrated, accessible, and equitable health care by interprofessional teams who are accountable for addressing the majority of an individual's health and wellness needs across settings and through sustained relationships with patients, families, and communities.

To make this vision a reality for everyone in the United States, the committee recommends specific actions, detailed below, that fall under five critical implementation objectives:

1. **Pay for primary care teams to care for people, not doctors to deliver services.**
   - The nation gets what it pays for, and payment reform that supports and encourages high-quality primary care, rather than actively discouraging it, is fundamental to the committee's vision of high-quality primary care.
2. **Ensure that high-quality primary care is available to every individual and family in every community.**
   - Everyone in the country should have easy access to high-quality primary care that is person centered, relationship oriented, and responsive to the needs of its community.

3. **Train primary care teams where people live and work.**
   - When primary care training is interprofessional and located in community settings, it is more effective at developing the skills that will keep people connected and healthy.
4. **Design information technology that serves the patient, family, and interprofessional care team.**
   - New health information technology standards should prioritize and facilitate integrated care that is person centered, supports relationships, and is responsive to the needs of its community.
5. **Ensure that high-quality primary care is implemented in the United States.**
   - Implementing high-quality primary care requires clear and meaningful measures of whole-person care, ongoing research, and leadership in the federal government to ensure federal policies support its development.

If clear recommendations supported by strong evidence were enough, the landmark 1996 Institute of Medicine (IOM) report *Primary Care: America's Health in a New Era* would have had a greater impact, and primary care in the United States would not be in its current weakened state. For this reason, the committee's scope of work calls for an implementation plan, not merely a set of recommendations.

The committee's implementation plan—comprising a set of actions for each implementation objective—is built on an implementation strategy consisting of three elements:

1. An implementation framework, one that accounts for the complexity of the U.S. health care system and its public- and private-sector actors.
2. An accountability framework, one that establishes a process for assessing the adequacy and completeness of implementation activities.
3. A public policy framework, one that prioritizes the development of government policy to implement high-quality primary care, consistent with its status as a common good.

These elements are fundamental to a strategy for overcoming the current barriers to implementing high-quality primary care in the United States. Of them, the third is most important. Health care is not a functioning market in the United States, and resource allocation is subject to the concentration of political and economic power. High-quality primary care—and the benefits it brings—will not thrive without supportive public policy.

Taken together, the actions recommended below comprise the committee's implementation plan. They attempt to build the necessary public support and political will; call for appropriately scaled actions by public- and private-sector actors at the macro, meso, and micro system levels; and create accountability structures to ensure the work gets done. Evidence supporting the value of primary care is ample, with extensive research identifying policies and practices that facilitate high-quality primary care. These activities focus on what is needed to promote and effectively scale them. See Appendix D for a table that sorts the committee's recommended action by system level and actor.

OBJECTIVE ONE: PAY FOR PRIMARY CARE TEAMS TO CARE FOR PEOPLE, NOT DOCTORS TO DELIVER SERVICES

Action 1.1: Payers—Medicaid, Medicare, commercial insurers, and self-insured employers—should evaluate and disseminate payment models based on the ability of those models to promote the delivery of high-quality primary care, as defined by the committee, and not on their ability to achieve short-term cost savings.

Action 1.2: Payers—Medicaid, Medicare, commercial insurers, and self-insured employers—using a fee-for-service (FFS) payment model for primary care should shift primary care payment toward hybrid (part FFS, part capitated) models, making them the default method for paying for primary care teams over time. For risk-bearing contracts with population-based health and cost accountabilities, such as those with accountable care organizations, payers should ensure that sufficient resources and incentives flow to primary care. Hybrid reimbursement models should:
   a. pay prospectively for interprofessional, integrated, team-based care, including incentives for incorporating non-clinician team members and for partnerships with community-based organizations;
   b. be risk adjusted for medical and social complexity;
   c. allow for investment in team development, practice transformation, and the infrastructure to design, use, and maintain necessary digital health technology; and
   d. align with incentives for measuring and improving outcomes for attributed populations.

Action 1.3: The Centers for Medicare & Medicaid Services should increase the overall portion of spending going to primary care by:
   a. accelerating efforts to improve the accuracy of the Medicare physician fee schedule by developing better data collection and valuation tools to identify overpriced services, with the goal of increasing payment rates for primary care evaluation and management services

by 50 percent and reducing other service rates to maintain budget
neutrality; and
b.   restoring the Relative Value Scale Update Committee to the advisory nature as originally intended by developing and relying on
additional independent expert panels and evidence derived directly
from practices.

Action 1.4: States should implement primary care payment reform by:
a.   using their authority to facilitate multi-payer collaboration on primary care payment and fee schedules and
b.   measuring and increasing the overall portion of health care spending in their state going to primary care.

Any effort to implement high-quality primary care must begin with
a commitment to pay primary care more and differently because of its
demonstrated and superior capacity among health care services to improve population health and health equity for all society, not because of
any ability to achieve short-term return on investment for a specific payer.
High-quality primary care is not a commodity service whose value needs to
be demonstrated in a competitive marketplace but rather a common good
to be promoted by responsible public policy and supported by private-
sector action. Implementation of primary care spending policies should
attend to the characteristics and practice of what constitutes primary care
in accordance with the committee's definition. As the largest payer in the
country, Medicare creates payment policies that set the standard for other
public and commercial payers, and it merits priority. In exchange, primary
care must be accountable for developing additional capacities consistent
with the committee's definition and garner additional merit for superior
performance.

The actions recommended here are tested. Hybrid capitation and FFS
arrangements, paired with practice transformation resources and aligned
across payers as set forth in Action 1.2, have been shown to build primary care capacity consistent with the committee's definition. Medicare fee
schedule changes have been discussed widely and recommended previously
and are actions well within the current purview of the U.S. Department of
Health and Human Services (HHS).

Many health systems providing primary care services through employed
or contracted models have accepted global capitated payments but continue
to operate and compensate primary care on an FFS model, blunting the effects of payment models intended to strengthen primary care. Health systems
in these arrangements should honor the intentions of payers and evidence
of superior performance, seeing that new payment models allocate sufficient
management authority and resources to the practice of primary care.

Because primary care makes up a small proportion of overall health care spending, the reduction in other service prices noted in Action 1.3 will be minimal and will help to equilibrate compensation between primary care and other specialties, making primary care a more attractive choice for medical graduates. Changes to the fee schedule are necessary because capitation, budget rates, and compensation within health care systems typically rely on calculations powered by the fee schedule. In addition, the Medicare fee schedule is the basis for relative prices set by other payers. States and local markets that have implemented Action 1.4 have seen benefits in terms of reduced cost trends and improved quality. More states should follow their lead.

Self-insured employers with in-state employment bases should follow the lead of their home states and participate in these efforts. Employers with a geographically dispersed workforce should follow Medicare's lead and recognize the need to prioritize and pay for high-quality primary care.

These recommended actions, while supported by evidence, have not been scaled and widely implemented for two reasons. First, high-quality primary care requires additional resources. These payment reform innovations have been evaluated against the wrong standard: short-term savings, rather than promoting high-quality primary care, which is a value in and of itself. The focus on repeatedly testing new primary care payment models with a few clinicians, in search of "a better mousetrap" to achieve these short-term savings, has left most primary care clinicians to languish in underpaying FFS arrangements with the wrong incentives. Attention should be focused on moving more clinicians to existing models rather than testing new ones.

Second, budget neutrality or premium stability requirements mean increasing the investments in primary care, redistributing funds, and prioritizing it over other health care services, which is what the committee is calling for in designating it as a common good. Achieving this rebalancing requires leadership, particularly in the public sector. The COVID-19 pandemic's further weakening of primary care has opened the policy window and leadership opportunity for the Centers for Medicare & Medicaid Services (CMS), employers, and more state officials to act without delay.

OBJECTIVE TWO: ENSURE THAT HIGH-QUALITY PRIMARY CARE IS AVAILABLE TO EVERY INDIVIDUAL AND FAMILY IN EVERY COMMUNITY

Action 2.1: To facilitate an ongoing primary care relationship, all individuals should have the opportunity to have a usual source of primary care.

    a.   Payers—Medicaid, Medicare, commercial insurers, and self-insured employers—should ask all covered individuals to declare a usual source of primary care annually and should assign non-responding enrollees using established methods, track this information, and use it for payment and accountability measures.

b. Health centers, hospitals, and primary care practices should assume and document an ongoing clinical relationship with the uninsured people they are treating.

Action 2.2: To improve access to high-quality primary care for underserved populations, and to facilitate empanelment of uninsured people, the U.S. Department of Health and Human Services, enabled by congressional appropriations, should target sustained investment in the creation of new health centers (including federally qualified health centers, look-alikes, and school-based health centers), rural health clinics, and Indian Health Service facilities in federally designated shortage areas.

Action 2.3: To improve access to high-quality primary care services for Medicaid beneficiaries, the Centers for Medicare & Medicaid Services should:

a. Revise and enforce its fee-for-service (section 1902) and managed care (section 1937) access standards for primary care for Medicaid beneficiaries, ensuring them adequate access to primary care as defined by the committee, and

b. Provide technical assistance resources to state Medicaid agencies for implementing and attaining these standards, and measure and publish state performance on these standards.

Action 2.4: The Centers for Medicare & Medicaid Services should permanently support the COVID-era rule revisions and Medicaid and Medicare benefits interpretations that have facilitated integrated team-based care, enabled more equitable access to telephone and virtual visits, provided equitable payment for non-in-person visits, eased documentation requirements, expanded the role of interprofessional care team members, and eliminated other barriers to high-quality primary care.

Action 2.5: Primary care practices should move toward a community-oriented model of primary care by:

a. Including community members with lived experience in their governance, practice design, and practice delivery and

b. Partnering with community-based organizations.

Accreditation bodies should encourage practices to be more community oriented by revising their standards to facilitate these changes.

Successfully implementing high-quality primary care means everyone should have access to the "sustained relationships" primary care offers. The committee recognizes this access is more likely to happen when everyone has adequate health insurance with no financial barriers to primary care. Absent that, payers can improve and reinforce access by taking a page from public health and making "the right choice the easy choice": encouraging, formalizing, and administratively supporting the existing relationships between their enrollees and primary care teams. Declaring their usual source of care is a reasonable expectation of enrollees in exchange for insurer benefits. Aligned payer action will reinforce the value of primary care as a common good and reduce beneficiaries' misperceptions that access to specialty care is somehow being limited by any one payer. While private primary care practices are not obligated to treat the uninsured, those that do and are able should assume an ongoing clinical relationship with them.

Primary care cannot be accessible if it is not available or has financial barriers to its use. The Health Resources and Services Administration (HRSA) Health Center Program now provides care to 1 in 11 Americans and has proven to be effective at improving the ability of people without insurance or in medically underserved urban and rural communities to access high-quality primary care. As an organized system of primary care, it merits additional scaling.

As the second-largest payer in the country, with disproportionate numbers of children and high-needs beneficiaries, Medicaid needs a primary care strategy, one led by CMS and implemented and enforced by its state partners, that results in addressing the documented low rates for primary care that are paid by state Medicaid agencies and their contractors and that particularly limit children's access to high-quality primary care. This strategy should be led by CMS and implemented and enforced by its state partners. A Medicaid program that is reformed to mirror Medicare in terms of payment standards and federal responsibility may be the most straightforward path to ensuring equitable access to high-quality primary care for its beneficiaries (Perrin et al., 2020). However, short of such a complete reform of Medicaid, federal access-to-care standards for state Medicaid programs can be readily modified to catalyze state and managed care organization payment and coverage policies to prioritize high-quality primary care. Meeting federal access standards and those from accrediting bodies will require states and their contracted managed care organizations to take the actions needed, including increasing Medicaid rates for primary care and expanding primary care provider networks.

Primary care accessibility should not be limited by the walls of the practice, however. The COVID-19 pandemic forced Medicare and other payers to quickly scale the ability to access primary care teams virtually by video and telephone. The benefits of these forms of care have been shown to extend well beyond improved infection control, and payment and regulatory barriers to their use need to be minimized.

Finally, much of what improves health has little to do with medical care, and efforts by primary care teams to build health-improving relationships with community organizations and public health agencies should be fostered. This will require action from practices and systems themselves but should also be incorporated into accreditation standards. In keeping with the team-based, relational nature of high-quality primary care, these efforts should place patients, their families, and community members at the center of the design and accountability efforts for successful implementation.

OBJECTIVE THREE: TRAIN PRIMARY CARE TEAMS WHERE PEOPLE LIVE AND WORK

Action 3.1: Health care organizations and local, state, and federal government agencies should expand and diversify the primary care workforce, particularly in federally designated shortage areas, to strengthen interprofessional teams and better align the workforce with the communities they serve.

a.   Public and private health care organizations should ensure inclusion, support, and training for family caregivers, community health workers, and other informal caregivers as members of the interprofessional primary care team.

b.   The U.S. Department of Education and the U.S. Department of Health and Human Services should partner to expand educational pipeline models that would encourage and increase opportunities for students who are under-represented in health professions.

c.   The Health Resources and Services Administration, state and local government, and health care systems should redesign and implement economic incentives, including loan forgiveness and salary supplements, to ensure that interprofessional care team members, especially those who reflect the diverse needs of the local community, are encouraged to enter primary care in rural and underserved areas.

d.   Health systems and organizations should develop a data-driven approach to customizing interprofessional teams to meet the needs of the population they serve.

Action 3.2: The Centers for Medicare & Medicaid Services, the U.S. Department of Veterans Affairs, the Health Resources and Services Administration (HRSA), and states should redeploy or augment funding to support interprofessional training in community-based, primary care practice environments. The revised funding model should be sufficient in size to improve access to primary care and ensure that training programs can adequately support primary care pipeline needs of the future.

    a.   HRSA funding (via Title VII and Title VIII programs) for other health professions training should be increased and prioritized for interprofessional education.

    b.   The U.S. Department of Health and Human Services, enabled by Congress as needed, should redesign the graduate medical education (GME) payment to support training primary care clinicians in community settings and expand the distribution of training sites to better meet the needs of communities and populations, particularly in rural and underserved areas. Effective HRSA models (e.g., Teaching Health Centers, Rural Training Tracks) should be prioritized for existing GME funding redistribution and sustained discretionary funding.

    c.   GME funding should be modified to support the training of all members of the interprofessional primary care team, including but not limited to nurse practitioners, pharmacists, physician assistants, behavioral health specialists, pediatricians, and dental professionals.

Black, Hispanic, American Indian and Alaska Native, and Native Hawaiian and other Pacific Islander people are currently under-represented in nearly every clinical health care occupation. For care teams to address well-documented disparities in treatment based on race and ethnicity, its members must reflect the lived experience of the people and families they serve. Primary care is no exception, and organizations that train, hire, and finance primary care clinicians bear a responsibility to ensure that the demographic composition of its primary care workforce reflects the communities and that the care delivered is culturally appropriate.

More fundamentally, developing a workforce able to deliver the committee's definition of primary care will require reshaping what is expected of training programs and the clinical settings in which that training occurs. Continuing to train individual primary care clinicians in inpatient settings, as is commonplace today, will not accomplish this. Many examples exist of team-based training in community settings, but they can only be scaled if financial incentives, mostly in the form of GME payments, are recalibrated to support all members of the primary care team. This reshaping will not be accomplished quickly and, recognizing the significance of this task (IOM, 2014), the committee also recommends broader adoption of alternative financing sources for HRSA-developed, community-based primary care training.

OBJECTIVE FOUR: DESIGN INFORMATION TECHNOLOGY THAT SERVES THE PATIENT, FAMILY, AND INTERPROFESSIONAL CARE TEAM

Action 4.1: The Office of the National Coordinator for Health Information Technology and the Centers for Medicare & Medicaid Services should develop the next phase of digital health, including electronic health record, certification standards to:

    a. Align with the functions of primary care—supporting the relationship between clinicians, care teams, and patients; providing access and continuous contact over time; collecting and understanding the patient's story; and focusing on the patient and family rather than the disease;

    b. Account for the user experience of clinicians and patients (e.g., clicks and time spent using system, data transferred without manual review, and improvements in care delivery and health outcomes) to ensure that health systems are truly interoperable;

    c. Ensure equitable access and use of digital health systems that support equitable care and deliver national standards, including guidelines, measures, and decision-making functions, while allowing local tailoring;

    d. Include highly usable sensemaking functionality, such as automated tools that make sense of data, identify clinically important data, and inform care;

    e. Ensure base products meet certification standards with minimal need for local modification to meet requirements; and

    f. Hold health information technology vendors and state and national support agencies financially responsible for failing to achieve benchmarks.

Action 4.2: The Office of the National Coordinator for Health Information Technology (ONC) and the Centers for Medicare & Medicaid Services (CMS) should plan for and adopt a comprehensive aggregate patient data system to enable primary care clinicians and interprofessional teams to easily access comprehensive patient data needed to provide whole-person care.

    a. This data source needs to be usable by any certified digital health tool for patients, families, clinicians, and care team members.

    b. ONC and CMS could accomplish this through a centralized data warehouse, individual health data card, or distributed sources connected by a real-time, functional health information exchange. Each approach has its own challenges, and an initial effort would need to decide on the right national approach.

Digital health, and electronic health records (EHRs) in particular, represent both the opportunities for improving care coordination and person-centeredness and the risks of clinical burden. Digital health is a major source of professional dissatisfaction and clinician burnout (NASEM, 2019). The committee supports federal standards setting for this field, but it has determined that current certification requirements are a significant barrier to high-quality primary care. The recommended elements for new certification requirements suggested here will require additional planning before adoption as well as new policies and authorizations to enforce standards. Creating and implementing these changes requires innovation by vendors and state and national support agencies and accomplishing these goals will not be easy to ascertain.

Similarly, aggregated patient data systems, planned for and adopted by federal entities, can both ensure high-quality primary care and reduce the chances of patient data being used for personal or organizational profit. The experience of local and regional health information exchanges and other nations' approach to solving this common problem can inform this effort. The committee acknowledges that digital health and the shortcomings of current EHRs is an issue that affects all of health care, but believes that high-functioning, user-friendly health information technology (HIT) can produce outsized benefits for primary care specifically by enabling primary care's coordinating functions. Improved EHR functionality and a comprehensive data system can facilitate the aggregation of information across all settings, including the community, and make that information usable by the entire primary care team to promote access to care, care coordination, strong relationships, and integration with population health.

OBJECTIVE FIVE: ENSURE THAT HIGH-QUALITY PRIMARY CARE IS IMPLEMENTED IN THE UNITED STATES

Action 5.1: The U.S. Department of Health and Human Services (HHS) Secretary should establish a Secretary's Council on Primary Care to enable the vision of primary care captured in the committee's definition.

    a. Council members should include the Centers for Medicare & Medicaid Services Administrator; the Directors of the Center for Medicare & Medicaid Innovation, the Health Resources and Services Administration, and the Agency for Healthcare Research and Quality; the Assistant Secretary for Planning and Evaluation at HHS; and the National Coordinator for the Office of the National Coordinator for Health Information Technology.

    b. The council should coordinate primary care policy across HHS agencies with attention to the following responsibilities: (1) assess federal primary care payment sufficiency and policy; (2) monitor primary care workforce sufficiency including training financing, production and preparation, incentives for federally designated shortage areas, and federal clinical assets/investments (health centers, rural health clinics, the Indian Health Service, and the U.S. Department of Veterans Affairs); (3) coordinate and assess the adequacy of the federal government's research investment in primary care; (4) address primary care's technology, data, and evidence needs, including interagency collaboration in the use of multiple data sources; (5) promote alignment of public and private payer policies in support of high-quality primary care; and (6) establish meaningful metrics for assessing the quality of primary care that embrace person-centeredness and health equity goals. Additionally, the council should coordinate implementing the committee's recommended actions that target federal agencies.

c. As part of its coordination role, the council should verify adequate budgetary resources are allotted in respective agencies for fulfilling these responsibilities.

d. The council should annually report to Congress and the public on the progress of its implementation plan and performance on each of these six responsibilities.

e. In all its work, the Secretary's Council on Primary Care should be informed through regular guidance and recommendations provided by a Primary Care Advisory Committee, created by the HHS Secretary under the Federal Advisory Committee Act, that includes members from national organizations that represent significant primary care stakeholder groups, such as patients, certifying boards, professional organizations, health care worker organizations, payers, and employers.

Action 5.2: The U.S. Department of Health and Human Services should form an Office of Primary Care Research at the National Institutes of Health and prioritize funding of primary care research at the Agency for Healthcare Research and Quality, via the National Center for Excellence in Primary Care Research.

Action 5.3: To improve accountability and increase chances of successful implementation, primary care professional societies, employers, consumer groups, and other stakeholders should assemble, and regularly compile and disseminate a "high-quality primary care implementation scorecard," based on the five key implementation objectives identified in this report. One or more philanthropies should assist in convening and facilitating the scorecard development and compilation.

Table 12-1 summarizes the committee's proposed scorecard, which aggregates a small number of already-compiled, state- and national-level measures for each implementation objective in this report. (See Appendix E for a discussion of measurement sources and considerations related to the scorecard.)

Successfully implementing a set of recommendations or a plan rests in part on clear accountability. Lack of accountability hampered efforts to implement many aspects of the recommendations in the 1996 IOM report. For these reasons, the committee's task would be incomplete if it did not

TABLE 12-1 The Health of Primary Care: A Proposed U.S. Scorecard (Summary)

Objective 1: Pay for primary care teams to care for people, not doctors to deliver services

Measure 1.1: Percentage of total spend going to primary care—commercial insurance

Measure 1.2: Percentage of total spend going to primary care—Medicare

Measure 1.3: Percentage of total spend going to primary care—Medicaid

Measure 1.4: Percentage of primary care patient care revenue from capitation

Objective 2: Ensure that high-quality primary care is available to every individual and family in every community

Measure 2.1: Percentage of adults without a usual source of health care

Measure 2.2: Percentage of children without a usual source of health care

Measure 2.3: Primary care physicians per 100,000 people in medically underserved areas

Measure 2.4: Primary care physicians per 100,000 people in areas that are not medically underserved

Objective 3: Train primary care teams where people live and work

Measure 3.1: Percentage of physicians trained in community-based settings, rural areas, Critical Access Hospitals, Medically Underserved Areas

Measure 3.2: Percentage of physicians, nurses, and physician assistants working in primary care

Measure 3.3: Percentage of new physician workforce entering primary care each year

Measure 3.4: Residents per 100,000 population by state

Objective 4: Design information technology that serves the patient, family, and interprofessional care team

The committee is not aware of adequate measures or data sources that capture the use or availability of person-centered digital health in primary care (or any health care) settings, underscoring the urgency for further research in this area

Objective 5: Ensure that high-quality primary care is implemented in the United States

Measure 5.1: Investment in primary care research by the National Institutes of Health in dollars spent and percentage of total projects funded

---

assign accountability for implementation. While state-level and private-sector innovations can provide valuable examples, the committee believes federal leadership and responsibility is essential to scaling its vision of high-quality primary care:

- As the only health care service positively associated with improved population health status and equity, primary care constitutes a common good. Therefore its strength and viability make it a public policy priority.
- As the first- and second-largest payers in the country, Medicare and Medicaid payments shape our health care delivery system. Medicare payment policy's incompatibility with high-quality primary care has weakened primary care.
- Federal payments and policy determine health care workforce training priorities.
- Federal funding determines medical and health care services research priorities.

For these reasons, a Secretary's Council on Primary Care at HHS is the appropriate accountable entity for coordinating the significant federal role and agency activity called for in these actions. The council should also be accountable for monitoring and aligning private-sector activities in support of primary care and ensuring that the committee's vision for primary care is supported by future administration policy. Senior secretary–level coordination is necessary because of the various and widespread agency-level activities that affect primary care, including workforce training and safety net funding within HRSA, payment and benefits policy at CMS, HIT within the Office of the National Coordinator for Health Information Technology, and research at the Agency for Healthcare Research and Quality (AHRQ) and the National Institutes of Health (NIH). No one HHS agency can take on the task of coordination, which will continue to be in the public interest beyond the scope or term of a special task force, another accountability mechanism the committee considered and rejected.

This council, to be effective, should be given authority by the secretary to ensure adequate budgetary expenditures are made in appropriate agencies for implementing the actions in this report. Public reporting will also increase its accountability. A key task for the council, in addition to coordinating federal policies and receiving input and guidance from a Primary Care Advisory Committee, will be overseeing the establishment of clear accountability measures for providing primary care consistent with the committee's definition. Done judiciously and with stakeholder input; a focus on core, evidence-based, high-value primary care functions; uniform guidelines that allow for flexible application based on contextual population need, care delivery setting, and community input; and attention to what has been learned in the field of quality measurement, these measures can change expectations for what constitutes high-quality primary care and also facilitate learning and catalyze improved population health.

Just as the financing of primary care delivery has suffered relative to other health services, so has the financing of research on the field of primary care. The country has defunded this research at its peril, as it seeks how to have a rational, just, cost-effective health care system. To address this shortcoming, the committee recommends establishing an NIH Office of Primary Care Research, with functions similar to its Office of Emergency Care Research. This new entity, coupled with the funding of AHRQ's National Center for Excellence in Primary Care Research, could foster a much-needed system of learning and improvement in primary care that would help make the committee's vision of high-quality primary care a reality for everyone in the United States.

Finally, to increase the chances for successful implementation, designated actors must be held publicly accountable for their responsibilities. Ample evidence exists for what is necessary for high-quality primary care. Health service researchers regularly generate a variety of measures related to aspects of primary care delivery in the United States, which to date have not been organized and regularly compiled to assess performance and progress. Organized capacity for this work of accountability is profoundly absent: the professional diversity of the high-quality primary care team is its clinical strength but its political and economic weakness. While a single voice to advocate for public policy change exists for other health care services, such as hospitals, the pharmaceutical industry, and nursing homes, primary care has no similar voice and as a result suffers in the policy-making process. The committee's recommended Federal Advisory Committee to the Secretary's Council on Primary Care could serve this function. Organizing primary care clinicians, consumer groups, and other interested stakeholders (from the variety of settings in which primary care is delivered) to measure the implementation of the critical activities recommended by the committee using the proposed scorecard will not only hold the designated actors accountable and increase the likelihood of successful implementation but also catalyze a common agenda for a vital common good.

CONCLUSION

High-quality primary care for everyone in the United States will deliver benefits for individuals and society. It will make the nation healthier and enable outcomes to be shared more fairly. This is not a new insight, and it was core to the IOM's 1996 report. The nation, however, has turned its collective back to this evidence, and the state of primary care—the heart of our health system—has weakened at a time when the nation needs it more than ever.

We know how to have high-quality primary care; indeed, examples of it around the country have shown it is possible to:

- Pay for primary care teams to care for people, not doctors to deliver services.
- Ensure that high-quality primary care is available to every individual and family in every community.
- Train primary care teams where people live and work.
- Design HIT that serves the patient, family, and primary care team.

The nation should systematically implement and scale these possibilities for everyone in the United States. The nation deserves nothing less, but doing so requires leadership, accountability, and clear steps to accomplish this work. The committee hopes the work captured in this report helps realize this vision sooner rather than later.

REFERENCES

IOM (Institute of Medicine). 1996. *Primary care: America's health in a new era.* Washington, DC: National Academy Press.

IOM. 2014. *Graduate medical education that meets the nation's health needs.* Washington, DC: The National Academies Press.

Martin, S., R. L. Phillips, Jr., S. Petterson, Z. Levin, and A. W. Bazemore. 2020. Primary care spending in the United States, 2002–2016. *JAMA Internal Medicine* 180(7):1019–1020.

NASEM (National Academies of Sciences, Engineering, and Medicine). 2019. *Taking action against clinician burnout: A systems approach to professional well-being.* Washington, DC: The National Academies Press.

PCPCC (Patient-Centered Primary Care Collaborative). 2018. *Fact sheet: Spending for primary care.* Washington, DC: Patient-Centered Primary Care Collaborative.

Perrin, J. M., G. M. Kenney, and S. Rosenbaum. 2020. Medicaid and child health equity. *New England Journal of Medicine* 383(27):2595–2598.

Reiff, J., N. Brennan, and J. Fuglesten Biniek. 2019. Primary care spending in the commercially insured population. *JAMA* 322(22):2244–2245.

Appendix A

Committee Member, Fellow, and Staff Biographies

COMMITTEE MEMBERS

Linda McCauley, R.N., Ph.D., FAAN, FAAOHN (*Co-Chair*), is a global leader in environmental health and the dean of the Emory University School of Nursing. She co-chairs the National Academies of Sciences, Engineering, and Medicine's Committee on Implementing High-Quality Primary Care and previously served on the National Academies' Board on Population Health and Public Health Practice, and the Environmental Roundtable, and the National Academy of Medicine Membership Committee. In 2020, she was named to the U.S. Environmental Protection Agency's (EPA's) Children's Health Protection Advisory Committee. For more than 20 years, Dr. McCauley has been consistently funded for innovative research on children's environmental health, vulnerable workers and occupational health, environmental justice, and the impacts of climate change on human health. She leads large multi-disciplinary research projects and research centers that are conducted in partnerships with vulnerable communities. Her work has been supported with funding from the Centers for Disease Control and Prevention, the National Institutes of Health, EPA, the U.S. Department of Defense, and the U.S. Department of Veterans Affairs. This year, Dr. McCauley was awarded an Honorary Fellowship in the Royal Academy of Nursing for the international impact of her work. She was inducted into the Sigma Theta Tau International Nursing Hall of Fame in 2016 and is a fellow of the American Academy of Nursing and the American Academy of Occupational Health Nurses. Her research has resulted in more than 150 publications, ongoing consultations, leadership on occupational and environmental advisory panels, testimony to government oversight bodies, and international presentations on interprofessional practice and the advancement of nursing science.

Robert L. Phillips, Jr., M.D., M.S.P.H. (*Co-Chair*), is the founding executive director of the Center for Professionalism and Value in Health Care. From 2012 to 2018, he was the vice president for research and policy, where he led the launch of a national primary care clinical registry and a Measures That Matter research and development program for primary care. He is a graduate of the Missouri University of Science and Technology (1990) and the University of Florida College of Medicine (1995; with honors for special distinction). He completed training in family medicine at the University of Missouri in 1998, followed by a 2-year fellowship in health services research and public health (M.S.P.H., 2000). After his fellowship, Dr. Phillips became the assistant director of the Robert Graham Center in Washington, DC, from 2004 to 2012, and he served as its director. Dr. Phillips currently practices part time in a community-based residency program in Fairfax, Virginia, and is a professor of family medicine at Georgetown University and Virginia Commonwealth University. He served on the American Medical Association's Council on Medical Education and as the president of the National Residency Matching Program. Dr. Phillips has been on several Federal Advisory Committees, including as the vice chair of the Council on Graduate Medical Education, the National Committee on Vital and Health Statistics, and the Negotiated Rule-Making Committee for Shortage Area Designation. A nationally recognized leader on primary care policy and health care reform, Dr. Phillips was elected to the National Academy of Medicine (NAM) in 2010 and is currently the chair of the Membership Committee. He previously was the NAM Membership Committee Section 08 chair and a member of three consensus studies for the National Academies of Sciences, Engineering, and Medicine: Committee on Depression, Parenting Practices, and the Health Development of Young Children; Committee on Integrating Primary Care and Public Health; and Committee on Assessing Progress on Implementing the Recommendations of the Institute of Medicine Report *The Future of Nursing: Leading Change, Advancing Health*. He has also been a reviewer for several studies, is a frequent participant in NAM/National Academies workshops and roundtables, and was a member of the NAM Vital Directions writing committee in 2016.

Asaf Bitton, M.D., M.P.H., is the executive director of Ariadne Labs, a health systems innovation center at Brigham and Women's Hospital and the Harvard T.H. Chan School of Public Health, and an associate professor of medicine and health care policy at Harvard Medical School. He is a national and global expert on primary care policy, financing, and delivery. He previously served as the director of Ariadne Labs' Primary Health Care Program, leading primary care measurement and improvement work in more than a dozen countries along with previous work directing regional medical home learning collaboratives in Massachusetts. He is a core founder and the leader of the Primary Health Care Performance Initiative, a partnership that includes the World Bank, the World Health Organization, and the Bill & Melinda Gates Foundation and is dedicated to transforming the global state of primary health care. Currently, this partnership is scaling the launch and use of country-level dashboards on primary care performance across more than 20 countries, with a goal of 60 countries by 2022. He is a senior advisor for primary care policy at the Center for Medicare & Medicaid Innovation since 2012; he helped design and test three major comprehensive primary care payment and delivery initiatives, now active in 18 states, with more than 70 payers and 3,000 practices that serve more than 3 million Medicare beneficiaries and 15 million total patients. These initiatives represent the largest tests of combined primary care payment and clinical practice transformation work in the United States. He is a primary care physician at a medical home practice in Jamaica Plain, Massachusetts, that he helped to found in 2011. He currently serves on the National Advisory Council for Healthcare Research at the Agency for Healthcare Research and Quality. He is an elected member of the International Academy of Quality and Safety and a fellow of the American College of Physicians.

Tumaini Rucker Coker, M.D., M.B.A., is an associate professor of pediatrics at the University of Washington School of Medicine, the director of research at the Seattle Children's Center for Diversity & Health Equity, and the principal investigator (PI) at the Seattle Children's Research Institute Center for Child Health, Behavior, and Development. Dr. Coker's research focuses on community-engaged design and evaluation of innovative interventions to reduce socioeconomic disparities of care among children and on primary care practice redesign for children in low-income communities. She is the PI for two large, multi-year, National Institutes of Health–funded projects that focus on developing, adapting, and testing interventions to improve the delivery of care to children in low-income communities: a multi-site trial of a parent coach-led model for preventive care and a trial of a parent text messaging program to enhance parent–provider communication about chronic disease management. As the PI, she recently completed a project funded by the Patient-Centered Outcomes Research Institute using telehealth to improve access to mental health services for children in low-income communities. Dr. Coker's work has been published widely, in journals such as *JAMA*, *Pediatrics*, and the *American Journal of Public Health*, and covered by media outlets, including *The Wall Street Journal*, CNN, *USA Today*, and NBC. Dr. Coker was commissioned to complete technical reviews for two National Academies of Sciences, Engineering, and Medicine reports: *Parenting Matters: Supporting Parents of Children Ages 0–8* and *Adolescent Health Services: Missing Opportunities*. She also served as a panelist for the public session for the National Academies report *Intersecting Professions in the Birth Through Age 8 Continuum*.

Carrie Colla, Ph.D., is a professor at the Dartmouth Institute for Health Policy and Clinical Practice at the Geisel School of Medicine. A health economist, Dr. Colla focuses on physician payment, health insurance markets, and insurance benefit design. Her work is aimed at improving the quality, accessibility, and cost of health care. Dr. Colla's research is dedicated to examining health system performance and the effectiveness of payment and delivery system reforms, including accountable care organizations. Her empirical studies include the effects of changes in Medicare reimbursement for physicians and institutional providers on vulnerable populations; the prevalence and drivers of low-value health care services; and the effects of care management and coordination in physician practices. Dr. Colla has been the principal investigator for the annual National Survey of Accountable Care Organizations since its inception, and she is a lead investigator in Dartmouth's Agency for Healthcare Research and Quality Center of Excellence to Study High-Performing Health Care Systems. Dr. Colla is a member of the Physician-Focused Payment Model Technical Advisory Committee, which makes recommendations to the Secretary of the U.S. Department of Health and Human Services on payment model proposals. Dr. Colla participated in the National Academy of Medicine (NAM) Robert Wood Johnson Foundation Health Policy Fellowship, spending time as a congressional Fellow and working as a senior advisor at the Center for Medicare & Medicaid Innovation. She is an Emerging Leader in Health and Medicine Scholar at NAM. Dr. Colla received her Ph.D. in health policy and her M.A. in economics from the University of California, Berkeley.

Molly Cooke, M.D., MACP, FRCP, is a professor of medicine at the University of California, San Francisco, where she is a practicing general internist and teaches primary care internal medicine. Her medical practice focuses on the care of patients with HIV and other chronic illnesses. Dr. Cooke's academic focus is health professions education, with a particular emphasis on educational initiatives addressing patient outcomes and cost of care in complex, chronically ill patients. Her papers have been published in the *New England Journal of Medicine*, the *Annals of Internal Medicine*, *Academic Medicine*, *JAMA*, and *Science*. She is an author of *Educating Physicians: A Call for Reform of Medical School and Residency* (2010), winner of the PROSE award for distinction in scholarly publication in 2011. In additional to her own experience as a primary care physician, Dr. Cooke has considered primary care from national and international perspectives. Beginning in 2004, she served in a number of leadership roles in the American College of Physicians (ACP), which is the professional association for internal medicine physicians in the United States, comprising 154,000 members; she was president of ACP from 2013 to 2014. She has a broad understanding of health care in the United States and the perspective of generalist clinicians, including non-physician health professionals, in rural and underserved areas. Internationally, she has worked and/or consulted in China, Cuba, India, and Uganda and visited many other countries, including Canada, Japan, Mexico, New Zealand, the United Arab Emirates, and the United Kingdom, to learn about their health care systems and health professions workforce.

Jennifer E. DeVoe, M.D., D.Phil., is a practicing family physician, health services researcher, and national primary care leader based in Portland, Oregon. As the John & Sherrie Saultz Professor and Chair of the Oregon Health & Science University (OHSU) Department of Family Medicine, she oversees nearly 200 faculty, 72 resident physicians, and several of OHSU's primary care clinics. Dr. DeVoe also serves as the inaugural director of OHSU's new Center for Primary Care Research and Innovation. She was the first chief research officer and executive director of the OCHIN practice-based research network from 2010 to 2016, where she led the development of a unique community laboratory, linking together electronic health record (EHR) data from more than 400 community health center clinics across multiple states to build the most robust safety net research database in the country. She is the past president of the North American Primary Care Research Group, the premiere international professional organization for primary care researchers. Dr. DeVoe studies access to health insurance coverage and health care services, disparities in care, and how policy and practice changes affect the health of children and families. She and her team pioneered the use of EHR data in research, studying health care use by uninsured and underinsured populations, which has garnered her national attention, particularly relating to the Children's Health Insurance Program and the Patient Protection and Affordable Care Act. She served as a National Academy of Medicine (NAM)/American Board of Family Medicine Puffer Fellow from 2012 to 2014 and was elected to the NAM in 2014. She is the inaugural chair of the NAM's primary care interest group (2017–2019). Dr. DeVoe serves on the board of governors for the Patient-Centered Outcomes Research Institute.

Rebecca S. Etz, Ph.D., is an associate professor of family medicine and population health at Virginia Commonwealth University (VCU) and the co-director of The Larry A. Green Center—Advancing Primary Health

Care for the Public Good. Dr. Etz has deep expertise in qualitative research methods and design, primary care measures, practice transformation, and engaging stakeholders. Dr. Etz received her Ph.D. in cultural anthropology from Rutgers University in 2004. Her career has been dedicated to learning the heart and soul of primary care. Her work has resulted in iterative research cycles that expose and reflect on the tacit norms and principles of primary care in which clinicians, thought leaders, and patients are equally invested. Her work follows three main lines of inquiry: (1) bridging the gap between the business of medicine and the lived experience of the human condition; (2) making visible the principles and mechanisms on which the unique strength of primary care is based; and (3) exposing the unintended, often damaging consequences of policy and transformation efforts applied to primary care but not informed by primary care concepts. As a member of the VCU Department of Family Medicine and Population Health and the previous co-director of the ACORN PBRN, Dr. Etz has been the principal investigator of several federal and foundation grants, contracts and pilots, all directed toward making the pursuit of health a humane experience. She often serves on expert panels and as a board member for national primary care organizations. Recent research activities have included studies in primary care measures, behavioral health, care coordination, preventive care delivery, simulation modeling, care team models, organizational change, community-based participatory research, the study of exemplars, and adaptive use of health technologies. Dr. Etz has presented to the National Academies study committees, written a National Academy of Medicine discussion paper, and participated in planning meetings.

Susan Fisher-Owens, M.D., is a clinical professor of pediatrics in the University of California, San Francisco (UCSF), School of Medicine and preventive and restorative dental sciences in the UCSF School of Dentistry. She practices at Zuckerberg San Francisco General, the county public hospital, and created an award-winning and sustainable oral health clinic embedded in its pediatric outpatient clinic. Dr. Fisher-Owens works with physicians on how to prevent oral disease in children or control it in adults (particularly pregnant women) and with dentists on how to work with children and incorporate context of care. Her research on a conceptual model of children's oral health is cited internationally, and her current research focuses on children's oral health disparities. She serves on the California State Oral Health Plan and the California Perinatal and Infant Oral Health Quality Advisory Board and leads the integration effort of CavityFreeSF. She recently was an executive committee member on the American Academy of Pediatrics Committee on Oral Health. In addition to her clinical and research interests of oral health, she is a champion of interprofessional/team-based care and centering supportive services in primary care to best meet people's needs, including integrating in primary care supports for social determinants of health, through several venues. She also leads a public health effort on vaccinations.

Jackson Griggs, M.D., FAAFP, is the chief executive officer of the Heart of Texas Community Health Center, a 14-site federally qualified health center serving 59,000 patients in Central Texas. Dr. Griggs is a family physician who has trained more than 150 primary care residents. He is the president of the McLennan County Medical Education and Research Foundation, overseeing the Waco Family Medicine Residency Program and fellowships in hospice and palliative care medicine, sports medicine, and clinical informatics. His research has included topics in primary care, population health, and mental illness. Through community engagement and collaboration, Dr. Griggs inaugurated an award-winning integrated behavioral health program, a wellness center for low-income families, a medical–legal partnership, and a produce prescription program for community health center patients.

Shawna Hudson, Ph.D., is a professor and the research division chief in the Department of Family Medicine and Community Health and the founding director of the Center Advancing Research and Evaluation for Patient-Centered Care at the Rutgers Robert Wood Johnson Medical School. She is a medical sociologist and has a joint faculty appointment in the Rutgers School of Public Health in the Department of Health Behavior, Society, and Policy. Dr. Hudson holds research memberships in the Rutgers Institute for Translational Medicine and Science, the Rutgers Cancer Institute of New Jersey, and the Institute for Health, Healthcare Policy, and Aging Research. She is a mixed methods researcher and the principal investigator (PI) and co-PI on multiple National Institutes of Health (NIH)-funded studies. She has published extensively on the role of primary care in long-term follow-up care for cancer survivors. Dr. Hudson is a community-engaged primary care researcher working with vulnerable populations at the intersections of community health, primary care, and specialty care. She is the director for the Community Engagement Core of the New Jersey Alliance for Clinical and Translational Science, which is a Clinical and Translational Science Awards consortium. She leads its $5 million NIH-funded Rapid Acceleration of Diagnostics for Underserved Populations initiative to improve outreach and access to COVID-19 testing within New Jersey vulnerable and underserved communities.

Shreya Kangovi, M.D., is the founding executive director of the Penn Center for Community Health Workers and an associate professor at the University of Pennsylvania Perelman School of Medicine. She is a leading expert on improving population health through evidence-based community health worker programs. Her research also highlights the perspectives of socially disadvantaged patients, who are often left out of health care design. Dr. Kangovi led the team that designed IMPaCT, a standardized, scalable program that leverages community health workers—trusted laypeople from local communities—to improve health. IMPaCT has been tested in three randomized controlled trials and improves chronic disease control, mental health, and quality of care while reducing total hospital days by 65 percent. It has a $2:1 annual return on investment to payers and has been delivered to more than 10,000 high-risk people in the Philadelphia region. In the past 3 years, IMPaCT has become the most widely disseminated community health worker program in the United States; it is being replicated by organizations across 18 different states, including the Veterans Health Administration; state Medicaid programs; integrated health care organizations; and even retailers such as Walmart. Dr. Kangovi founded the Penn Center for Community Health Workers, a national center of excellence dedicated to advancing health in low-income populations through effective community health worker programs. Dr. Kangovi has authored numerous scientific publications and received more than $25 million in funding, including federal grants from the National Institutes of Health and the Patient-Centered Outcomes Research Institute. She is the recipient of the 2019 Robert Wood Johnson Foundation Health Equity Award, an elected member of the American College of Physicians, and a member of the National Academies of Sciences, Engineering, and Medicine's Roundtable on the Promotion of Health Equity.

Christopher F. Koller, M.A., M.P.P.M., is the president of the Milbank Memorial Fund, a 115-year-old operating foundation that improves population health by connecting leaders with the best information and experience. Before joining the fund, he served the state of Rhode Island as the country's first health insurance commissioner between 2005 and 2013. Under Mr. Koller's leadership, the Rhode Island Office of the Health Insurance Commissioner was nationally recognized for its rate review process and its efforts to use insurance regulation to promote payment reform, primary care revitalization, and delivery system transformation. The office was also one of the lead agencies in implementing the Patient Protection and Affordable Care Act in Rhode Island. Prior to serving as health insurance commissioner, Mr. Koller was the chief executive officer of the Neighborhood Health Plan of Rhode Island for 9 years. In this role, he was the founding chair of the Association of Community Affiliated Plans. Mr. Koller has a bachelor's degree (summa cum laude) from Dartmouth College and master's degrees in social ethics and public/private management from Yale University. He was a member of the National Academies of Sciences,

Engineering, and Medicine's Board on Health Care Services from 2014 to 2019 and served on the National Academies' Committee on Essential Health Benefits and Committee on Integrating Social Needs Care and in numerous national and state health policy advisory capacities. Mr. Koller is also a professor of practice in the Department of Health Systems Policy and Practice in the School of Public Health at Brown University. Mr. Koller serves on the boards of the Primary Care Development Corporation, Fair Health, and the Commonwealth Care Alliance of Massachusetts.

Alex H. Krist, M.D., M.P.H., is a professor of family medicine and population health at Virginia Commonwealth University and an active clinician and teacher at the Fairfax Family Practice Residency. He is the director of the Virginia Ambulatory Care Outcomes Research Network, director of community-engaged research at the Center for Clinical and Translational Research, and the current chairperson for the United States Preventive Services Task Force. Dr. Krist's areas of interest include implementation of preventive recommendations, patient-centered care, shared decision making, cancer screening, and health information technology. He is the primary author of numerous peer-reviewed publications and has presented to a wide range of audiences at national and international conferences. Dr. Krist was elected to the National Academy of Medicine in 2018.

Luci K. Leykum, M.D., M.B.A., M.Sc., is the executive associate chair for the Department of Internal Medicine and a professor in the Department of Internal Medicine at the Dell Medical School at The University of Texas at Austin. She is also a health services researcher in the South Texas Veterans Health Care System and the principal investigator (PI)/center lead for the Elizabeth Dole Center of Excellence for Veteran and Caregiver Research. She completed residency training in internal medicine at the Columbia-Presbyterian Medical Center, joining the Columbia faculty in 2002. In 2004, she accepted a clinician-investigator position at the University of Texas Health Science Center at San Antonio and the South Texas Veterans Health Care System, and she earned an M.Sc. in clinical investigation from The University of Texas in 2007. In 2019, she became the associate chair for clinical innovation in the Department of Medicine at the Dell Medical School. Dr. Leykum's research has focused on applying the lens of complexity science to clinical systems. She has served as a co-PI in studies of learning in primary care teams and led and contributed to clinical systems improvement and change publications on a variety of care settings. Her most recent studies use a complexity science framework to understand how relationships and sensemaking differ between physician teams and how these differences relate to patient outcomes.

Benjamin Olmedo, M.M.Sc., PA-C, works in family medicine and urgent care for Dignity Pacific Central Coast Health Centers, where he is also involved in clinical informatics, quality measures, and equitable health outcomes. Following his distinguished Army service, Mr. Olmedo earned his PA-C through the Yale School of Medicine Physician Associate Program, after which he commissioned in the U.S. Public Health Service, where he worked in rural Alaska for 3 years with the Indian Health Service. While in Alaska, Mr. Olmedo furthered his experience by serving on the board of directors for the Mat-Su Healthcare Foundation and was honored through Save the Children's REAL Award in 2014 for community outreach, improving patient outcomes, and increasing use of clinic services. Mr. Olmedo served as the president of the Public Health Service Academy of Physician Assistants from 2015 to 2016, was the chief clinical consultant for physician assistants for the Indian Health Service from 2017 to 2019, and worked in California with a rural tribal health clinic from 2015 to 2019, where he was the emergency preparedness coordinator, on the California Tribal Epidemiology Center advisory council, and the chair of the Clinical Education Committee, in addition to providing same-day access to health care services. He is currently an officer in the U.S. Navy Reserves and in the Executive M.P.H. Program through the University of California, Los Angeles, Fielding School of Public Health.

Brenda Reiss-Brennan, Ph.D., APRN, is a medical anthropologist and a psychiatric nurse practitioner working in primary care for more than 40 years. As a principal investigator, she leads the Intermountain Healthcare (IH) adoption, diffusion, and evaluation of clinical integration for mental health and medical care. The cost and quality evidence of the Mental Health Integration (MHI) innovation has transformed primary care culture and spread rapidly over 120 IH medical clinics, including uninsured, rural, and specialty, and 45 non-IH community clinics throughout the United States. MHI provides a proven integrated team-based culture that has effectively improved quality and patient experience while reducing costs. Dr. Reiss-Brennan holds a long-standing faculty appointment at the University of Utah College of Nursing. She serves as a local, national, and international consultant for cultural innovation, implementation science, and scaling of MHI cost, quality, and patient and staff experience research to improve population health and well-being.

Hector P. Rodriguez, Ph.D., M.P.H., is a professor, the Kaiser Permanente Endowed Chair in Health Policy and Management, and the director of the Center for Healthcare Organizational and Innovation Research at the University of California, Berkeley. He is an expert in organizational analysis and performance management in health care organizations and public health systems. Prior to his academic career, he was a management consultant for the Permanente Medical Group, where he worked with leaders and clinicians in northern California to implement primary care practice redesign and evaluate their impact on patient care. He has more than 100 peer-reviewed publications, including key articles focused on measuring and improving patients' experiences of care and patient-reported outcomes, primary care teamwork, implementation fidelity, and multi-level organizational analyses. Dr. Rodriguez is an elected member of the National Academy of Medicine and a recipient of the John D. Thompson Investigator Award from the Association of University Programs in Health Administration.

Mary Roth McClurg, Pharm.D., M.H.S., is a professor and the executive vice dean—chief academic officer at the University of North Carolina (UNC) Eshelman School of Pharmacy. Dr. Roth McClurg spent 12 years as a clinical pharmacist in primary care practice within the VA Health System and in the interdisciplinary geriatric clinic within the Department of Geriatrics at UNC Healthcare, providing direct care as part of an interprofessional care team. She has focused her research efforts on advancing comprehensive medication management and the role of the clinical pharmacist as an integral member of the primary care team, with the goal of optimizing medication use and improving care in people with multiple chronic diseases. Dr. Roth McClurg is a fellow of the American College of Clinical Pharmacy.

Robert J. Weyant, M.S., D.M.D., Dr.P.H., serves as the associate dean of dental public health and community outreach and a professor and the chair of the Department of Dental Public Health at the School of Dental Medicine. He is also a professor of epidemiology at the Graduate School of Public Health. He received a master's degree in public health, a dental degree from the University of Pittsburgh School of Dental Medicine, and a doctoral degree in epidemiology from the University of Michigan. Dr. Weyant is a former Navy dental officer and VA dentist. He has been a diplomate of the American Board of Dental Public Health since 1987, is a past president of the American Association for Public Health Dentistry, and is the editor in chief of the *Journal of Public Health Dentistry*. He currently serves on numerous local, state, and national committees aimed at reducing oral health disparities, increasing the dental workforce, and improving access to oral care. Dr. Weyant's research involves basic and social epidemiological research related to oral health disparities. Presently, he is the principal investigator (PI) or co-PI on several National Institutes of Health–funded studies of oral disease etiology. Dr. Weyant also directs the Center for Oral Health Research in Appalachia and oversees the joint degree program in public health.

FELLOWS

National Academy of Medicine Fellows

Kameron Matthews, M.D., J.D., FAAFP, is a board-certified family physician, advocate, and policy maker, with a career focus on underserved patient populations. She serves as the assistant undersecretary for health for clinical services and the chief medical officer of the Veterans Health Administration. In 2017, she was named one of National Minority Quality Forum's 40 Under 40 Leaders in Minority Health. She served as the 2018–2020 National Academy of Medicine (NAM)—American Board of Family Medicine James C. Puffer Fellow and was elected to the membership of the NAM in 2020.

Lars Peterson, M.D., Ph.D., is a family physician and a health services researcher who serves as the vice president of research for the American Board of Family Medicine. He also has an appointment as an associate professor in the Department of Family and Community Medicine at the University of Kentucky, where he provides direct clinical care and teaches students and residents. Dr. Peterson, a native of Utah, received his medical and graduate degrees from Case Western Reserve University in Cleveland, Ohio, and completed his family medicine residency at the Trident/Medical University of South Carolina family medicine residency program. Dr. Peterson leads a research team focused on elucidating the outcomes of family medicine certification, in particular the impact that certification activities have on the quality of care delivered by family physicians. Additionally, Dr. Peterson and his team seek to understand the ecology of family medicine over time—what physicians do in practice and their contribution to high-quality health care. His personal research interests also include investigating associations between area-level measures of health care and socioeconomics with health and access to health care, rural health, primary care, and comprehensiveness of primary care. Dr. Peterson has authored more than 100 peer-reviewed publications and made more than 100 national/international conference presentations.

Dima M. Qato, Pharm.D., M.P.H., Ph.D., is a pharmacist and a pharmacoepidemiologist and currently serves as the Hygeia Centennial Chair and an associate professor (with tenure) in the Titus Family Department of Clinical Pharmacy at the University of Southern California (USC) School of Pharmacy. She has also been appointed as a senior fellow with the USC Leonard D. Schaeffer Center for Health Policy and Economics. Dr. Qato has been selected as a National Academy of Medicine Pharmacy Fellow for 2018–2020. She received her Pharm.D. from the University of Illinois at

Chicago, an M.P.H. from the Johns Hopkins Bloomberg School of Public Health, and a Ph.D. in public health from the University of Illinois School of Public Health. Dr. Qato's research focuses on access and safe use of medications in vulnerable populations in the United States and abroad. She uses population-based methods to better understand the underlying mechanisms responsible for the use, underuse, and unsafe use of medications, how these patterns may influence health outcomes and health disparities, and what can be done from a community and policy perspective to address these growing public health problems. Dr. Qato's research has been published in leading peer-reviewed journals, including *JAMA* and *Health Affairs*. Her work has received widespread media coverage, including in *The New York Times*, NPR, PBS News, *The Washington Post*, *The Atlantic*, CNN, BBC, and *National Geographic* and is funded by various agencies, including the National Institutes of Health and the Robert Wood Johnson Foundation. She has also influenced national and state policy around medication access and safety. Dr. Qato's goal is to promote public accountability in ensuring access to and safe use of medications at the national, state, and local levels. In an effort to achieve this goal, Dr. Qato is interested in incorporating polypharmacy and the role of pharmacies in ongoing health care reform.

National Academies Christine Mirzayan Fellow

Jennifer Puthota is a medical student at the CUNY School of Medicine in New York. She received her bachelor's degree in 2017 after studying biomedical sciences at the City College of New York's Sophie Davis School. Working closely with her school's Humanities in Medicine program, Ms. Puthota participates in the practice of Narrative Medicine, is compelled by the storytelling and listening component of health care, and is on track to graduate with distinction in this practice. During her undergraduate years, Ms. Puthota worked in a cell biology laboratory at the City College of New York; she investigated epithelial cell polarization and the specific role of kinesins within cell architecture. She performed clinical research during her first 2 years of medical school at the Icahn School of Medicine at Mount Sinai, where she was a research assistant for a laboratory examining the possible genetic factors underlying mental illnesses, such as schizophrenia and bipolar disorder. Her most recent research project focused on climate change and how increasing air temperatures may be negatively affecting birth outcomes both in the United States and across the globe. She was interested in the intersectionality of disciplines, so she was very much encouraged to apply for the Mirzayan Fellowship Program. She hopes to better understand how policy works with the sciences to bolster health.

STAFF

Marc Meisnere, M.H.S., is a program officer on the National Academies of Sciences, Engineering, and Medicine's Board on Health Care Services. Since 2010, Mr. Meisnere has worked on a variety of National Academies consensus studies and other activities that have focused on mental health services for service members and veterans, suicide prevention, primary care, and clinician well-being. Before joining the National Academies, Mr. Meisnere worked on a family planning media project in northern Nigeria with the Johns Hopkins Center for Communication Programs and on a variety of international health policy issues at the Population Reference Bureau. He is a graduate of Colorado College and the Johns Hopkins Bloomberg School of Public Health.

Tracy A. Lustig, D.P.M., M.P.H., is a senior program officer with the Health and Medicine Division of the National Academies of Sciences, Engineering, and Medicine. Dr. Lustig was trained in podiatric medicine and surgery and spent several years in private practice. In 1999, she was awarded a congressional fellowship with the American Association for the Advancement of Science and spent 1 year working in the office of U.S. Senator Ron Wyden. Dr. Lustig joined the National Academies in 2004. She was the study director for consensus studies on the geriatrics workforce, oral health, ovarian cancer research, and the report *Social Isolation and Loneliness in Older Adults: Opportunities for the Health Care System*. She has also directed workshops on the allied health workforce, the use of telehealth to serve rural populations, assistive technologies, and hearing loss. In 2009, she staffed a National Academies–wide initiative on the "Grand Challenges of an Aging Society" and helped to launch the Forum on Aging, Disability, and Independence, which she currently directs. Dr. Lustig has a doctor of podiatric medicine degree from Temple University and an M.P.H. with a concentration in health policy from The George Washington University.

Sarah K. Robinson is a research associate with the Board on Health Care Services. Prior to her time at the National Academies of Sciences, Engineering, and Medicine, she worked in health care market research, focusing on first-in-class medications, implantable devices, and telehealth platforms. She has led numerous primary research initiatives on a wide variety of topics, including patient–clinician communication barriers, treatment algorithms and decision making, and insurance transparency. Ms. Robinson received her B.A. in political science and English from the University of Chicago.

Samira Abbas is a senior program assistant on the Board on Health Care Services. She serves on the Social Security Administration study on diagnosing and treating adult cancers and the study on implementing high-quality primary care. Ms. Abbas recently worked with Visionary Consulting Partners as an administrative assistant and was previously in eye care, where she accumulated extensive experience as an optician, optometric/ophthalmic technician, and vision insurance specialist. She attended Virginia Commonwealth University in Richmond, Virginia, majoring in biology and minoring in chemistry.

Sharyl Nass, Ph.D., serves as the director of the Board on Health Care Services and director of National Academies of Sciences, Engineering, and Medicine's National Cancer Policy Forum (NCPF). To enable the best possible care for all patients, the board undertakes scholarly analysis of the organization, financing, effectiveness, workforce, and delivery of health care, with emphasis on quality, cost, and accessibility. NCPF examines policy issues pertaining to the entire continuum of cancer research and care. For two decades, Dr. Nass has worked on a broad range of health and science policy topics, including the quality and safety of health care and clinical trials, developing technologies for precision medicine, and strategies for large-scale biomedical science. She has a Ph.D. in cell biology from Georgetown University and undertook postdoctoral training at the Johns Hopkins University School of Medicine and a research fellowship at the Max Planck Institute in Germany. She also holds a B.S. and an M.S. from the University of Wisconsin–Madison. She has received the Cecil Medal for Excellence in Health Policy Research, a National Academies Distinguished Service Award, and the Institute of Medicine staff team achievement award (as team leader).

Appendix B

Primary Care: America's Health in a New Era Report Recommendations

The Institute of Medicine's (IOM's) 1996 report *Primary Care: America's Health in a New Era*[1] was foundational and represented an ambitious plan to strengthen primary care in the United States. The Committee on Implementing High-Quality Primary Care's deliberations and the resulting report were highly influenced by it. The complete text of the recommendations put forth in 1996 is below.

RECOMMENDATIONS

2.1 *To Adopt the Committee's Definition*
This committee has defined primary care as the provision of integrated, accessible health care services by clinicians who are accountable for addressing a large majority of personal health care needs, developing a sustained partnership with patients, and practicing in the context of family and community. The committee recommends the adoption of this definition by all parties involved in the delivery and financing of primary care and by institutions responsible for the education and training of primary care clinicians.

5.1 *Availability of Primary Care for All Americans*
The committee recommends development of primary care delivery systems that will make the services of a primary care clinician available to all Americans.

---

[1] IOM (Institute of Medicine). 1996. *Primary care: America's health in a new era.* Washington, DC: National Academy Press.

5.2 *Health Coverage for All Americans*
To assure that the benefits of primary care are more uniformly available, the committee recommends that the federal government and the states develop strategies to provide health coverage for all Americans.

5.3 *Payment Methods Favorable to Primary Care*
The committee recommends that payment methods favorable to the support of primary care be more widely adopted.

5.4 *Payment for Primary Care Services*
The committee recommends that when fee-for-services is used to reimburse clinicians for patient care, payments for primary care be upgraded to reflect better the value of these services.

5.5 *Practice by Interdisciplinary Teams*
The committee believes that the quality, efficiency, and responsiveness of primary care are enhanced by the use of interdisciplinary teams and recommends the adoption of the team concept of primary care wherever feasible.

5.6 *The Underserved and Those with Special Needs*
The committee recommends that public or private programs designed to cover underserved populations and those with special needs include the provision of primary care services as defined in this report. It further recommends that the agencies or organizations funding these programs carefully monitor them to ensure that such primary care is provided.

5.7 *Primary Care and Public Health*
The committee recommends that health care plans and public health agencies develop specific written agreements regarding their respective roles and relationships in (a) maintaining and improving the health of the communities they serve and (b) ensuring coordination of preventive services and health promotion activities related to primary care.

5.8 *Primary Care and Mental Health Services*
The committee recommends the reduction of financial and organizational disincentives for the expanded role of primary care in the provision of mental health services. It further recommends the development and evaluation of collaborative care models that integrate primary care and mental health services more effectively. These models should involve both primary care clinicians and mental health professionals.

5.9 *Primary Care and Long-Term Care*
To improve the continuity and effectiveness of services for those requiring long-term care, the committee recommends that third-party payers (including Medicare and Medicaid), health care organizations, and health professionals promote the integration of primary care and long-term care by coordinating or pooling financing and removing regulatory or other barriers to such coordination.

5.10 *Quality of Primary Care*
The committee recommends the development and adoption of uniform methods and measures to monitor the performance of health care systems and individual clinicians in delivery primary care as defined in this report. Performance measures should include cost, quality, access, and patient and clinician satisfaction. The results should be made available to public and private purchasers of care, provider organizations, clinicians, and the general public.

5.11 *Primary Care in Academic Health Centers*
The committee recommends that academic health centers explicitly accept primary care as one of their core missions and provide leadership in the development of primary care teaching, research, and service delivery programs.

6.1 *Programs Regarding the Primary Care Workforce*
The committee recommends (a) that the current level of effort to increase the supply of primary care clinicians be continued and (b) that these primary care training programs and delivery systems focus their efforts on improving the competency of primary care clinicians and on increasing access for populations not now receiving adequate primary care.

6.2 *Monitoring the Primary Care Workforce*
The committee recommends that state and federal agencies carefully monitor the supply of and requirements for primary care clinicians.

6.3 *Addressing Issues of Geographic Maldistribution*
The committee recommends that federal and state governments and private foundations fund research projects to explore ways in which managed care and integrated health care systems can be used to alleviate the geographic maldistribution of primary care clinicians.

6.4 *State Practice Acts for Nurse Practitioners and Physician Assistants*
The committee recommends that state governments review current restrictions on the scope of practice of primary care nurse practitioners and

physician assistants and eliminate or modify those restrictions that impede collaborative practice and reduce access to quality primary care.

7.1 *Training in Primary Care Sites*
All medical schools should require their undergraduate medical students to experience training in settings that deliver primary care as defined by this committee.

7.2 *Common Core Competencies*
The committee recommends that common core competencies for primary care clinicians, regardless of their disciplinary base, be defined by a coalition of appropriate educational and professional organizations and accrediting bodies.

7.3 *Emphasis on Common Core Competencies by Accrediting and Certifying Bodies*
The committee recommends that organizations that accredit primary care training programs and certify individual trainees support curricular reforms that teach the common core competencies and essential elements of primary care.

7.4 *Special Areas of Emphasis in Primary Care Training*
The committee recommends that the curricula of all primary care education and training programs emphasize communication skills and cultural sensitivity.

7.5 *All-Payer Support for Primary Care Training*
The committee recommends the development of an all-payer system to support health professions education and training. A portion of this pool of funds should be reserved for education and training in primary care.

7.6 *Support for Graduate Medical Education in Primary Care Sites*
The committee recommends that a portion of the funds for graduate medical education be reallocated to provide explicit support for the direct and overhead costs of primary care training in nonhospital sites, such as health maintenance organizations, community clinics, physician offices, and extended care facilities.

7.7 *Interdisciplinary Training*
The committee recommends that (a) the training of primary care clinicians include experience with the delivery of health care by interdisciplinary teams; and (b) academic health centers work with health maintenance

organizations, group practices, community health centers, and other health care delivery organizations using interdisciplinary teams to develop clinical rotations for students and residents.

7.8 Experimentation and Evaluation

The committee recommends that private foundations, health plans, and government agencies support ongoing experimentation and evaluation of interdisciplinary teaching of collaborative primary care to determine how such teaching might best be done.

7.9 Retraining

The committee recommends that (a) curricula of retraining programs in primary care include instruction in the core competencies proposed for development in Recommendations 7.2 and 7.3 and (b) certifying bodies in the primary care disciplines develop mechanisms for testing and certifying clinicians who have undergone retraining for primary care.

8.1 Federal Support for Primary Care Research

The committee recommends that (a) the Department of Health and Human Services identify a lead agency for primary care research and (b) the Congress of the United States appropriate funds for this agency in an amount adequate to build both the infrastructure required to conduct primary care research and fund high-priority research projects.

8.2 National Database and Primary Care Data Set

The committee recommends that the Department of Health and Human Services support the development of and provide ongoing support for a national database (based on a sample survey) that reflects the majority of health care needs in the United States and includes a uniform primary care data set based on episodes of care. This national survey should capture data on the entire U.S. population, regardless of insurance status.

8.3 Research in Practice-Based Primary Care Research Networks

The committee recommends that the Department of Health and Human Services provide adequate and stable financial support to practice-based primary care research networks.

8.4 Data Standards

The committee recommends that the federal government foster the development of standards for data collection that will ensure the consistency of data elements and definitions of terms, improve coding, permit analysis of episodes of care, and reflect the content of primary care.

8.5 *Study of Specialist Provision of Primary Care*
The committee recommends that the appropriate federal agencies and private foundations commission studies of (a) the extent to which primary care, as defined by the IOM, is delivered by physician specialists and subspecialists, (b) the impact of such care delivery on primary care workforce requirements, and (c) the effects of these patterns of health care delivery or such care on the costs and quality of and access to health care.

9.1 *Establishment of a Primary Care Consortium*
The committee recommends the formation of a public–private, nonprofit primary care consortium consisting of professional societies, private foundations, government agencies, health care organizations, and representatives of the public.

Appendix C

Committee's Calculations to Determine the Impact of the Decreased Density of Primary Care Physicians Between 2005 and 2015

Assumptions:
Rural population: 46 million (Cromartie et al., 2020)
U.S. total population: 331 million (U.S. Census Bureau, 2021)
Life expectancy: 78.6 years (Arias and Xu, 2019)

Loss of primary care physicians (PCPs) from rural counties between 2005 and 2015: –7.0 per 100,000 population (Basu et al., 2019)

Loss of PCPs in the United States overall between 2005 and 2015: –5.2 per 100,000 population (Basu et al., 2019)

+10 PCPs per 100,000 population is associated with an increase of 51.5 days of life expectancy per person (Basu et al., 2019)

IMPACT OF LOSS OF PRIMARY CARE PHYSICIANS IN RURAL COUNTIES, 2005–2015

If +10 PCPs per 100,000 population = 51.5 days of gained life per person

–7 PCPs per 100,000 population = 51.5 × .7 = 36.05 days of potential life lost per person

46 million people × 36.05 days = 1,658,300,000 days of potential life lost between 2005 and 2015

1,658,300,000 days / 365 = 4,543,287 years of potential life lost between 2005 and 2015

4,542,287 / 10 = 454,328 years of potential life lost per year

454,328 years of lost life per year / 365 days = 1,245 years of potential life lost per day

454,328 years of life lost per year; 1,245 years of potential life lost per day

If the average life expectancy is 78.6 years, 454,328/78.6 = 5,780 potential lives lost per year 1,245 per day / 78.6 = 15.84 potential lives lost per day

IMPACT OF LOSS OF PRIMARY CARE PHYSICIANS IN THE UNITED STATES, 2005–2015

If +10 PCPs per 100,000 population = 51.5 days of gained life per person

–5.2 PCPs per 100,000 population = 51.5 × .52 = 26.78 days of potential life lost per person

331 million people × 26.78 days = 8,864,180,000 days of potential life lost between 2005 and 2015

8,864,180,000 / 365 = 24,285,425 years of potential life lost between 2005 and 2015

24,285,425 / 10 = 2,428,543 years of potential life lost per year between 2005 and 2015

2,428,543 / 365 days = 6,654 years of potential life lost per day

2,428,543 years of potential life lost per year; if the average life expectancy is 78.6 years, 2,428,543 / 78.6 = 30,897 lives lost per year; 6,654 / 78.6 = 85 lives lost per day

A typical commuter plane carries 200 passengers (180 passengers in a Boeing 757; 250 passengers in an Airbus); 200 passengers / 85 lives lost per day = roughly one 200-person plane crashing every 2–3 days

REFERENCES

Arias, E., and J. Xu. 2019. *National vital statistics reports: United States life tables, 2017 (vol. 68, no. 7).* Hyattsville, MD: National Center for Health Statistics.

Basu, S., S. A. Berkowitz, R. L. Phillips, Jr., A. Bitton, B. E. Landon, and R. S. Phillips. 2019. Association of primary care physician supply with population mortality in the United States, 2005–2015. *JAMA Internal Medicine* 179(4):506–514.

Cromartie, J., E. A. Dobis, T. P. Krumel, D. McGranahan, and J. Pender. 2020. *Rural America at a glance: 2020 edition.* Washington, DC: U.S. Department of Agriculture.

U.S. Census Bureau. 2021. *U.S. and world population clock.* https://www.census.gov/popclock (accessed January 13, 2021).

Appendix D

Three System-Level Tables of Actors and Actions

Macro System Level	
Actor	**Action**
Congress	2.2: Create new health centers, rural health clinics, Indian Health Service facilities, etc. 3.2.B: Support community-based training with graduate medical education payment
Accrediting organizations	2.5: Help practices embrace community-oriented care models
Primary care professional societies, consumer groups, and philanthropies	5.3: Regularly track progress and disseminate a "high-quality primary care scorecard"

Meso System Level	
Actor	**Action**
State governments (including state Medicaid programs)	1.4: Implement payment reform 2.3: Publish performance on Medicaid standards 3.1.C: Incentivize care team diversity 3.2: Increase support for training in community practices

Actor	Action
U.S. Department of Health and Human Services	2.2: Create new health centers, rural health clinics, Indian Health Service facilities, etc. 3.1.B: Partner with the U.S. Department of Education to increase opportunities for under-represented students 3.2.B: Support community-based training with graduate medical education payment 3.2.C: Expand graduate medical education funding beyond physicians 5.1: Establish a Secretary's Council on Primary Care 5.2: Form an Office of Primary Care Research at the National Institutes of Health and prioritize research funding at the Agency for Healthcare Research and Quality
Health Resources and Services Administration	3.1.C: Incentivize care team diversity 3.2: Increase support for training in community practices
Office of the National Coordinator for Health Information Technology	4.1: Develop the next phase of electronic health record certification standards 4.2: Adopt an aggregate patient data system
Centers for Medicare & Medicaid Services	1.1: Support payment models that promote the delivery of high-quality primary care 1.2: Shift from fee-for-service to hybrid reimbursement 1.3: Increase portion of primary care spending 2.1.A: Help beneficiaries declare a usual source of primary care 2.3: Ensure adequate access for Medicaid beneficiaries and provide assistance to agencies 2.4: Make permanent the COVID-era rule revisions 3.2: Increase support for training in community practices 4.1: Develop the next phase of digital health certification standards 4.2: Adopt an aggregate patient data system
U.S. Department of Veterans Affairs	3.2: Increase support for training in community practices
U.S. Department of Education	3.1.B: Partner with the U.S. Department of Health and Human Services to increase opportunities for under-represented students
Commercial payers	1.1: Support payment models that promote the delivery of high-quality primary care 1.2: Shift from fee-for-service to hybrid reimbursement 2.1.A: Help beneficiaries declare a usual source of primary care
Publicly and privately owned health care organizations	2.1.B: Empanel uninsured patients in the system 3.1.A: Support and train non-clinician team members, including caregivers 3.1.C: Incentivize care team diversity 3.1.D: Develop a data-driven approach for tailoring to community needs

Micro System Level

Actor	Action
Individual primary care practices	2.1.B: Empanel uninsured patients in the system 2.5: Embrace community-oriented care models 3.1.A: Support and train non-clinician team members, including caregivers
Patients	2.1.A and 2.1.B: Declare a usual source of primary care

Appendix E

The Health of Primary Care: A U.S. Scorecard

The committee was given the task of creating an implementation plan in addition to the typical task of developing recommendations. An implementation plan needs a set of metrics to track how well it is going and whether its aims are achieved over time. To that end, the committee offers this scorecard of selected measures that would meet both purposes and could be managed by one or more of the sponsoring organizations, federal agencies, or other interested stakeholders. The scorecard covers most report recommendations as objectives and offers data sources and example data, where possible, for dimension-related measures for each objective.

Very few of the 1996 report recommendations, or those for most past Institute of Medicine reports about primary care, have ever been actualized. Tracking on these scorecard dimensions will help achieve the intentions of the report sponsors and stakeholders and the committee's recommendations, strengthening the foundation of America's health care system.

SCORECARD PRINCIPLES

The committee proposes suggested measures for this scorecard using the following principles:

- The measures should be previously developed—as opposed to proposed new measures—and each should track the committee's objectives, either directly or indirectly.

- The measures should be few, easily understood by the general public, and consistent over time.
- Data for the measures must be collected regularly, comprehensively, and reliably for producing assessment at relevant scope or geography; preferably, data will be publicly available and non-proprietary.
- Accountable unit—the measure should be available at the national and state levels, so as to engage advocates and policy makers.

These principles result in a small number of measures and do not address all the committee's recommendations. Assessing the implementation status of a number of recommendations cannot currently be reliably accomplished. Additional research to accomplish this is a different task from monitoring: the work of developing and testing additional measures is not as important to implementation accountability as effectively deploying existing measures.

For each measure, the committee lists data sources and sample performance from those data sources. The committee does not propose a single data source for those measures where multiple are available. Despite the committee's emphasis on team-based care and training throughout the report, robust data sources for non-physician team members and team-based care itself continue to pose a challenge. This reality is reflected in the proposed measures below.

The scorecard development process (see Action 5.3 in Chapter 12) should include selecting the appropriate data, prioritizing the frequency and reliability of source data. A comment section for each objective discusses the proposed measures, data sources, and where additional measures are needed.

The committee is not proposing targets for each measure. Establishing a baseline and documenting changes over time are critical to assessing implementation efforts.

THE HEALTH OF PRIMARY CARE:
A PROPOSED U.S. SCORECARD

Objective 1: Pay for primary care teams to care for people, not doctors to deliver services.

Measure 1.1: Percentage of total spend going to primary care—commercial insurance

Potential data sources:	Sample performance:
Medical Expenditure Panel Survey (MEPS) (AHRQ, 2021)	MEPS data (2011–2016): 6.0 percent (narrow definition[1] of primary care) 10.2 percent (broad definition[2] of primary care) State-level analysis also available (Jabbarpour et al., 2019)
Health Care Cost Institute (HCCI) (HCCI, 2020)	HCCI data (2017): 4.35 percent (narrow definition)[3] 8.04 percent (broad definition)[4] (Reiff et al., 2019)
Truven Health MarketScan (IBM, 2020) (proprietary)	Truven Health MarketScan data (2018) 5.95 percent (The Commonwealth Fund, 2020b)

Measure 1.2: Percentage of total spend going to primary care—Medicare

Potential data sources:	Sample performance:
MEPS (AHRQ, 2021)	MEPS data (2011–2016): 4.4 percent (narrow definition) 6.9 percent (broad definition) State-level analysis also available (Jabbarpour et al., 2019)
Medicare Master Beneficiary Summary File (MMBSF) (CMS, 2020c)	MMBSF data (2015): 2.12 percent (narrow definition)[5] 4.88 percent (broad definition)[6] (Reid et al., 2019)
Centers for Medicare & Medicaid Services (CMS) Limited Data Set (LDS) (CMS, 2020b)	The Commonwealth Fund (2017) 5.66 percent (The Commonwealth Fund, 2020a)

Measure 1.3: Percentage of total spend going to primary care—Medicaid	
Potential data source:	Sample performance (2011–2016):
MEPS (AHRQ, 2021)	6.0 percent (narrow definition) 11.2 percent (broad definition) State-level analysis also available (Jabbarpour et al., 2019)

Measure 1.4: Percentage of primary care patient care revenue from capitation	
Potential data source:	Sample performance:
National Ambulatory Medical Care Survey (NAMCS) (CDC, 2020a)	
MEPS (AHRQ, 2021)	MEPS (2013): 5.3 percent of office-based visits (Zuvekas and Cohen, 2016)

Comments:

Definitions are important when calculating the percentage of total health care spending directed to primary care; differences in the definitions used are listed below. The source data also differ, sometimes even within a source; for example, The Commonwealth Fund estimates for Medicare spending derive from the CMS LDS file, which is easier to access and analyze than the MMBSF. The LDS and the MMBSF estimates are not too dissimilar, but the difference may be related to nuanced definitional choices that are more readily assessed using the MMBSF. The percentage of total health spending in primary care for children is typically higher, as children have less chronic care and lower use of high-cost care settings. Medicaid data are important for this assessment of federal payments to primary care, but access to aggregate, national Medicaid data has been difficult until recently.

The scorecard measures related to paying for team-based care and moving away from fee-for-service, volume-based funding focuses on the current insufficiency of funding, points to sources of data about primary care investment across payer types, and also creates a tracking mechanism for capitated, or population-based, payment. The MEPS is a reliable source for longitudinally tracking primary care investment and claims data that are useful for looking at particular sectors, such as the investment made in caring for children (Medicaid) versus older persons (Medicare). The NAMCS also has relevant questions about practice financing and organization. While these data elements are captured by the MEPS and the NAMCS, they are not typically reported by federal agencies and are currently dependent on outside researchers to produce them from the data.

Apart from the survey sources listed here, with the large number of private and public payers in the United States, no reliable comprehensive source yet exists for more detailed information for how primary care physicians are paid, a key recommendation of the committee.

[1] Jabbarpour et al.'s narrow definition of primary care is restricted to physicians practicing family medicine, general practice, geriatrics, general internal medicine, and general pediatrics.
[2] Jabbarpour et al.'s broad definition includes the narrow definition plus nurses and nurse practitioners, physician assistants, obstetrician-gynecologists, general psychiatrists, psychologists, and social workers.
[3] Reiff et al.'s narrow definition includes evaluation and management visits, vaccinations, care planning, "and other related services" rendered by family practice, geriatric medicine, gynecology, internal medicine, or pediatric physicians; physician assistants; or nurse practitioners.
[4] Reiff et al.'s broad definition includes all services rendered by those same primary care clinicians.
[5] Reid et al.'s narrow definition involves services to Healthcare Common Procedure Coding System codes on professional claims, including evaluation and management visits, preventive visits, care transition or coordination services, and in-office preventive services, screening, and counseling rendered by physicians practicing family medicine, general practice, general internal medicine, and general pediatrics.
[6] Reid et al.'s broad definition includes all services rendered in the narrow definition plus nurses and nurse practitioners, physician assistants, obstetrician-gynecologists, and geriatricians.

Objective 2: Ensure that high-quality primary care is available to every individual and family in every community.

Measure 2.1: Percentage of adults without a usual source of health care

Potential data source:	Sample performance:
National Health Interview Survey (NHIS) (CDC, 2021)	14.6 percent (2018) (CDC, 2018)

Measure 2.2: Percentage of children without a usual source of health care

Potential data source:	Sample performance:
NHIS (CDC, 2021)	4.3 percent (2018) (CDC, 2020b)

Measure 2.3: Primary care physicians per 100,000 people in medically underserved areas	
Data sources:	No known score
Health Resources and Services Administration (HRSA) area resource file (HRSA, 2019), HRSA Medically Underserved Area (MUA) shape files (HRSA, 2020a)	

Measure 2.4: Primary care physicians per 100,000 people in areas that are not medically underserved	
Data sources:	No known score
HRSA area resource file (HRSA, 2019), HRSA MUA shape files (HRSA, 2020a)	

Comments:
While reliably predictive, these measures do not fully address a key goal of this objective, which is to ensure access to *high-quality* primary care when needed.

Several efforts have been made to measure high-quality primary care, and this report offers several related recommendations. The committee offers a new definition for high-quality primary care, but there are no established measures to assess its availability.

Regarding need, as discussed in Chapter 3, some recent studies based on national health surveys suggest that visits to primary care have declined significantly in recent years, often associated with a rise in high-deductible health plans (Chou et al., 2019; Ganguli et al., 2019, 2020; Rao et al., 2019; Ray et al., 2020). This reduction is a source of concern if it is also associated with not receiving care when needed, avoiding preventive care, or seeking care in more expensive settings. Wait times for sick and new care-seeker visits could be another way to assess access; however, outside of the U.S. Department of Veterans Affairs, the committee is not aware of any measures that meet its criteria to be included in this scorecard.

Measures 2.3 and 2.4 require further analysis to determine performance; however, this could be done by overlaying HRSA's MUA shape file over HRSA's area resource file.

Objective 3: Train primary care teams where people live and work.

Measure 3.1: Percentage of physicians trained in community-based settings, rural areas, Critical Access Hospitals (CAHs), MUAs

Potential data sources:	Sample performance:
Medicare Claims Public Use Files (CMS, 2020a) American Medical Association (AMA) Physician Masterfile (AMA, 2021)	More than 3,400 physicians in residency training were identified as having spent time during residency in federally qualified health centers (FQHCs), rural health clinics (RHCs), or CAHs while training between 2001 and 2005, or 2009 using Medicare claims data and the AMA Physician Masterfile (Phillips et al., 2013). While this study did not do so, the AMA Physician Masterfile could be used to determine the total number of residents in a given year to calculate the percentage who trained in FQHCs, RHCs, or CAHs

Measure 3.2: Percentage of physicians, nurses, and physician assistants (PAs) working in primary care

Potential data sources:	Sample performance:
AMA Physician Masterfile (AMA, 2021)	Physicians (2017): 31.9 percent (Petterson et al., 2018)
HRSA National Sample Survey of Registered Nurses (HRSA, 2020b)	Nurses (2018): 14.5 percent of registered nurses, 28.8 percent of advanced practice registered nurses (HHS et al., 2020)
National Commission on Certification of Physician Assistants (NCCPA) Statistical Profile of Certified Physician Assistants (NCCPA, 2020b)	PAs (2019): 25.0 percent (NCCPA, 2020a)

Measure 3.3: Percentage of new physician workforce entering primary care each year

Potential data source:	Sample performance:
AMA Physician Masterfile (AMA, 2021)	25.2 percent (2006–2008) (Chen et al., 2013)

Measure 3.4: Residents per 100,000 population by state

Potential data source:	Sample performance:
Medicare Provider Cost Report Public Use Files (CMS, 2019)	New York (2010): 77.1 residents in training per 100,000 population North Dakota (2010): 11.5 per 100,000 (Mullan et al., 2013)

Comments:
The funding for physician training is closely tied to hospitals and not to community-based settings, where most primary care is delivered. No single measure captures training in community-based settings, but Measure 3.1 highlights data sources that could be used together to estimate the proportion of trainees who train in safety net settings. The committee is not aware of comparable data sources for other professions, highlighting the difficulty of measuring progress across the primary care workforce. Measure 3.3's sample score includes hospitalists and is thus an overestimate. Measure 3.4 highlights the uneven distribution of physician trainees relative to the population. While not primary care specific, this is important because trainees are more likely to practice in locations where they trained.

Objective 4: Design information technology that serves the patient, family, and interprofessional care team.

The committee is not aware of adequate measures or data sources that capture the use or availability of person-centered digital health in primary care (or any health care) settings, underscoring the urgency for further research in this area.

Objective 5: Ensure that high-quality primary care is implemented in the United States.

Measure 5.1: Investment in primary care research by the National Institutes of Health (NIH) in dollars spent and percentage of total projects funded.

Potential data source:	Sample performance:
NIH RePORT database (NIH, 2020)	Family medicine received $71 million, 0.22 percent of total funding from NIH (2011–2014) (Cameron et al., 2016)
	Seven hundred and fifty projects related to primary care, approximately 1 percent of the total, were funded by NIH (fiscal years 2012–2018) (Mendel et al., 2020)

Comments:

As the committee recommends in Chapter 12, using this scorecard will itself be a way to track progress of the implementation of this committee's five objectives. However, Measure 5.1 above gets to the committee's recommended research action. While this report has cited numerous examples of best practices and presented an evidence-based vision for implementing high-quality primary care, primary care research is woefully underfunded and underdeveloped. Enhancing the evidence base could propel the field, to the benefit of all Americans.

REFERENCES

AHRQ (Agency for Healthcare Research and Quality). 2021. *Medical expenditure panel survey.* https://www.meps.ahrq.gov/mepsweb (accessed January 13, 2021).

AMA (American Medical Association). 2021. *AMA physician masterfile.* https://www.ama-assn.org/practice-management/masterfile/ama-physician-masterfile (accessed January 13, 2021).

Cameron, B. J., A. W. Bazemore, and C. P. Morley. 2016. Lost in translation: NIH funding for family medicine research remains limited. *Journal of the American Board of Family Practice* 29(5):528–530.

CDC (Centers for Disease Control and Prevention). 2018. *Summary health statistics tables: National Health Interview Survey, 2018 (Table A-16).* Atlanta, GA: Centers for Disease Control and Prevention.

CDC. 2020a. *Ambulatory health care data.* https://www.cdc.gov/nchs/ahcd/datasets_documentation_related.htm#data (accessed January 13, 2021).

CDC. 2020b. *National health interview survey: Interactive summary health statistics for children*. https://www.cdc.gov/nchs/nhis/KIDS/www/index.htm (accessed November 23, 2020).

CDC. 2021. *National health interview survey*. https://www.cdc.gov/nchs/nhis/index.htm (accessed January 13, 2021).

Chen, C., S. Petterson, R. L. Phillips, Jr., F. Mullan, A. Bazemore, and S. D. O'Donnell. 2013. Towards graduate medical education (GME) accountability: Measuring the outcomes of GME institutions. *Academic Medicine* 88(9):1267–1280.

Chou, S.-C., A. K. Venkatesh, N. S. Trueger, and S. R. Pitts. 2019. Primary care office visits for acute care dropped sharply in 2002–15, while ED visits increased modestly. *Health Affairs* 38(2):268–275.

CMS (Centers for Medicare & Medicaid Services). 2019. *Medicare provider cost report public use files*. https://www.cms.gov/Research-Statistics-Data-and-Systems/Statistics-Trends-and-Reports/Medicare-Provider-Cost-Report (accessed December 21, 2020).

CMS. 2020a. *Basic stand alone (BSA) Medicare claims public use files (PUFs)*. https://www.cms.gov/Research-Statistics-Data-and-Systems/Downloadable-Public-Use-Files/BSAPUFS (accessed December 21, 2020).

CMS. 2020b. *Limited data set (LDS) files*. https://www.cms.gov/Research-Statistics-Data-and-Systems/Files-for-Order/LimitedDataSets (accessed December 21, 2020).

CMS. 2020c. *Master beneficiary summary file: Limited data set*. https://www.cms.gov/Research-Statistics-Data-and-Systems/Files-for-Order/LimitedDataSets/MBSF-LDS (accessed Novermber 6, 2020).

Ganguli, I., T. H. Lee, and A. Mehrotra. 2019. Evidence and implications behind a national decline in primary care visits. *Journal of General Internal Medicine* 34(10):2260–2263.

Ganguli, I., Z. Shi, E. J. Orav, A. Rao, K. N. Ray, and A. Mehrotra. 2020. Declining use of primary care among commercially insured adults in the United States, 2008–2016. *Annals of Internal Medicine* 172(4):240–247.

HCCI (Health Care Cost Institute). 2020. *Commercial data*. https://healthcostinstitute.org/data (accessed November 6, 2020).

HHS (U.S. Department of Health and Human Services), HRSA (Health Resources and Services Administration), and NCHWA (National Center for Health Workforce Analysis). 2020. *Characteristics of the U.S. nursing workforce with patient care responsibilities: Resources for epidemic and pandemic response*. Rockville, MD: Health Resources and Services Administration.

HRSA (Health Resources and Services Administration). 2019. *Area health resource files*. https://data.hrsa.gov/topics/health-workforce/ahrf (accessed January 13, 2021).

HRSA. 2020a. *Medically underserved areas (MUA) find*. https://data.hrsa.gov/tools/shortage-area/mua-find (accessed November 6, 2020).

HRSA. 2020b. *Nursing workforce survey data*. https://data.hrsa.gov/topics/health-workforce/nursing-workforce-survey-data (accessed November 6, 2020).

IBM. 2020. *IBM marketscan (Truven Health)*. https://marketscan.truvenhealth.com (accessed December 21, 2020).

Jabbarpour, Y., A. Greiner, A. Jetty, M. Coffman, C. Jose, S. Petterson, K. Pivaral, R. Phillips, A. Bazemore, and A. Neumann Kane. 2019. *Investing in primary care: A state-level analysis*. Washington, DC: Patient-Centered Primary Care Collaborative.

Mendel, P., C. A. Gidengil, A. Tomoaia-Cotisel, S. Mann, A. J. Rose, K. J. Leuschner, N. S. Qureshi, V. Kareddy, J. L. Sousa, and D. Kim. 2020. *Health services and primary care research study: Comprehensive report*. Santa Monica, CA: RAND Corporation.

Mullan, F., C. Chen, and E. Steinmetz. 2013. The geography of graduate medical education: Imbalances signal need for new distribution policies. *Health Affairs* 32(11):1914–1921.

NCCPA (National Commission on Certification of Physician Assistants). 2020a. *2019 statistical profile of certified physician assistants: An annual report of the National Commission on Certification of Physician Assistants*. Johns Creek, GA: National Commission on Certification of Physician Assistants.

NCCPA. 2020b. *NCCPA research*. https://www.nccpa.net/research (accessed November 6, 2020).

NIH (National Institutes of Health). 2020. *Research portfolio online reporting tools (report)*. https://report.nih.gov (accessed January 13, 2021).

Petterson, S., R. McNellis, K. Klink, D. Meyers, and A. Bazemore. 2018. *The state of primary care in the United States: A chartbook of facts and statistics*. Washington, DC: Robert Graham Center.

Phillips, R. L., Jr., S. Petterson, and A. Bazemore. 2013. Do residents who train in safety net settings return for practice? *Academic Medicine* 88(12):1934–1940.

Rao, A., Z. Shi, K. N. Ray, A. Mehrotra, and I. Ganguli. 2019. National trends in primary care visit use and practice capabilities, 2008–2015. *Annals of Family Medicine* 17(6):538–544.

Ray, K. N., Z. Shi, I. Ganguli, A. Rao, E. J. Orav, and A. Mehrotra. 2020. Trends in pediatric primary care visits among commercially insured U.S. children, 2008–2016. *JAMA Pediatrics* 174(4):350–357.

Reid, R., C. Damberg, and M. W. Friedberg. 2019. Primary care spending in the fee-for-service Medicare population. *JAMA Internal Medicine* 179(7):977–980.

Reiff, J., N. Brennan, and J. Fuglesten Biniek. 2019. Primary care spending in the commercially insured population. *JAMA* 322(22):2244–2245.

The Commonwealth Fund. 2020a. *Primary care spending as share of total, age 65 and older*. https://datacenter.commonwealthfund.org/topics/primary-care-spending-share-total-age-65-and-older (accessed January 13, 2021).

The Commonwealth Fund. 2020b. *Primary care spending as share of total, ages 18–64*. https://datacenter.commonwealthfund.org/topics/primary-care-spending-share-total-ages-18-64 (accessed January 13, 2021).

Zuvekas, S. H., and J. W. Cohen. 2016. Fee-for-service, while much maligned, remains the dominant payment method for physician visits. *Health Affairs* 35(3):411–414.